AF322996

CANCER SCREENING

CANCER SCREENING

Edited by

DOUGLAS S. REINTGEN, M.D.

Associate Professor of Surgery,
University of South Florida College of Medicine;
Program Leader, Cutaneous Oncology,
H. Lee Moffitt Cancer Center and Research Institute,
Tampa, Florida

ROBERT A. CLARK, M.D.

Professor of Radiology,
University of South Florida College of Medicine;
Chief, Diagnostic Radiology Service,
H. Lee Moffitt Cancer Center and Research Institute,
Tampa, Florida

With 24 illustrations and 3 color plates

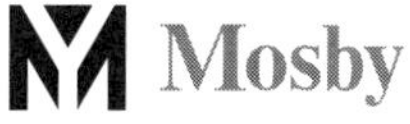

St. Louis   Baltimore   Boston   Carlsbad   Chicago   Naples   New York   Philadelphia   Portland
London   Madrid   Mexico City   Singapore   Sydney   Tokyo   Toronto   Wiesbaden

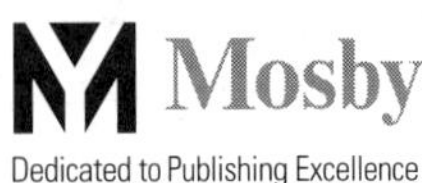

Publisher: Anne S. Patterson
Editor: Susie Baxter
Developmental Editor: Anne Gunter
Project Manager: Patricia Tannian
Senior Production Editor: Suzanne C. Fannin
Book Design Manager: Gail Morey Hudson
Cover Designer: Teresa Breckwoldt
Manufacturing Supervisor: Karen Lewis

Printed in the United States of America
Composition by The Clarinda Company
Color separations by Color Dot Graphics, Inc.
Printing/binding by Maple-Vail Book Mfg. Group

Mosby-Year Book, Inc.
11830 Westline Industrial Drive
St. Louis, Missouri 63146

Library of Congress Cataloging in Publication Data

Cancer screening / edited by Douglas Reintgen, Robert A. Clark.
    p.   cm.
    Includes bibliographical references and index.
    ISBN 0-8151-7142-0 (alk. paper)
    1. Cancer–Dignosis.   2. Medical screening.   I. Reintgen,
Douglas Scott. II. Clark, Robert A. (Robert Alan), 1947-
    [DNLM: 1. Neoplasms–prevention & control.   2. Mass Screening.
QZ 26 C217143 1996]
RA645.C3C3647 1996
362.1'96994–dc20
DNLM/DLC
for Library of Congress   95-33562
                                             CIP

96 97 98 99 00 / 9 8 7 6 5 4 3 2 1

CONTRIBUTORS

JOHN ALBERTINI, M.D.
Department of Surgery,
University of South Florida,
Tampa, Florida

WILLIAM J. CATALONA, M.D.
Professor and Chief,
Division of Urologic Surgery,
Washington University School of Medicine,
St. Louis, Missouri

DENIS CAVANAGH, M.D.
Professor of Obstetrics and Gynecology,
Director, Division of Gynecologic Oncology,
University of South Florida College of Medicine;
Tampa General Hospital,
Tampa, Florida

ROBERT A. CLARK, M.D.
Professor of Radiology,
University of South Florida College of Medicine;
Chief, Diagnostic Radiology Service,
H. Lee Moffitt Cancer Center and Research
    Institute,
Tampa, Florida

JAMES V. FIORICA, M.D.
Assoicate Professor of Obstetrics and
    Gynecology,
University of South Florida College of Medicine;
Division of Gynecologic Oncology,
H. Lee Moffitt Cancer Center and Research
    Institute,
Tampa, Florida

JUDY E. GARBER, M.D.
Assistant Professor of Medicine
Harvard Medical School;
Director of Cancer Risk and Prevention Clinics
Dana-Farber Institute,
Boston, Massachusetts

ALAN GELLER, R.N., M.P.H.
Melanoma Research Coordinator,
Department of Dermatology,
Boston University School of Medicine,
Boston, Massachusetts

MITCHEL S. HOFFMAN, M.D.
Associate Professor of Obstetrics and
    Gynecology,
Division of Gynecologic Oncology,
University of South Florida College of Medicine;
Director of Women's Cancer Screening Center,
Tampa General Hospital,
Tampa, Florida

RICHARD C. KARL, M.D.
Juan C. Bolivar Professor of Surgical Oncology,
University of South Florida College of Medicine;
Program Leader, Gastrointestinal Oncology,
H. Lee Moffitt Cancer Center and Research
    Institute,
Tampa, Florida

HOWARD K. KOH, M.D.
Professor of Dermatology,
    Medicine and Public Health,
Boston University School of Medicine;
Director, Cancer Prevention and Control Center,
Boston University Medical Center,
Boston, Massachusetts

STEPHEN L. LUTHER, Ph.D.
Adjunct Assistant Professor,
Health Policy and Management,
University of South Florida College of Public
  Health;
Director, Lifetime Cancer Screening Program,
H. Lee Moffitt Cancer Center and Research
  Institute,
Tampa, Florida

CONNIE MACK
United States Senator, Florida

RONA M. MACKIE, M.D., DSc.
Professor of Dermatology and Head of
  Department,
Department of Dermatology,
University of Glasgow;
Chairman, UK Skin Cancer Working Party,
Glasgow, Scotland

JACK S. MANDEL, Ph.D., M.P.H.
Assistant Professor
Professor and Head,
Division of Environmental and Occupational
  Health,
School of Public Health,
University of Minnesota,
Minneapolis, Minnesota

SOFIA D. MERAJVER, M.D., Ph.D.
Division of Hematology and Oncology,
University of Michigan Medical Center,
Ann Arbor, Michigan

DOUGLAS S. REINTGEN, M.D.
Associate Professor of Surgery,
University of South Florida College of
  Medicine;
Program Leader, Cutaneous Oncology,
H. Lee Moffitt Cancer Center and Research
  Institute,
Tampa, Florida

BARBARA K. RIMER, Dr.P.H.
Professor, Department of Community and Family
  Medicine,
Duke University Medical Center;
Director, Cancer Prevention, Detection and
  Control Research,
Duke Comprehensive Cancer Center,
Durham, North Carolina

WILLIAM S. ROBERTS, M.D.
Associate Professor of Obstetrics and
  Gynecology,
University of South Florida College of Medicine;
H. Lee Moffitt Cancer Center and Research
  Institute,
Tampa, Florida

JOHN C. RUCKDESCHEL, M.D.
Professor of Medicine,
University of South Florida College of Medicine;
Center Director,
H. Lee Moffitt Cancer Center and Research
  Institute,
Tampa, Florida

HENRY WAGNER, Jr., M.D.
Associate Professor of Radiology,
University of South Florida College of Medicine;
Program Leader, Thoracic Oncology Program,
H. Lee Moffitt Cancer Center and Research
  Institute,
Tampa, Florida

BARBARA L. WEBER, M.D.
Associate Professor and Director of Breast Cancer
Program
Department of Internal Medicine and Genetics,
University of Pennsylvania School of Medicine,
Philadelphia, Pennsylvania

TIMOTHY J. YEATMAN, M.D.
Assitant Professor of Surgery,
University of South Florida,
Tampa, Florida

PREFACE

Almost everything about cancer screening is controversial. Issues related to cancer screening are intensely investigated and hotly debated, often more so than in other areas of medicine. This environment of controversy and debate is appropriate because cancer screening carries the promise of great expectations with the burden of potentially great expense.

Cancer screening subjects otherwise healthy individuals to a medical test for a disease that most of them do not have and will never develop. Yet these individuals may be subjected to invasive diagnostic procedures, anxiety, costs, and perhaps even mobidity related to false positive test results. Why consider doing this? It is because screening offers the potential benefit of fewer cancer deaths in the group of individuals screened. This apparent conflict, between the incurred risks and costs to *individuals* and the benefits to a *group,* is one of the main reasons that clinicians debate intensely the value of cancer screening.

Clinicians are advocates for their individual patients. A physician offers the best possible diagnostic and treatment recommendations to a patient, based on available medical information and the unique needs of that patient. Cancer screening, however, often forces clinicians to make recommendations to an individual based on perceived benefits to an anonymous group; the benefits may or may not accrue to the individual considered. Moreover, because recommendations for screening practice are usually made based on cost-effectiveness analyses, a clinician directly faces the conflict between recommendations made to an individual and the overall costs to the anonymous group.

Clinicians are usually uncomfortable with the questions, "What is the value of saving a human life?," and "What price should be paid to prevent death?" These are difficult questions, but they are pertinent to the cancer screening discussion. Detecting a curable cancer in a 35-year-old women with a productive life ahead of her may be worth a higher price than detecting a similar cancer in a 70-year-old woman—but maybe not. What is a "productive life"?

Studies have shown that up to 75% of the health care dollar may be spent in the last year of life, prolonging briefly the inevitable death of the patient. Yet this extra time of life may be quality time for which a person would pay dearly. Who determines who pays and what price is right? There is no solid tumor at the stage-4 level that is currently curable. Should funds currently spent to treat stage-4 cancer be diverted to prevention and early detection programs? Certainly, this is a viable thesis if benefit to the group, rather than the individual, is the only measure of value. Yet most clinicians and patients would balk at this thought.

Other parallels can be drawn. It is estimated that the national expenditures for automobile seat belts is $600,000 for every life saved. Most states have laws that stipulate the use of seat belts; noncompliance subjects a person to risk of fines and loss of driver's license. The addition of air bags to all automobiles would cost the American public over $1 million for every life saved. Few seriously question whether these policies are correct or if this money is well spent because of the public demand for safety. Yet for calculations of medical cost-effectiveness, and particularly for analyses of cancer screening, values of $50,000 per year of life saved are considered expensive.

Clinical trials to assess cancer screening efficacy are difficult and expensive to conduct and analyze. Often the best information available for a given cancer screening strategy is incomplete at best. This book is an attempt to consolidate this information, imperfect as it is, in one source. The authors assembled here are knowledgeable and opinionated; it is hoped that fact and opinion are clearly discernible. More important, it is hoped that this book may provide a framework for the continuing debate about cancer screening. The inherent conflicts between the public health and medical approaches to cancer screening may not be entirely resolvable, but the issues deserve our attention. This book is an attempt to describe the current state of cancer screening, to bring information to the debate, and to bring attention to these issues. If cancer prevention and screening are to be useful strategies in the twenty-first century, these issues must be addressed squarely and honestly.

Douglas S. Reintgen
Robert A. Clark

CONTENTS

CANCER SCREENING

PRINCIPLES OF CANCER SCREENING

1

Robert A. Clark
Douglas S. Reintgen

EVALUATION OF A PROPOSED SCREENING STRATEGY
   Systematic method for evaluation
   Potential pitfalls and biases in evaluation
      Lead time bias
      Length bias
      Overdiagnosis bias

It seems intuitive that cancer screening is beneficial. Detecting cancer early, when it is small and has not spread from its primary site, rather than late, when it has metastasized to other vital organs, certainly seems reasonable.

> *Yet despite being an intuitive or reasonable concept, cancer screening remains difficult, controversial, and often confusing.*

Why not screen everyone to detect cancer early? Why not recommend screening for the most common, or the most lethal, cancers? On the other hand, how can screening be considered useful, when most screened individuals never get the disease, yet may incur screening costs and the anxiety of false positive tests? Why is cancer screening so controversial, so debated, and so seldom clearly recommended as valuable?

The answers to these questions are the contents of this book and are often different for specific cancers. However, many general principles of cancer screening are common to the different cancers and different screening strategies. The purposes of this chapter are to outline these principles of cancer screening, define terms common to all types of screening, articulate the expected benefits and potential risks of screening, offer criteria for assessment of proposed screening programs, delineate the potential sources of bias and error in evaluation, and propose systematic methods for evaluation of cancer screening.

> *These principles should be considered ideals; few, if any, cancer screening strategies fulfill all the degrees of proof outlined here.*

However, on reading the remainder of this book and while evaluating the rationale for new screening tests or proposed strategies, these principles should be kept in mind. The farther the rationale for a new screening strategy wanders from these principles, the less justification there is for its adoption. Each of us must, in the end, make our own decisions about cancer screening; this chapter allows a framework to be developed on which to make these decisions.

DEFINITIONS
Cancer Screening

> *Cancer screening is the application of a test to detect a potential cancer in a person who has no signs or symptoms of the cancer.*

There are at least two different types of cancer screening.[1,2] The first type is more traditional: a test to detect cancer before it is clinically apparent, early in its natural history, before it has become systemic, when treatment may be more effective, or less expensive, or both. An abnormal screening test in this situation leads to further diagnostic evaluation, including other diagnostic tests or biopsy, to determine if cancer is present, and to subsequent treatment if cancer is detected.

The second type of cancer screening may become more prevalent in the future: screening for risk factors or other markers, such as genetic or molecular, that put one at high risk for developing cancer. It is not yet clear what an abnormal screening test in this situation means or what recommendations should follow.[3,4] If a high-risk marker is identified but no cancer is detectable, genetic counseling may be appropriate. Alternatively, if options exist to lower the risk, education about these choices would be appropriate. Recommendations for more frequent or intensive screening tests of the first type might be considered, as might prophylactic removal of target tissue.

> *Cancer screening is a secondary form of cancer prevention. Primary prevention is the prevention of the formation of cancer.*

Cessation of cigarette smoking is primary prevention for lung cancer; avoidance of sunburns and use of sunscreens are primary prevention strategies for skin cancer. Because the causes of most cancers are unknown, primary prevention of most cancers is not possible. Detection of cancer early, before its clinical manifestations, is secondary prevention.

The term *cancer screening* is essentially synonymous with other terms, such as *early detection*.[1] The term *cancer screening* may be modified by some authors as mass, routine, regular, or selective cancer screening. However, these modifiers have no universally accepted definitions. Every cancer screening strategy must identify its target population, the proposed screening test, and frequency of the screening tests. Knowledge of these parameters for any screening strategy makes other modifier terms moot.

Cancer Screening Test

The cancer screening test is the method proposed to detect a specific target cancer.[1,2] A cancer screening test may be a single modality or a combination of tests. Laboratory tests of blood or body fluids, physical examinations, invasive procedures, and imaging tests are examples of screening tests.

Asymptomatic

A goal of cancer screening is to detect cancer before it is clinically apparent, before a person has known signs or symptoms of the disease. The definition of *asymptomatic* therefore must be placed in the perspective of the person being screened; he or she has no known signs or symptoms of cancer before the screening test. For example, consider a man with no known signs or symptoms who goes to his physician for a physical examination; his physician feels a prostate nodule during a digital rectal examination of the gland. The man now has a sign of cancer detected by the physician and the screening test; nevertheless the person was asymptomatic before the screening, and the cancer was detected by screening. This example of asymptomatic holds even if the man had symptoms related to another condition, such as benign prostate hypertrophy. Similarly, a woman without knowledge of a breast lump, who has a mass detected during a clinical breast examination by her physician, was asymptomatic before the screening test. This concept is valid but less clear in the model of skin cancer screening, where the screening test is inspection of a skin lesion. Individuals are more aware of their skin moles, freckles, and changes in skin pigmentation than they are of the texture of their prostate glands. *Asymptomatic* means that before the application of the screening test, the screened individual and the person doing the screening are unaware of any signs or symptoms of cancer in the individual, regardless of signs or symptoms of other conditions.

Screened Individual

Screened individuals may be identified in this book and in other cancer screening literature as *patients.* However, ideally they are not patients.

> *Screening involves application of a test to an asymptomatic person, an otherwise healthy individual. A screened individual does not become a patient until his or her screening test is abnormal.*

A new set of concerns, anxieties, costs, and discomforts begins when one becomes a patient. Potential benefits of screening must outweigh the potential risks because any harm to an asymptomatic person is not to be considered lightly. The terms *individual, person,* and *screenee* are used interchangeably in this chapter to denote the screened individual.

Target Population

The individual to be screened has certain characteristics that identify him or her as a candidate for cancer screening. For example, women do not have prostate glands and therefore are not candidates for prostate cancer screening. Similarly, prostate cancer is exceedingly rare, if not unheard of, in teenage boys, and therefore screening is inappropriate in this age group. The target population of a proposed screening strategy defines the characteristics of individuals appropriate to receive the screening test. Typical defining characteristics of a target population include sex, family history, specific known risk factors, geographic region of birth or residence, race or ethnicity, and age.

Screening Practitioner

The screening practitioner is the health care professional who applies the cancer screening test to the individual being screened.[1] The screening test may be applied by any of many types of health care professionals: primary care physicians, specialist physicians, nurses, physician assistants, technicians, and others.

Diagnosis

> *Screening is not diagnosis. The cancer screening test is not diagnostic, but rather identifies those asymptomatic individuals with a high likelihood of having cancer.*

The results of the screening test separate the screened individuals into two groups: those with normal and those with abnormal tests. Some individuals with normal screening tests subsequently are found to have cancer (a false negative screening test) with diagnostic tests, such as biopsy; all individuals with abnormal screening tests require some diagnostic evaluation. Some of those with an abnormal screening test and further diagnostic evaluation do not have cancer (a false positive screening test). Diagnosis is the clinical problem-solving process applied to patients, that is, symptomatic people, or those asymptomatic people with abnormal screening tests.[1,2,5]

Symptomatic individuals need diagnostic evaluation to determine the cause of symptoms. A screening test applied to a symptomatic person cannot be considered a cancer screening event because the person requires diagnostic evaluation regardless of the results of the screening test. Moreover, the value of a screening strategy cannot be assessed if symptomatic people are included in the target population because these people may already have advanced disease that needs diagnostic evaluation.

Screening Strategy or Protocol

A cancer screening strategy or protocol defines the operational parameters of a cancer screening program: who, how, what, where, and when. The screening strategy or protocol defines the target population to be screened, the screening test to be applied, when the screening test should be applied, and how often the screening test should be applied. It may also define who should apply the screening test, the conditions under which it should be applied, and the criteria for an abnormal test. There are at least two separate uses for strategies or protocols.[1] A screening strategy or protocol has its first use in designing clinical trials and interpreting scientific data about screening. The second, separate use of screening strategies or protocols is to make recommendations to individuals or groups about cancer screening.

It is important to clearly understand the screening protocol design when interpreting scientific evidence about cancer screening. The protocol of a screening clinical trial is often limited by the ability to recruit subjects to the trial, resources available to conduct the trial, and the best estimates of the parameters by the investigators.

> *The results obtained by the trial are valid only for the conditions of the protocol studied.*

For example, assume that a cancer screening protocol studies a target population of white European women ages 50 to 69 years, applies a screening test every 2 years for 10 years, and finds 40% fewer cancer deaths in screened women than in unscreened women. Although this is strong evidence of the effectiveness of cancer screening, it may not be applicable to women over age 70 years, younger than age 49 years, or Japanese women. The results of this protocol may not be enough evidence alone, for example, to justify recommending cancer screening annually for all African-American women over age 40 years.

Alternatively, consider the example of a cancer screening test applied to men between ages 65 and 75 years that finds no benefit to the screened group when compared with unscreened men. This does not mean there is no potential benefit to screening men younger than age 65 years; it only means that no information is available about screening younger men.

The scientific literature about cancer screening is replete with clinical trials that have different screening strategies and protocols for the same target cancer. It is difficult to compare or combine the data from these trials to answer scientific questions that were not posed before the design of the clinical trial.

However, this does not mean that screening strategies for clinical practice are limited to those studied by clinical trials. Cancer screening strategies or protocols may be recommended by individual practitioners, professional medical societies, public health agencies, or health maintenance organizations. Their recommendations are based on their best assessment of the available scientific evidence and their best estimate of applicability to individuals or target populations not included in the original scientific protocols. This best estimate of applicability to individuals or groups not included in the original scientific protocols varies among makers of policy, groups, and practitioners. It should not be surprising then that guidelines for cancer screening may vary among various organizations and among practitioners.

Outcomes

The scientific evidence of the value of screening requires first that outcomes of a screening protocol be measured.

> *Outcomes are the health and economic results that occur related to screening.*

Outcomes include the benefits, harms, and costs of screening and its incurred diagnostic evaluations.[1,6,7] These outcomes are measures by tracking the detailed clinical results of screened individuals. Specific important outcome measures in cancer screening are listed in Table 1-1.

Effectiveness

The effectiveness of cancer screening is determined by comparing outcomes to determine whether the benefits outweigh the harms and whether the health outcomes (benefits and harms) are worth the costs.[1,6,7] Moreover, the outcomes and effectiveness measures of the screened population must be compared with those of a similar unscreened group to ensure the effectiveness of screening. For example, for a screening program to be judged effective, the stage distribution of detected cancers in screenees should be shifted toward lower stage can-

---

TABLE 1-1

OUTCOME MEASURES IN CANCER SCREENING

Short-term Measures
- Number of individuals in the target population offered screening
- Number and proportion of individuals in target population who received screening
- Number and proportion of target population examined by multiple screens
- Number or prevalence of preclinical cancers detected
- Proportion of abnormal screenees brought to definitive diagnosis or follow-up
- Cost per cancer detected
- Sensitivity and specificity of the screening test
- Positive and negative predictive values of the screening test

Long-term Measures
- Stage distribution of detected cancers
- Case fatality rate of screened individuals
- Site-specific cancer mortality rate of screened target population
- Total costs

cers in the screened vs. unscreened population. Similarly, the case fatality rate for screenees should be significantly less than for the unscreened group, and, most important, the site-specific mortality rate for the screened population should be significantly less than for the unscreened group.

Cost-effectiveness

Ideally, the costs of the screening program (screening costs, diagnostic evaluations, treatment costs of detected cancers, and value of years of life lost to cancer deaths) should be less than the costs in the unscreened group (diagnostic evaluations, treatment costs of detected cancers, and value of years of life lost to cancer deaths). Relevant costs to be considered in this evaluation are listed in Table 1-2.

> *It has been notoriously difficult, however, to document cost savings as a result of screening programs.*

Since demonstration of overt cost savings as a result of screening may not be possible,[8] other types of cost analysis are usually performed. There are several levels of such analysis: cost-determination, cost-minimization, cost-effectiveness, cost-benefit, and cost-utility analyses.[1,9-13]

Cost determination depends on the perspective of the evaluation, the purpose, and the time frame of the study. For example, if costs are evaluated

---

TABLE 1 - 2

RELEVANT COSTS TO BE MEASURED IN A CANCER SCREENING PROGRAM

- Costs of screening tests
    Direct costs or charges
    Indirect costs (time and anxiety)
- Costs incurred by abnormal screening tests
    Direct costs or charges (diagnostic evaluation or biopsy)
    Indirect costs (complications, morbidity, anxiety, time, and loss of work)
- Costs related to false positive screening tests
    Direct costs or charges (diagnostic evaluation or biopsy)
    Indirect costs (complications, morbidity, anxiety, time, and loss of work)
- Costs related to false negative screening tests
    False sense of security
    Delay in diagnosis as a result of ignoring clinical symptoms
- Costs related to treatment and rehabilitation
    Direct costs or charges (treatment and rehabilitation)
    Indirect costs (complications, morbidity, anxiety, time, and loss of work)
- Costs related to death
    Direct costs or charges related to death
    Indirect costs (years of life lost)

from the viewpoint of a screening facility, only costs (not charges) related to the screening examination would be included. If a more comprehensive societal viewpoint is taken, costs would include charges for screening plus incurred charges for all screening-induced procedures and expenses. If differences exist in treating screening-detected cancers as compared with clinically detected cancers, such costs might also be included in an evaluation.

Cost-minimization analysis is the simplest type of complete economic evaluation. In cost-minimization analysis two or more programs with equivalent outcomes are compared. The classic example of this type of analysis is the comparison of the same surgical procedure performed on an inpatient and an outpatient basis. Because the outcomes are identical, this type of evaluation simply compares the costs of the programs compared. It does not directly relate to a screening program because there is not usually another identifiable program that has an equal outcome.

Cost-effectiveness analysis defines outcomes in natural units, such as cancers detected, survival rates, years of life gained, or tumor response to treatment. To compare two programs, their outcomes must be measured in equivalent units. The costs of each program may then be identified, and the incremental or additional cost of one program relative to the other is compared with the incremental change in outcome for that program relative to the other. The results are expressed as a ratio. When one program is more effective and less costly than another, the choice is obvious. When one program is more costly and more effective than another (such as screening versus usual clinical care), its value is less obvious without such a cost-effectiveness analysis.

Cost-benefit analysis defines the outcomes of programs in monetary units. Programs are compared by subtracting the incremental costs from the incremental benefits and calculating a net cost for one program over another. This technique is difficult because natural units, such as years of life gained, must be valued in dollars.

> *Wide disagreements exist among health professionals, actuaries, economists, and lawyers over the monetary value of a year of life.*

Difficulties arise when considering differences such as employed versus unemployed people, race, men versus women, homemakers versus those employed outside the home, elderly versus young, and high-income versus low-income earners. If the disease occurs with different frequencies in different subgroups, discrimination may occur in this type of valuation. Moreover, the impact of the disease and its treatment on quality of life are not evaluated with this type of analysis. Because of these limitations, cost-benefit analysis of programs has not commonly been done.

Cost-utility analysis defines outcomes in terms of quality of life without a monetary value. The outcomes are expressed in units of time, for example, years, and are adjusted for quality using utility techniques. This analysis calculates a cost per quality-adjusted life year (QALY) gained. The costs of different programs may then be compared directly because their outcomes may be defined in equivalent terms. Measurement of quality of life is a rapidly evolving field. Many approaches exist, and the approach taken in a research study is often different from that in a clinical setting. Common standards and reconciliation of different types of measurement are now evolving, but to date few studies have used this type of analysis to evaluate screening.

Prevalence

> *The prevalence of cancer is the number of cancers that exist in a defined population at a given point in time.*

The prevalence rate is commonly expressed as number of cancers per 100,000 individuals in the population.[1,2]

> *The ideal screening test would detect all the prevalent cases of cancer in the first screen of a previously unscreened population. Subsequent screening examinations would detect incidence cases developing in the population since the prior screen.*

Incidence

> *The incidence of cancer is the number of cancers that develop in a population during a defined period.*

The incidence rate is commonly expressed as number of cancers per year per 100,000 individuals in the population.[1,2] The incidence rate for a given cancer is lower than the prevalence rate. Theoretically, in a defined population of individuals who all received three cancer screens at yearly intervals, the first screen would detect all prevalence cases (developing for several years before the first screening). The second and third screens would detect incidence cases, that is, only those cases that had developed since the first screen.

MEASURES OF VALIDITY OF A SCREENING TEST
True Positive Test

A true positive (TP) screening test is an abnormal test for cancer in an individual who is subsequently found to have cancer within a defined period after the test.[14,15]

True Negative Test

A true negative (TN) screening test is a normal test for cancer in an individual who is subsequently found not to have cancer within a defined period after the test.[14,15]

False Positive Test

A false positive (FP) screening test is an abnormal test for cancer in an individual who is subsequently found not to have cancer within a defined period after the test.[14,15]

False Negative Test

A false negative (FN) screening test is a normal test for cancer in an individual who is subsequently found to have cancer within a defined period after the test.[14,15]

Sensitivity

The sensitivity of a screening test is its ability to detect those individuals with cancer in the population.[2,14,15] The sensitivity of the test is the TP ratio, that is, the proportion of positive tests in all individuals with disease. It is defined as the number of TP cases divided by the total number of cancer cases (sum of TP and FN cases) (Table 1-3).

$$\text{Sensitivity} = \frac{\text{TP}}{\text{TP} + \text{FN}}$$

Specificity

The specificity of the test is its ability to identify those free from cancer in the population.[2,14,15] The specificity of the test is the TN ratio, that is, the

---

T A B L E   1 - 3

EXAMPLE OF VALIDITY MEASURES OF A SCREENING TEST

	True characteristics in the population	
Results of screening test	**Have the disease**	**Do not have the disease**
Positive test	80	100
Negative test	20	800
TOTAL	100	900

True positive tests = 80.
True negative tests = 800.
False positive tests = 100.
False negative tests = 20.
Sensitivity = 80/(80 + 20) = 0.80.
Specificity = 800/(800 + 100) = 0.89.
Positive predictive value = 80/(80 + 100) = 0.44.
Negative predictive value = 800/(800 + 20) = 0.98.

proportion of negative tests in all individuals without disease. It is defined as the number of TN cases divided by the total number of people without the disease (sum of TN and FP cases) (see Table 1-3).

$$\text{Specificity} = \frac{\text{TN}}{\text{TN} + \text{FP}}$$

Positive Predictive Value

The positive predictive value is the measure of the validity of a positive test, that is, the proportion of positive tests that are TP cases (see Table 1-3).

$$\text{Positive predictive value} = \frac{\text{TP}}{\text{TP} + \text{FP}}$$

The predictive value of a test depends on the disease prevalence (Table 1-4). As the prevalence of cancer increases in the population, the positive predictive value of the screening test increases, even though its sensitivity and specificity remain unchanged.[16-18] Therefore for maximum efficiency and cost-effectiveness, screening should be focused on the highest risk (highest prevalence) populations.

TABLE 1-4

RELATIONSHIP OF PREDICTIVE VALUE OF THE SCREENING TEST TO THE PREVALENCE OF CANCER IN THE POPULATION*

Test results	Has disease	Does not have disease
Prevalence of Cancer = 1%†		
Positive	99	495
Negative	1	9405
TOTAL	100	9900
Prevalence of Cancer = 5%‡		
Positive	495	475
Negative	5	9025
TOTAL	500	9500

*Sensitivity of screening test = 0.99.
Specificity of screening test = 0.95.
†TP = 99.
FP = 495.
TN = 9405.
FN = 1.
Sensitivity = 99/(99 + 1) = 0.99.
Specificity = 9405/(9405 + 495) = 0.95.
Positive predictive value = 99/594 = 0.17.
‡TP = 495.
FP = 475.
TN = 9025.
FN = 5.
Sensitivity = 495/(495 + 5) = 0.99.
Specificity = 9025/(9025 + 475) = 0.95.
Positive predictive value = 495/970 = 0.51.

Negative Predictive Value

The negative predictive value is the measure of the validity of a negative test, that is, the proportion of negative tests that are true negative cases (see Table 1-3).

$$\text{Negative predictive value} = \frac{TN}{TN + FN}$$

GOVERNING PRINCIPLES OF CANCER SCREENING

Several governing principles should be met for a cancer screening program to be worthwhile (Table 1-5). These principles define characteristics of the disease being screened, the screening test applied, and the outcomes measured.[1,2,19]

Disease

The disease considered for screening should have a high prevalence and incidence and should have serious clinical consequences measured in mortality, morbidity, and costs. The biology and natural history of the disease should be known. Ideally the cancer should exist for a long time in a preclinical phase amenable to screening, and this preclinical phase should have a high prevalence in the screened population. The disease should have an effective treatment of early-stage disease, and this treatment should be more effective than treatment of late-stage disease. When a disease has no effective treatment or when treatment in its early stage is no more effective than in its advanced states, screening is problematic unless counseling is shown to be useful.

Screening Test

An effective screening test should be able to detect cancer in its preclinical phase, with acceptable sensitivity, specificity, and predictive values. Moreover, the test should be safe. Screened individuals are asymptomatic and should not suffer complications of a screening examination. To be applied efficiently in

---

TABLE 1-5

GOVERNING PRINCIPLES OF A WORTHWHILE CANCER SCREENING PROGRAM

Characteristics of the disease	Characteristics of the screening test
High morbidity, mortality, and costs	Able to detect disease in preclinical phase
High prevalence and incidence	Effective (that is, sensitive and specific)
Known natural history and biology	Safe
Preclinical phase with high prevalence	Simple and inexpensive
Effective treatment of early stage disease	Acceptable to individuals

large populations, the screening test should be simple, inexpensive, and accessible. Finally, if compliance with repeated screens is expected, the test must be acceptable to the screened individuals.

Outcomes Measured

Table 1-1 lists the outcome measures to be evaluated in a proposed screening program.

> *The most important measure of the effectiveness of a screening strategy is demonstration that the mortality rate from the disease is significantly lower in the total population offered screening compared with the cancer mortality rate in an equivalent population of unscreened people.*

The ultimate proof of effectiveness of a screening strategy usually requires a randomized, controlled, defined population clinical trial in which the appropriate outcome measures, including site-specific mortality rate, are compared in equivalent screened and unscreened groups.

Expected Benefits of Screening

The expected benefits of screening are reduction in the death rate from the target cancer, reduced morbidity from the disease, and savings of health care costs. Additional benefits may include improved length and quality of life and reduced pain, anxiety, and disability.

Expected benefits of screening derive from the true positive results of a screening test. A true positive screening test result holds promise for the potential benefits of screening, that is, possible reduction in cancer morbidity and mortality. A true negative screening test result can provide reassurance, but this is not the benefit that makes screening effective.

Potential Harms of Screening

The potential harms of screening include harms related to the test itself or to its results. Potential harms related to the test itself are the costs, inconvenience, anxiety, and discomfort associated with the screening test. There may also be potential risks (complications) related to invasive screening tests.

The possible harms of the screening results are related to false positive and false negative tests. A false positive test result may cause anxiety and incurs a diagnostic evaluation, with its attendant costs, potential risks, and side effects. A false negative test result may lead to a false sense of security. Subsequent clinical signs or symptoms of cancer may be dismissed because of a prior negative screening test, resulting in further delay in detection.

EVALUATION OF A PROPOSED SCREENING STRATEGY
Systematic Method for Evaluation

A systematic approach to cancer control research has been developed[20,21] that provides a framework for the evaluation of a proposed screening strategy (Table 1-6).

The first step in evaluating a proposed screening strategy begins with knowledge about the basic biology and epidemiology of the cancer. A proposed strategy must incorporate information about characteristics of the populations at high risk, cancer prevalence and incidence rates, tumor growth rates, mortality rates, and costs of care and disability. The second step, hypothesis development, must synthesize the available scientific information and propose possible interventions to be applied to the cancer problem. Cancer screening may not always be the appropriate intervention; primary prevention, if possible, is desired. The proposed intervention strategy should be expressed as a testable hypothesis that can be evaluated in an objective, scientific fashion.

Next, methodologic research is necessary to characterize the variables to be controlled or monitored in subsequent clinical trials. This phase might include pilot studies to identify target populations or compliance rates of screened individuals, to evaluate application or acceptability of screening tests, or to estimate the efficacy of the screening test. When the methods have been adequately tested and proven, they may be incorporated into clinical intervention trials. Initial trials may be uncontrolled, but ideally these interventions should be controlled. Cohort studies or case-control trials may be used to estimate benefits from a screening intervention; however, randomized, controlled trials are likely to give the most convincing results.

The next phase of evaluation of a proposed screening strategy consists of defined population studies. The purpose of a defined population study is to measure quantitatively the impact of a screening intervention. This study also identifies barriers to widespread adoption of the intervention and methods for overcoming these barriers. This type of study is conducted in a large, well-characterized population, chosen in such a way that the study subjects and results are representative of, and generalizable to, the ultimate target population. The defined population must be large enough to show a significant intervention benefit. The screening strategy is beneficial if the defined population studies dem-

---

TABLE 1 - 6

CANCER CONTROL PHASES: A SYSTEMATIC EVALUATION PROCESS FOR PROPOSED SCREENING STRATEGIES

Basic research and epidemiology
Hypothesis development
Methods development
Controlled intervention trials
Defined population studies
Demonstration and implementation projects
Nationwide dissemination programs

onstrate a significant reduction in disease-specific mortality rate in the entire population offered screening, when compared with the unscreened group.

When screening is shown to be beneficial in defined population studies, demonstration and implementation programs are appropriate. The purpose of these programs is to apply the proven intervention in a community at large with measurement of the public health impact.

> *A surveillance system should be in place to ensure that the application, accuracy, and effectiveness of screening in the community are equal to that demonstrated in clinical trials.*

It is pointless to promote widespread screening unless a measurement system can document its community-wide use. Quality control processes may be developed during this phase, using the short-term outcome measures identified during prior phases as parameters of adequate quality. This phase also permits assessment of the adequacy of diagnostic evaluation and treatment in the community.

> *Screening itself is of no value without the necessary diagnosis and treatment capabilities.*

Finally, when demonstration and implementation programs ensure that community dissemination can be achieved, nationwide screening programs and policy recommendations may be developed. These nationwide programs and recommendations may be based on the best scientific information available from the prior phases of evaluation.

Potential Pitfalls and Biases in Evaluation

The systematic evaluation process outlined here is not always completed. Various pressures may urge researchers, physicians, and individuals to bypass certain steps of this process. These pressures include immediate clinical acceptance and dissemination of a new screening test, expense of defined population studies, and preliminary recommendations for screening from professional organizations. However, without the assurance of this process, an incompletely evaluated screening strategy may deliver more harms and costs than benefits. Moreover, without the demonstrated benefit of a screening intervention in a defined population trial, the potential benefit of a screening strategy may be overestimated and invalid.

Almost invariably, individuals with cancer identified by screening have longer survival times than those diagnosed with usual clinical detection. However, these apparent increased survival times are not necessarily equivalent to reduction in mortality from cancer. At least three concepts—biases—contribute to this apparent survival increase and potentially mask the lack of screening benefit: lead time bias, length bias, and overdiagnosis bias. Randomized, controlled clinical trials minimize these biases and more accurately identify and quantify the benefits of a screening strategy.

Lead Time Bias

Lead time bias[1,18] refers to clinical outcome observations that are not adjusted for the timing of the diagnosis.

> *The time by which screening advances the diagnosis of cancer compared with the usual clinical detection is the lead time.*

In an uncontrolled clinical trial this lead time appears to increase survival time because survival is measured from the time of diagnosis to the time of death. However, despite this apparent increase in survival time, the natural history of the disease and the time of death are unchanged (Figure 1-1).

> *This apparent increase in survival time without the benefit of mortality reduction is lead time bias.*

A beneficial screening strategy detects cancer before its systemic spread, alters the natural history of the disease, and defers the time of death. This alter-

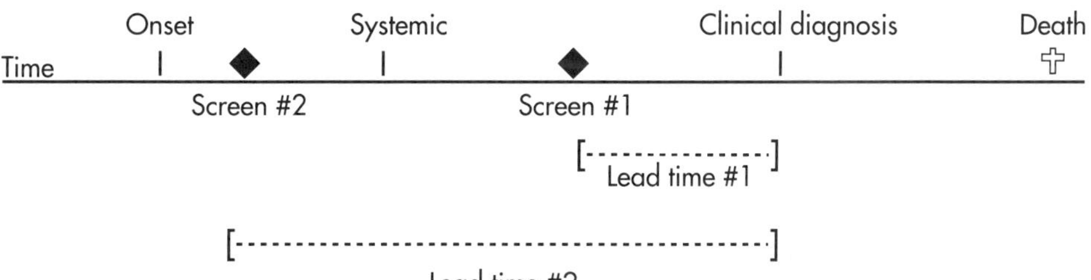

Figure 1-1 Lead time bias. The time line extends from left to right, depicting onset of cancer, its systemic spread, the subsequent clinical diagnosis, and finally, death. The diamonds represent applications of screening tests. If a screening test is applied at screen #1, the time of diagnosis is advanced from the time of usual clinical diagnosis by lead time #1. Survival time is apparently increased by this lead time, even though the natural history of the disease is unchanged. If a screening test is applied at screen #2, the lead time is increased (lead time #2). If screen #2, applied before the systemic spread of the cancer, alters the natural history of the disease, the time of death is deferred, or moved to the right. This alteration of the natural history of the disease, with prolongation of life, cannot be recognized without comparison of the screened group to controls. A randomized, controlled trial is necessary to control for lead time bias.

ation of the natural history of the disease, with prolongation of life, cannot be recognized without comparison of the screened group to controls. A randomized, controlled trial is necessary to control for lead time bias.

Length Bias

Length bias refers to clinical outcome observations that are not adjusted for the rate of progression of disease.[1,18] The probability that a cancer will be detected by screening is directly proportional to the length of its detectable preclinical phase, which is inversely related to its rate of progression. Individuals with rapidly progressive cancers—those with short preclinical phases—are more likely than average to die of their disease and are less likely to be identified by screening.

> *Individuals with slowly progressive cancers, that is, those with long preclinical phases, are less likely than average to die of their disease and are more likely to be identified by screening.*

Therefore screening tends to detect cancer subsets with long preclinical phases, less aggressive progression, and perhaps better inherent prognosis (Figure 1-2).

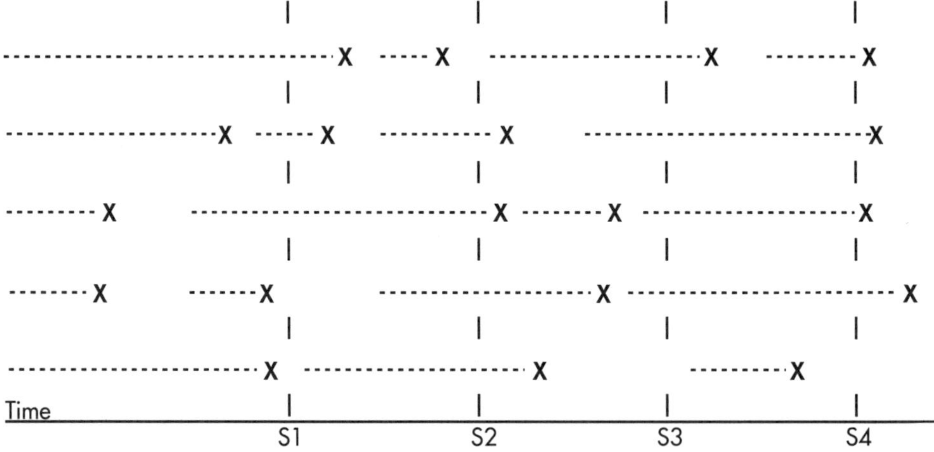

Figure 1-2   Length bias sampling. The time line extends from left to right. Each *X* signifies a cancer death, and the *horizontal dashed lines* indicate the duration the cancer has been present before death. The entire group of dashed lines and Xs represents a heterogeneous population of cancers, with varied rates of progression. The application of four screening tests is represented by *S1 to S4*. The *vertical lines* represent the times of screening; if the vertical line intersects a horizontal line, the cancer is detected by screening. The four screening examinations tend to detect those cancers with the longest horizontal lines, that is, those with the longest detectable phase or the slowest progression. Those cancers with the slowest progression (the longest horizontal lines) offer two opportunities for screening detection before death. Note that at virtually any time, a one-time screening is more likely to select patients who live with the disease for the longest time. This is length bias sampling.

> *If, in an uncontrolled clinical screening trial, the outcomes of individuals with screening-detected cancers are compared with a general population of clinically detected cancers, the screened group may demonstrate an artificially higher survival rate because of this length bias sampling effect.*

A randomized, controlled trial obviates this bias. The benefit of screening is recognized by the disease-specific reduction in mortality for the total population offered screening, compared with the unscreened control group, not just for the individuals with screening-detected cancers.

Overdiagnosis Bias

Length bias effect may be magnified as the screening test threshold is lowered and the least aggressive tumors are detected.

> *Among this group of neoplasms may be cases that would regress, remain stable, or progress too slowly to ever have become clinically apparent during the individual's lifetime.*

This effect has been termed *overdiagnosis bias,* or *pseudodisease.*[1,18]

Overdiagnosis bias is compounded by the difficulty in defining pathologically the distinct lines between benign hyperplasia, atypical hyperplasia, dysplasia, and carcinoma. As a screening strategy detects less aggressive tumors, at earlier stages in the progression of disease, some cases of benign conditions are classified as cancers, artificially elevating the apparent survival benefit. Again, randomized, controlled trials offset the effects of this error by controlling for this bias.

REFERENCES

1. Eddy DM: *Common screening tests,* Philadelphia, 1991, American College of Physicians.
2. Hulka BS: Cancer screening: degrees of proof and practical application, *Cancer* 62:1776, 1988.
3. Hoskins KF et al: Assessment and counseling for women with a family history of breast cancer: a guide for clinicians, *JAMA* 273:577, 1995.
4. Shattuck-Eidens D et al: A collaborative survey of 80 mutations in the *BRCA1* breast and ovarian cancer susceptibility gene: implications for presymptomatic testing and screening, *JAMA* 273:535, 1995.
5. Moskowitz M: Screening is not diagnosis, *Radiology* 133:265, 1979.
6. Ellwood PM: Shattuck lecture on outcomes management: a technology of patient experience, *N Engl J Med* 318:1549, 1988.

7. Wennberg JE: Outcomes research, cost containment, and the fear of health care rationing, *N Engl J Med* 323:1202, 1990.

8. Fries JF et al: Reducing health care costs by reducing the need and demand for medical services, *N Engl J Med* 329:321, 1993.

9. Doubilet P, Weinstein MC, McNeil BJ: Use and misuse of the term "cost-effective" in medicine, *N Engl J Med* 314:253, 1986.

10. Doubilet PM: "Cost-effective": a trendy, often misused term, *Am J Roentgenol* 148:827, 1987.

11. Eisenberg JM: Clinical economics: a guide to the economic analysis of clinical practice, *JAMA* 262:2879, 1989.

12. Detsky AS, Naglie G: A clinician's guide to cost-effectiveness analysis, *Ann Intern Med* 113:147, 1990.

13. Goodwin PJ: Economic evaluations of cancer care: incorporating quality-of-life issues. In Osoba D, editor: *Effect of cancer on quality of life,* Boca Raton, Fla, 1991, CRC Press.

14. McNeil BJ, Keeler E, Adelstein SJ: Primer on certain elements of medical decision making, *N Engl J Med* 293:211, 1975.

15. McNeil BJ, Adelstein SJ: Determining the value of diagnostic and screening tests, *J Nucl Med* 17:439, 1976.

16. Moskowitz M: Impact of *a priori* medical decisions on screening for breast cancer, *Radiology* 171:605, 1989.

17. Moskowitz M: Predictive value, sensitivity, and specificity in breast cancer screening, *Radiology* 167:576, 1988.

18. Black WC, Welch HG: Advances in diagnostic imaging and overestimations of disease prevalence and the benefits of therapy, *N Engl J Med* 1237, 1993.

19. Cadman D et al: Assessing the effectiveness of community screening programs, *JAMA* 251:1580, 1984.

20. Greenwald P, Cullen JW: The new emphasis in cancer control, *J Natl Cancer Inst* 74:543, 1985.

21. Greenwald P, Cullen JW, McKenna JW: Cancer prevention and control: from research through applications, *J Natl Cancer Inst* 79:389, 1987.

SCREENING FOR SPECIFIC CANCERS

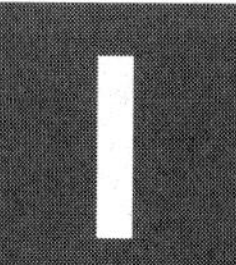

BREAST CANCER

2

Robert A. Clark

BREAST CANCER AS AN APPROPRIATE DISEASE FOR SCREENING

MAMMOGRAPHY AS AN APPROPRIATE SCREENING TEST

CONTROLLED INTERVENTION TRIALS: CASE-CONTROL STUDIES

DEFINED POPULATION STUDIES: RANDOMIZED, CONTROLLED TRIALS

DEMONSTRATION AND IMPLEMENTATION PROJECTS
  Quality assurance issues
  Cost issues
  Incurred costs of screening
  Cost-effectiveness studies
  Access issues

NATIONWIDE DISSEMINATION PROGRAMS AND POLICY RECOMMENDATIONS

Screening for breast cancer with mammography is the most extensively studied cancer screening program, yet it remains one of the most intensely debated.

Breast cancer screening has been undergoing evaluation for over 30 years and has been "proven effective" for over a decade, yet breast cancer screening remains controversial.

Important practical issues, such as when to start screening, when to stop screening, and how often to screen, remain hotly debated, and there are valid concerns about the cost-effectiveness of screening when compared with other health care choices.

> *To understand this apparent dichotomy, the inherent controversies that emerge when trying to balance the best medical advice given to an individual versus the public health policy recommendations given to a population must be understood.*

Moreover, the ongoing development of breast cancer screening, including (1) the continuation of basic research in the biology, genetics, and epidemiology of the disease, (2) the continuation of development of screening mammography technology, (3) the identification of target populations, (4) the design and results of clinical trials, (5) the results of community demonstration and implementation projects, and (6) the development of nationwide health policy programs and recommendations must be appreciated.

Chapter 1 defines the principles of cancer screening and proposes a framework for the evaluation of screening strategies. Breast cancer screening is the only cancer screening program that has been judged by both all the governing principles and all the phases of evaluation. Therefore this structure provides a framework for discussion of breast cancer screening with mammography.

BREAST CANCER AS AN APPROPRIATE DISEASE FOR SCREENING

Any disease considered for screening should have a high prevalence and incidence and should have serious clinical consequences measured in mortality, morbidity, and costs. The biology and natural history of the disease should be known; ideally, the cancer should exist for a long time in a *preclinical* phase amenable to screening, and this preclinical phase should have a high prevalence in the screened population. The disease should have an effective treatment of early-stage disease, and this treatment should be more effective than treatment of late-stage disease.

Breast cancer exhibits the characteristics of an appropriate disease to screen.

> *For women, breast cancer is the most common cancer and the second most common cause of cancer deaths.*

Currently there are over 180,000 new cases of breast cancer annually and more than 46,000 deaths each year from the disease.[1] In the United States alone, treatment of breast cancer consumes over $6 billion annually, more than any other cancer.[2]

The incidence of breast cancer has been increasing at a rate of 1% to 2% a year for the past several decades,[3,4] with a 4% annual increase between 1982 and 1986.[3] The recent, acute rise in incidence has been attributed to increased use of mammographic screening,[3] since most of this increase has been in early-stage disease. However, the reason for the long-term rise in incidence, greatest in older women, is unknown.

Breast cancer incidence and prevalence increase with age.[1,5,6] For women older than age 50, the prevalence of disease is about six cancers per 1000 women screened; for women over age 65, the prevalence is about nine cancers per 1000 women screened. The annual incidence of disease for women over age 50 is about three to four cancers per 1000 women screened. The probability of American women ages 40 to 59 years developing invasive breast cancer is 1 in 26, whereas for women ages 60 to 79 years it is 1 in 15.[1]

Although breast cancer is a heterogeneous disease, with a wide range of growth patterns, most breast cancer has a long preclinical phase.[7-11]

> *The mean doubling time for breast cancer may be 100 to 200 days, and the preclinical lead time gained by screening is on the order of 2 to 4 years compared with clinical detection.*

Moreover, treatment of early-stage disease is more effective than treatment of late-stage disease. The most powerful predictors of prognosis and survival in breast cancer are size of tumor and status of tumor in regional axillary lymph nodes.[3,9,10] When the detected tumors are small, treatment is more effective and more treatment options are available. Breast conservation therapy is equivalent to mastectomy for the treatment of early-stage breast cancer,[12] and women with smaller tumors are better candidates for breast preservation.

MAMMOGRAPHY AS AN APPROPRIATE SCREENING TEST

An effective screening test should be able to detect the disease in its preclinical phase, with acceptable sensitivity, specificity, and predictive values. Moreover, the test should be safe. Screened individuals are asymptomatic and should not suffer complications of a screening examination. To be applied to large populations efficiently, the test should be simple, inexpensive, and accessible. Finally, if compliance with repeated, periodic screens is expected, the test must be acceptable to the screened individuals.

It has been evident for at least 40 years that mammography could detect breast cancer before it could be detected by a woman or her physician.[13,14] The mammographic signs of breast cancer were described a generation ago, and the signs of early breast cancer were explicitly defined over a decade ago.[15,16] The mammographic signs of early breast cancer are (1) tumor mass, usually irregularly marginated or spiculated, (2) grouped (clustered), small calcifications with or without a mass, (3) poorly defined, asymmetric breast density, especially if developed since a prior examination, and (4) distortion of the breast parenchymal architecture by scirrhous tumor.

Continued research has refined our knowledge about the findings, strengths, and limitations of this radiographic examination. Screening mammography has a sensitivity rate over 80%, a specificity rate over 95%, and a positive predictive value over 20%.[6,17-27] Also, mammography is safe, with a negligible risk of radiation-induced carcinogenesis.

> *Screening mammography is not a perfect screening test, however; it fails to detect 10% to 20% of cancers.*

It is uncomfortable and occasionally painful, and it is somewhat expensive for a screening test.[28]

The most problematic characteristic of screening mammography is its lack of standardization in interpretation. Recent strides have been made in technical quality and standardization of image production, due first to the American College of Radiology Mammography Accreditation Program in 1987,[29] and later to the National Mammography Quality Standards Act of 1992.[30] These programs have prescribed standards governing equipment, image quality, radiation dose, and qualifications of personnel.

However, the interpretation of the mammographic image is difficult and remains as much an art as a science, and variation exists in quality of interpretation.[31] Quality assurance programs are being developed to improve interpretation by radiologists and to monitor interpretation quality with outcome audits.[20,22,24,25] Nevertheless, variation in mammographic interpretive quality will always exist, just as variation exists in all types of clinical expertise.[32]

CONTROLLED INTERVENTION TRIALS: CASE-CONTROL STUDIES

There have been at least four major case-control studies, two conducted in The Netherlands and one each in the United Kingdom and Italy.[33-38] The study parameters of these trials are summarized in Table 2-1, and the results are summarized in Table 2-2.[38]

TABLE 2-1

CASE-CONTROL STUDIES OF BREAST CANCER SCREENING

Study	Start date	Ages enrolled*	Screening interval (months)	Screening rounds in study	Duration of follow-up (years)
DOM	1974	50-64	25.5	5	12
Nijmegen	1975	35-65	24	4	8
United Kingdom	1979	45-64	24	4	7
Florence, Italy	1977	40-70	30	3-7	10

*Age range of participants, in years, at start of mammography screening.
DOM, Diagnostisch Onderzoek Mammacarcinoom.

These trials all indicate a benefit of screening with mammography, with reductions of the relative risk of breast cancer death in screened women.

The Diagnostisch Onderzoek Mammacarcinoom (DOM) study[33] was begun in 1974 in Utrecht, The Netherlands, and enrolled women 50 to 64 years of age. The screening examination was two-view mammography and breast physical examination performed at 2-year intervals, with five rounds of screening. The results indicate that screening reduced the risk of dying of breast cancer compared to the control group: the relative risk was 0.52 (confidence interval [CI] 0.32 to 0.83). This implies a 48% reduction in mortality as a result of screening.

The Nijmegen project[34] was begun in The Netherlands in 1975 and enrolled women 35 to 65 years of age. The screening examination was single-view mammography alone without breast physical examination, done at 2-year intervals with four rounds of screening. The results showed that screening decreased breast cancer mortality compared with the control group. The relative risk of death from breast cancer in screened women was 0.51 (CI 0.26 to 0.99), implying a 49% reduction in mortality.

The case-control trial in the United Kingdom[35] began in 1979 and enrolled women 45 to 64 years of age. The trial studied three groups of women: one group was offered eight yearly screenings, alternating breast physical examination, and single-view mammography (therefore single-view mammography at 2-year intervals for four rounds of mammographic screening); a second group was offered instruction in breast self-examination; and a third control group was offered no intervention. The study demonstrated a reduction in the relative risk of dying of breast cancer in the group screened with mammography (relative risk was 0.76 [CI 0.54 to 1.08]), implying a 24% reduction in breast cancer mortality in the screened group.

The Italian case-control study[36] was begun in Florence in 1977 and enrolled women 40 to 70 years of age. The screening examination was two-view mammography every 2 ½ years. The results indicate a reduction in breast cancer

---

TABLE 2-2

RELATIVE RISKS, ODDS RATIOS, AND 95% CONFIDENCE INTERVALS IN CASE-CONTROL STUDIES OF BREAST CANCER SCREENING

	Relative risk		
Study	Women all ages	Women younger than 50 years	Duration of follow-up (years)
DOM	0.52 (0.32-0.83)	—	12
Nijmegen	0.51 (0.26-0.99)	1.23 (0.31-4.81)	8
United Kingdom	0.76 (0.54-1.08)	—	7
Florence, Italy	0.53 (0.33-0.85)	—	10

DOM, Diagnostisch Onderzoek Mammacarcinoom.

deaths in the screened group. The relative risk of breast cancer death was 0.53 (CI 0.33 to 0.85), implying a 47% reduction in mortality in the screened group.

DEFINED POPULATION STUDIES: RANDOMIZED, CONTROLLED TRIALS

In addition to the case-control studies, nine major randomized, controlled trials of breast cancer screening have been conducted, an unparalleled accomplishment in research on cancer detection.[27,38] These trials varied in age ranges of women screened, periodicity of screenings, screening modalities, study and control sample sizes, percentage of women screened, and times of follow-up. Nevertheless, there is convincing evidence that breast cancer screening with mammography reduces breast cancer mortality for screened women, compared with control group women.[27]

> *A recent meta-analysis of all the studies of breast cancer screening calculated an overall benefit to screened women of about 25%.*

The study parameters of these trials[27,38] are summarized in Tables 2-3 and 2-4, and the results are summarized in Table 2-5.

All the controlled studies and the summary meta-analysis studies indicate a significant mortality reduction benefit of about 25% to 30% for screened women ages 50 to 74 years at entry. The magnitude of benefit in this age group was similar regardless of the number of mammographic views per screen, screening interval, or duration of follow-up.

> *In contrast, these data from controlled trials consistently demonstrated no screening benefit for women ages 40 to 49 years in the first 5 to 9 years after study entry.*

After 10 to 12 years of follow-up, there was still no benefit demonstrated for younger women in any of the studies (Tables 2-5 and 2-6). However, a statistically insignificant benefit of 13% mortality reduction was observed for women in a combined analysis of all the Swedish studies. Only the Health Insurance Plan (HIP) trial has data beyond 12 years of follow-up, and its results show a 25% decrease in mortality at 10 to 18 years after entry.

DEMONSTRATION AND IMPLEMENTATION PROJECTS
Quality Assurance Issues

Quality assurance in screening mammography is currently demanded by consumers, radiologists, primary care physicians, regulatory agencies, health care third-party payers, and public health strategists.

RANDOMIZED, CONTROLLED TRIALS OF BREAST CANCER SCREENING

Study	Start date	Ages enrolled*	Screening interval (months)	Screening rounds in study	Duration of follow-up (years)
United States					
Health Insurance Plan	1963	40-64	12	4	10, 18
Sweden					
Kopparberg	1977	40-74	24-33†	6	12
Ostergotland	1977	40-74	24-33†	6	12
Malmo	1976	45-69	18-24	6	12
Stockholm	1981	40-64	28	2	8
Gothenberg	1982	40-59	18	2	7
United Kingdom					
Edinburgh	1979	45-64	12-24	4	10
Canada					
Canada 1	1980	40-49	12	5	7
Canada 2	1980	50-59	12	5	7

*Age range of participants, in years, at start of mammography screening.
†Twenty-four months for women ages 40 to 49; 33 months for ages 50 to 69.

RANDOMIZED, CONTROLLED TRIALS OF BREAST CANCER SCREENING

Study	Start date	Screening modality	Interval between screenings (months)	No. of women (study group plus control group)
United States				
Health Insurance Plan	1963	2-view MM and CBE	12	60,995
Sweden				
Kopparberg	1977	1-view MM	24-33	134,867*
Ostergotland	1977	1-view MM	24-33	
Malmo	1976	2-view MM	18-24	42,283
Stockholm	1981	1-view MM	28	59,107
Gothenberg	1982	2-view MM	18	49,533
United Kingdom				
Edinburgh	1979	2-view MM and CBE	12-24	45,130
Canada				
Canada 1	1980	2-view MM and CBE	12	50,430
Canada 2	1980	2-view MM and CBE	12	39,405

*Kopparberg and Ostergotland combined.
MM, Mammography; *CBE*, clinical breast examination.

TABLE 2-5

RELATIVE RISKS, ODDS RATIOS, AND 95% CONFIDENCE INTERVALS IN RANDOMIZED, CONTROLLED STUDIES OF BREAST CANCER SCREENING

Study	Relative risk		Duration of follow-up (years)
	Women all ages	Women younger than 50 years	
United States			
Health Insurance	0.71 (0.55-0.93)	0.77 (0.50-1.16)	10
Plan	0.77 (0.61-0.97)	—	18
Sweden			
Kopparberg	0.68 (0.52-0.89)	0.75 (0.41-1.36)	12
Ostergotland	0.82 (0.64-1.05)	1.28 (0.76-2.33)	12
Malmo	0.81 (0.62-1.07)	0.51 (0.22-1.17)	12
Stockholm	0.80 (0.53-1.22)	1.04 (0.53-2.05)	8
Gothenberg	0.86 (0.54-1.37)	0.73 (0.27-1.97)	7
All Sweden	0.76 (0.66-0.87)	0.87 (0.63-1.20)	7-12
United Kingdom			
Edinburgh	0.84 (0.63-1.12)	0.78 (0.46-1.51)	10
Canada			
Canadian 1	—	1.36 (0.84-2.21)	7
Canadian 2	0.97 (0.62-1.52)	—	7

TABLE 2-6

SUMMARY META-ANALYSIS OF BREAST CANCER SCREENING TRIALS: RELATIVE RISKS, ODDS RATIOS, AND 95% CONFIDENCE INTERVALS

Studies	Relative risk		
	Women all ages	Women younger than 50 years	Women ages 50 to 74 years
Case-control	0.62 (0.49-0.77)	1.23 (0.31-4.81)	0.45 (0.29-0.70)
Randomized, controlled	0.79 (0.71-0.87)	0.92 (0.75-1.13)	0.77 (0.69-0.87)
All studies	0.75 (0.68-0.83)	0.93 (0.76-1.13)	0.74 (0.66-0.83)

There are two types of quality assurance: *technical* and *professional.* Technical quality assurance evaluates the *performance* of the mammographic examination, with the end point being production of high-quality, low-dose mammographic film images. Professional quality assurance evaluates the patterns and accuracy of the *interpretations* of mammograms.

The technical quality of mammography is one of the most regulated parameters in medicine. At least five regulatory bodies (American College of Radiology, Health Care Financing Agency, Joint Commission on Accreditation of Healthcare Organizations, individual state health care agencies, and Food and Drug Administration [FDA]) claim quality assurance jurisdiction and prescribe different quality requirements. The National Mammography Quality Standards Act of 1992 was an attempt to consolidate the various quality assurance requirements into one regulatory effort.[30] As of October 1, 1994, only facilities accredited by the FDA, as the designee of the Secretary of the Department of Health and Human Services, may perform mammography. This accreditation process specifies that (1) equipment used be dedicated to mammography, (2) personnel performing mammography be licensed or certified, (3) physicians interpreting mammograms be certified, and (4) mammographic and film-processing equipment be inspected by a medical physicist at least annually. This law provides for an advisory committee of health professionals to assess quality standards and facility regulations.

None of the above technical regulations addresses professional interpretation performance or quality.

> *The most problematic characteristic of screening mammography is its lack of standardization in interpretation.*

Professional quality assurance requires an individual practice audit[17-20,22,24,25] to define the characteristics of the women examined, the interpretations given, the recommendations made, and follow-up of outcomes to define accuracy of interpretations and size of cancers detected.[31]

The controlled clinical trials previously noted use breast cancer mortality reduction as the primary measure of screening effectiveness. However, because so many data about breast cancer screening are available from these trials, intermediate or short-term measures that correlate with mortality reduction have been derived. Quality assurance guidelines have evolved from these measures by which a screening program can document its effectiveness.[20,27,39] By performing regular, periodic outcome audits of screening mammography practice, screening providers can ensure that their own practices conform to the standards of the defined population trials.

Measures of screening interpretation quality are listed in Table 2-7. These measures ensure accurate and effective mammography practice, and the stage distribution of cancers detected ensures a mortality benefit for screened women. Each screening mammography facility should monitor its outcomes to document its own effectiveness. The women being screened, as well as the clinicians who refer women for mammography, should insist that their local screening facilities meet these guidelines.

Cost Issues

A recent report reviewed the economic issues related to screening mammography.[28] The full economic impact of screening mammography has not been realized to date because only about half of eligible women receive regular screenings. Currently in the United States there are about 47 million women over age 40 who are eligible for screening mammography. The average charge for mammography in the United States is over $100.

T A B L E   2 - 7

OUTCOME MEASUREMENTS TO DOCUMENT PROFESSIONAL QUALITY ASSURANCE IN SCREENING MAMMOGRAPHY

Parameter	Proportion
Mammography Interpretation Patterns	
Positive test (abnormal mammography interpretation)	<0.15
Biopsies per 100 screening examinations	<0.02
Cancers detected by screening mammography (sensitivity)	>0.80
Cancers per recommended biopsy (positive predictive value)	>0.20
Stages of Cancers Detected	
In situ cancers	>0.15
Minimal cancers [stages $T_{is} + T_{1a} + T_{1b}$]	>0.40
Stage 1 cancers	>0.50
Stage 0 + stage 1	>0.65

> *If all women over age 40 were to receive annual mammograms, at an average charge of $100 per mammogram, the annual expenditures for screening mammography alone would be nearly $5 billion.*

This is double the expenditures for all cancer screening services in 1990, almost 1% of the total national health care expenditures for 1990, and about 25% of the total annual expenditures for diagnostic imaging.

The average charge for screening mammography in the United States is over $100, despite recent studies outlining methods to operate at high volume and reduced cost.[28,40-43] Essentially these reports have emphasized techniques to increase throughput of examinations and to maximize the use of resources. Because mammography service is characterized by high fixed costs (such as equipment and salaries) and negligible variable costs (such as film), the unit examination cost is minimized as throughput is maximized, and the marginal cost of each additional examination performed (until capacity is reached) is negligible.

Several techniques have been developed to improve screening efficiency and reduce costs: dedication to screening only, batch processing of films, loading of films on mechanical viewers for batch interpretations, simplified and standardized reporting of results either manually or by computer, and standardized follow-up and quality assurance.

> *High-volume screening has been proposed as the only feasible approach to low-cost screening.*

Not all screening facilities, however, may be able to duplicate these reported cost structures.[42] The largest difference in the cost structures of screening mammography facilities is a result of overhead allocation. When screening mammography is provided in a free-standing facility that does only screening (and not consultative or diagnostic examinations), without a radiologist in attendance and with no other assessment of overhead charges, efficiencies of high volume can be achieved and costs reduced. However, larger overhead costs are incurred if screening mammography is performed in a hospital or clinic setting, in a mobile unit, in combination with consultative studies, or with a radiologist in attendance. Barriers to high-volume, low-cost mammography then are the practice patterns of many mammography facilities and the expectations of many women receiving mammography and of their physicians.

Incurred Costs of Screening

> *The costs of diagnostic procedures incurred through screening are relevant to the economic impact of screening.*

As noted, there is variation in the interpretation practice of screening mammography. The percentage of abnormal interpretations requiring diagnostic evaluation can vary, and the diagnostic evaluation can include any combination of diagnostic mammography, sonography, magnetic resonance imaging (MRI), clinical physical examination, needle biopsy, or excisional biopsy. The prevailing charges, expenditures, and usage rates for these procedures in the community are not known.

Similarly, substantial variation in treatment patterns for breast cancer exist in the community.[12,44] The costs of mastectomy are different from those of breast-conserving surgery and radiation therapy, and therefore the usage rates of these therapies affect cost-effectiveness calculations. Few studies have addressed the cost-effectiveness of specific therapies for breast cancer. One example outlined the cost-effectiveness of adjuvant chemotherapy for node-negative breast cancer[45]; however, the usage rate of this therapy in the community is not known.

Cost-effectiveness Studies

Most analyses of breast cancer screening have been either mathematical models or related to clinical trials, and virtually all consider it a useful expenditure of resources.[28,37,46,47] In the reported studies great variation exists in the calculated cost per life-year saved. Brown and Fintor[47] have recently reviewed the relevant literature in this area and have shown how differences in assumptions and in considerations of incurred effects have resulted in such broad ranges of results. For example, many studies share a common assumption that has never been documented: large differentials between the treatment costs for early-stage and late-stage cancer.

Real expenditures (cost to society or the public health cost) and outcomes in the community may be different from those shown to exist in these studies. Variations in expenditures may be related to differences in underlying cost structures among facilities, to geographic differences in fee policies, or to differences in practice patterns of screening programs and treating physicians. Differences in practice patterns and costs probably exist within the United States for several reasons: geographic variations in health care expenditures, geographic variations in market penetration of managed care and health maintenance organizations, reimbursement differences, differences in expectations of women and physicians, malpractice trends, and local practice standards. For cost-effectiveness research to be useful in clinical practice, standards of practice patterns, expenditures, and outcomes must be defined and documented in the community.

Access Issues

An important component of any cancer screening program is demonstration of its successful dissemination into the community.

> *Although evidence of effectiveness in defined population trials is necessary, the public health benefits of a screening program are achieved only if it can be widely implemented.*

Numerous demonstration projects, community interventions, and educational programs have been developed to implement screening in the United States.[28] Currently about half of the eligible women in the United States receive regular mammographic screening. Various reasons that women do not receive screening include their knowledge and beliefs about screening, physician recommendations, access to medical care, and costs of mammography. In general, women with an underlying concern for health-related matters and women with strong family histories of breast cancer are more likely to participate in screening. Poor, uneducated, and older women are less likely to participate. Physicians may recommend screening mammography more often for women who are younger and better educated, and they are more likely to refer women for screening mammography when their own offices are well organized and when mammography services are easily scheduled and available. One of the most important determinants of a woman's participation in screening is the referral from her physician for a mammogram. Hence women's access to primary care physicians and their physicians' mammography referral practices are critical steps in screening use.

NATIONWIDE DISSEMINATION PROGRAMS AND POLICY RECOMMENDATIONS

Most public health authorities recommend breast cancer screening because screening significantly reduces mortality from the disease. Most industrialized countries with national health care systems recommend or provide mammography screening for breast cancer. In the United States most national public health agencies and medical professional organizations endorse breast cancer screening with mammography.

> *The National Cancer Institute cancer control goals for the year 2000 target participation of 80% of all eligible women in regular mammographic screening.*[48]

The Health Care Financing Agency, which administers Medicare, began reimbursing claims for screening mammography several years ago. Widespread consensus exists that screening mammography is a basic, essential element of health care for adult women.

However, despite the largest collection of data in the annals of screening research, there is continued debate about the fundamentals of clinical screening practice: Who should be screened? At what age should screening start? How often should screening occur? When should screening stop? The most widely disseminated American guidelines for screening mammography are summarized in Table 2-8. How could such learned organizations review the same data and fail to reach consensus about these practical matters?

The most conservative recommendations derive from a strict analysis of available combined data. The data demonstrate mortality reductions in screened women ages 50 to 69 years, and these breast cancer death rates were reduced by approximately 30% after 10 to 12 years. For women ages 40 to 49 years, no benefit from screening was found for the first 5 to 7 years, and mortality was insignificantly reduced by approximately 13% at 10 to 12 years after entry. No difference in benefit related to screening periodicity was apparent. Therefore the most conservative recommendation is annual or biennial screening mammography for women ages 50 to 69, or perhaps ages 50 to 74.[27,37,38]

Advocates for expanding the screening guidelines for the elderly note that breast cancer risk and incidence increase with age and that the efficacy and

---

TABLE 2 - 8

VARIOUS GUIDELINES FOR SCREENING MAMMOGRAPHY

Recommendations	Issuing or endorsing group
Annual or biennial mammography, ages 50 to 69 or 50 to 74	United States Preventive Services Task Force
	National Cancer Institute
Annual mammography, age 50 and older	American College of Physicians
Biennial mammography, age 65 and older	Health Care Financing Agency (Medicare)
Annual or biennial mammography, ages 40 to 49	American Cancer Society
	American College of Radiology
Annual mammography, age 50 and older	American Medical Association
	Seven other organizations

cost-effectiveness of screening increase as the incidence of disease increases. Moreover, screening mammography is technically easier to interpret and therefore is more sensitive for detection of cancer in elderly women because they are more likely to have fatty breasts than young women.

> *Because women over age 70 years still have a significant life expectancy, some experts argue that, even though there are no data to demonstrate benefit of screening in this age subgroup, it is extremely likely that benefit exists.*

Therefore advocates for screening of women age 70 years and older make their recommendations based on existing data and on their best estimate of a high likelihood of benefit.

> *The debate about screening women under age 50 is more intense than about screening elderly women. The incidence of cancer in this younger age subgroup is much lower, and the proportion of women with dense breast tissue, which limits the sensitivity of screening mammography, is much greater.*

Therefore without existing data one cannot expect a high likelihood of benefit in younger women as in older women. Moreover, if benefit exists in this age subgroup, it is smaller than in the older group, it is recognized later, and it is achieved at a higher cost.

However, the American Cancer Society, the American Medical Association, and the American College of Radiology remain firm in their recommendation of screening mammography for women ages 40 to 49 years.[49,50] These experts argue that, although breast cancer is less common in women ages 40 to 49 years than in older women, over 25% of all breast cancers occur in women under age 50 years. Moreover, the number of breast cancers in women ages 40 to 49 years is only 8% less than in women ages 50 to 59 years.

> *More than 40% of the years of life lost to breast cancer are from women diagnosed before age 50 years.*

Therefore these advocates argue that the problem of breast cancer in women ages 40 to 49 is significant.

These organizations conclude that available clinical trial data do not exclude the possibility of a benefit, but that information is insufficient to obtain meaningful results. They claim that the data suggest a benefit to screened women ages 40 to 49 years; five of the randomized, controlled trials demonstrate a mortality reduction with a mean value of approximately 17%. However, too few women were enrolled in the studies to make this benefit statistically significant. A new clinical trial to address this issue has begun in the United Kingdom, enrolling women ages 40 to 41 and screening them until age 49. The trial will not be completed for 15 years but will probably answer the question of screening benefit for women in this age subgroup.

Advocates for screening in this younger age subgroup also argue that mammography technology and experience have improved since the clinical trials were conducted. Mammography detects breast cancer with similar sensitivity in women ages 40 to 49 years and 50 to 59 years. There is no biologic or scientific reason for 50 years of age to be a critical point; rather it is a quirk of clinical trial study design and grouping data by decade that results in the current recommendations.

Advocates for expanding the screening age guidelines also argue that, if a physician is to be strict about screening mammography data, he or she also should be strict about recommending breast clinical examination and breast self-examination, for which there is much less information to support value in screening.

How should a woman and her physician interpret all this conflicting advice?

> *First, it is clear that screening mammography is worthwhile for women over the age of 50 years. Second, for women over age 70 years in otherwise good health, breast cancer screening is probably worthwhile. Third, a woman between the ages of 40 and 49 years should discuss screening with her physician.*

The decision to screen should take into account the information discussed here, as well as her risk factors, family history, desire for preventive health, and the economic burdens of screening. The decision should ideally be individualized in this area of controversy.

The ideal periodicity of screening examinations also is unclear. For women older than 50 years, no apparent difference in benefit exists between annual and biennial screening intervals. The intervals chosen should be based on the preferences and best judgment of the woman and her physician. However, if women ages 40 to 49 years are to be screened, the available data suggest annual intervals are more effective. The lead time gained for mammography for women ages 40 to 49 is approximately 2 years, shorter than that for older women. If women this age are screened every 2 years, the advantage of early detection is diminished. However, because biennial screening is effective in women ages 50 to 69 years and the benefit to be expected in women ages 40 to 49 years is probably less than the older age group, annual screening in the younger age subgroup is much less cost-effective than annual or biennial screening in the older group. Although an *individual woman* in her 40s and her physician may decide whether to screen, annual screening for women ages 40 to 49 is an expensive *public health policy* recommendation.

REFERENCES

1. Wingo PA, Tong T, Bolden S: Cancer statistics 1995, *CA Cancer J Clin* 45:8, 1995.
2. Zeigler J: New database allows researchers to evaluate cancer care costs, *J Natl Cancer Inst* 85:351, 1993.
3. Harris JR et al: Breast cancer. Part 1, *N Engl J Med* 327:319, 1992; Part 2, *N Engl J Med* 327:390, 1992; Part 3, *N Engl J Med* 327:473, 1992.
4. Miller BA, Feuer DJ, Hankey BF: Recent incidence trends for breast cancer in women and relevance of early detection: an update. *CA Cancer J Clin* 43:27, 1993.
5. Miller BA, Ries LA, Hankey BF: *Cancer statistics review: 1973-1989,* DHEW Pub No (NIH)92-2789, Bethesda, Md, 1992, National Cancer Institute.
6. Baker LH: Breast cancer detection demonstration project, *CA Cancer J Clin* 194, 1982.
7. Buchanan JB, Spratt JS, Heuser LS: Tumor growth, doubling times, and the inability of the radiologist to diagnose certain cancers, *Radiol Clin North Am* 21:115, 1983.
8. Fournier DV et al: Growth rate of 147 mammary carcinomas, *Cancer* 45:2198, 1980.
9. Tubiana M, Koscielny S: The natural history of breast cancer: implications for a screening strategy, *Int J Radiat Oncol Biol Phys* 19:1117, 1990.
10. Tubiana M, Koscielny S: Natural history of human breast cancer: recent data and clinical implications, *Breast Cancer Res Treat* 18:125, 1991.
11. Feig SA: Decreased breast cancer mortality through mammographic screening: results of clinical trials, *Radiology* 167:659, 1988.
12. Winchester DP, Cox JD: Standards for breast-conservation treatment, *CA Cancer J Clin* 42:134, 1992.
13. Gershon-Cohen J, Ingleby H: Roentgenography of cancer of the breast: a classified pathological basis for roentgenologic criteria, *Am J Roentgenol* 68:1, 1952.
14. Egan RL: Experience with mammography in a tumor institution: evaluation of 1,000 studies, *Radiology* 75:894, 1960.
15. Moskowitz M: Predictive value of certain mammographic signs in screening for breast cancer, *Cancer* 51:1007, 1983.
16. Sickles EA: Mammographic features of 300 consecutive nonpalpable breast cancers, *Am J Roentgenol* 146:661, 1986.
17. Bird RE: Low-cost screening mammography: report on finances and review of 21,716 consecutive cases, *Radiology* 171:87, 1989.
18. Bird RE: Professional quality assurance for mammography screening programs, *Radiology* 177:587, 1990.
19. Sickles EA et al: Medical audit of a rapid-throughput mammography screening practice: methodology and results of 27,114 examinations, *Radiology* 175:323, 1990.
20. Spring DB, Kimbrell-Wilmot K: Evaluating the success of mammography at the local level: how to conduct an audit of your practice, *Radiol Clin North Am* 25:983, 1987.
21. Gisvold JJ: Imaging of the breast: techniques and results, *Mayo Clin Proc* 65:56, 1990.
22. Linver MN et al: Improvement in mammography interpretation skills in a community ra-

diology practice after dedicated teaching courses: 2-year medical audit of 38,633 cases, *Radiology* 184:39, 1992.

23. Margolin FR, Lagios MD: Development of mammography and breast services in a community hospital, *Radiol Clin North Am* 25:973, 1987.

24. Murphy WA, Destouet JM, Monses BS: Professional quality assurance for mammography screening programs, *Radiology* 180:387, 1991.

25. Reinig JW, Strait CJ: Professional mammographic quality assessment program for a community hospital, *Radiology* 180:393, 1991.

26. Robertson CL: Private breast imaging practice: medical audit of 25,788 screening and 1,077 diagnostic examinations, *Radiology* 187:75, 1993.

27. Fletcher SW et al: Report of the International Workshop on Screening for Breast Cancer, *J Natl Cancer Inst* 85:1644, 1993.

28. Clark RA: Economic issues in screening mammography, *Am J Roentgenol* 158:527, 1992.

29. McLelland R et al: The American College of Radiology accreditation program, *Am J Roentgenol* 157:473, 1991.

30. Mammography Quality Standards Act of 1992, Pub No 102-539, Washington, DC, 1994, US Government Printing Office.

31. Elmore JG et al: Variability in radiologists' interpretations of mammograms, *N Engl J Med* 331:1493, 1994.

32. Kopans DB: The accuracy of mammographic interpretation, *N Engl J Med* 331:1521, 1994.

33. Collette HJA et al: Further evidence of benefits of a (non-randomized) breast cancer screening programme: the DOM project, *J Epidemiol Commun Health* 46:382, 1992.

34. Verbeek ALM et al: Mammographic screening and breast cancer mortality: age-specific effects in Nijmegen project, 1975-1982, *Lancet* 1:865, 1985.

35. Moss SM et al: A case-control evaluation of the effect of breast cancer screening in the United Kingdom trial of early detection of breast cancer, *J Epidemiol Commun Health* 46:362, 1992.

36. Palli D et al: Time interval since last test in a breast cancer screening programme: a case-control study in Italy, *J Epidemiol Commun Health* 43:241, 1989.

37. Eddy DM: Screening for breast cancer. In Eddy DM, editor: *Common screening tests,* Philadelphia, 1991, American College of Physicians.

38. Kerlikowske K et al: Efficacy of screening mammography: a meta-analysis, *JAMA* 273:149, 1995.

39. Sickles EA: Quality assurance: how to audit your own practice, *Radiol Clin North Am* 30:265, 1992.

40. Bird RE, McLelland R: How to initiate and operate a low-cost screening mammography center, *Radiology* 161:43, 1986.

41. Sickles EA et al: Mammographic screening: how to operate successfully at low cost, *Radiology* 160:95, 1986.

42. American Cancer Society workshop on strategies to lower the cost of screening mammography, *Cancer* 60 (suppl): 1669, 1987.

43. Evens RG: Mammographic screening: how to operate successfully at low cost, *Radiology* 161:850, 1986.

44. Welch WP et al: Geographic variation in expenditures for physicians' services in the United States, *N Engl J Med* 328:621, 1993.

45. Hillner BE, Smith TJ: Efficacy and cost-effectiveness of adjuvant chemotherapy of women with node-negative breast cancer, *N Engl J Med* 324:160, 1991.

46. Kattlove H et al: Benefits and costs of screening and treatment for early breast cancer: development of a basic benefits package, *JAMA* 273:142, 1995.

47. Brown ML, Fintor L: Cost-effectiveness of breast cancer screening: preliminary results of a systematic review of the literature, *Breast Cancer Res Treat* 25:113, 1993.

48. Greenwald PW, Sondik EJ: Cancer control objectives for the nation: 1985-2000, *National Cancer Institute Monograph* 2:1, 1986.

49. Sickles EA, Kopans DB: Deficiencies in the analysis of breast cancer screening data, *J Natl Cancer Inst* 85:1621, 1993.

50. Mettlin C, Smart CR: Breast cancer detection guidelines for women aged 40-49 years: rationale for the American Cancer Society reaffirmation of recommendations, *CA Cancer J Clin* 44:248, 1994.

3

CERVICAL CANCER

Mitchel S. Hoffman
Denis Cavanagh

EPIDEMIOLOGY

Using data from the National Cancer Institute's (NCI) SEER program it was estimated that there would be approximately 15,800 new cases of invasive cervical cancer in the United States in 1995 and 4800 related deaths.[1] In 1984 the estimates were 16,000 new cases and 6800 deaths, so the incidence and mortality have decreased.[2] However, this malignancy is still the seventh leading cause of cancer-related deaths in women in the United States and is the number one cause of cancer-related deaths in women in many developing countries.

The majority (85% to 90%) of cervical cancers show squamous cell origin histologically, with the remainder being adenocarcinomas. Most of the well-defined epidemiologic information relates to squamous cell carcinoma of the cervix.

Cervical cancers occur in women ages 35 to 55 years.

> *The cause of a large percentage of squamous cell cancers of the cervix appears to be a sexually transmitted factor or cofactor.*

Risk factors for these squamous cell tumors are similar to those for other sexually transmitted diseases and include early age at first coitus, multiple sexual partners, low socioeconomic status, and a history of a sexually transmitted disease. Smoking cigarettes may also be a risk factor.

Risk factors for adenocarcinoma are not as clear cut.[3] Sexual transmission does not appear to play a major role in the pathogenesis of this tumor. Oral contraceptive use has been associated with a slightly increased risk of cervical adenocarcinoma by some, but this is not an established risk factor. The proportion of adenocarcinomas to squamous cell carcinomas has increased over the past two decades, probably related to a decreasing incidence of the squamous cell carcinomas.[4] Adenocarcinoma of the cervix arises from the endocervical epithelium frequently within the endocervical canal. As a result, it may be missed by Papanicolaou (Pap) smear screening, tends to produce fewer early symptoms, and is more likely to be diagnosed at a later stage than squamous cell carcinoma.

Early symptoms of cervical cancer include a watery or blood-tinged vaginal discharge and irregular or postcoital bleeding. On examination, very early tumors are often occult but may be detectable with a colposcope. Beyond the microscopic or occult stage, the cancers may appear ulcerated or exophytic. Carcinomas arising in the endocervical canal may not be visible but cause the cervix to be palpably enlarged and hard.

PATHOGENESIS
Cancer Precursors

> *The majority of squamous cell carcinomas are thought to arise from a precancerous cervical condition.*

Such lesions have been termed *cervical dysplasia* or *cervical intraepithelial neoplasia (CIN)*. CIN is graded according to the degree of involvement of the epithelium as CIN I, II, or III, with CIN III representing full-thickness neoplastic change of the epithelium. The likelihood of progression to invasive cancer is much greater with CIN III. In one large study of patients with CIN I, 62% regressed to normal and 16% progressed to CIN III or invasive cancer.[5] A study of patients with CIN II reported regression in 54% and progression in 30%.[6] Based on limited site-specific information and on studies of carcinoma in situ at other sites, it is thought that the regression rate of CIN III is much lower and the risk of progression to invasive cancer much higher.[7-9]

Adenocarcinoma in situ is a well-described lesion arising from the endocervical epithelium. This lesion is much less common than CIN, and much less is known about its natural history.[10-16] There does, however, appear to be a definite association with the development of invasive adenocarcinoma.

CIN, regardless of severity, is generally asymptomatic and not grossly visible on examination. Risk factors for the development of CIN are essentially identical to those for invasive squamous cell carcinoma of the cervix.[17,18]

Possible Etiologic Factors

As previously discussed, the cause of the majority of precancerous and cancerous squamous lesions of the cervix appears to be a sexually transmitted factor or cofactor. A variety of agents, such as herpes simplex virus 2, have previously been implicated.[19]

> *The sexually transmitted factor currently considered most serious in the development of cervical squamous neoplasia is human papillomavirus (HPV).*

Over the past few decades an enormous amount of data has accumulated regarding this virus.

Through DNA technology approximately 70 different HPV types have been identified, with 20 of these affecting the human female genital tract. Only a few of these viruses have a strong association with high-grade CIN or invasive cancer and are therefore considered high-risk types (HPV 16, 18, 45, and 56).[20] Several HPV types have demonstrated an intermediate degree of risk, whereas others are associated with a low risk of cancer.

Cytopathic change (koilocytosis) resulting from the virus is recognized with light microscopy and is noted in a large percentage of low-grade CIN.[21] Considering low-grade CIN and early viral-type changes in the epithelium indistinguishable and basically the same disease process has now become generally accepted; the rationale for the new Bethesda cervical cytologic classification has been well stated by Kurman and associates.[22] This new classification is shown in Table 3-1. Although the Bethesda system has improved communications between cytopathologists and clinicians and all agree that the high-grade squamous epithelial lesion distinctions are clear cut, there is still considerable debate about the low-grade squamous epithelial lesions.[23] As the degree of CIN becomes more severe, the viral cytopathic changes are less pronounced and are generally not recognizable in invasive cancers. As DNA technology has advanced, incorporation of portions of the HPV DNA into the abnormal cells has been recognized.[24]

The majority of CIN and invasive squamous cell lesions have been shown to be associated with HPV. Low-grade CIN is positive for a mixture of low- and

---

T A B L E   3 - 1

BETHESDA SYSTEM FOR REPORTING CERVICAL CYTOLOGIC DIAGNOSES

Squamous Cell

Atypical squamous cells of undetermined significance
Low-grade squamous intraepithelial lesion
  • Cellular changes associated with human papillomavirus
  • Mild dysplasia
High-grade squamous intraepithelial lesion
  • Moderate dysplasia
  • Carcinoma in situ
Squamous cell carcinoma

Glandular Cell

Presence of endometrial cells in one of the following circumstances:
  • Out of phase in a menstruating woman
  • Postmenopausal woman
  • No menstrual history available
  • Atypical glandular cells of undetermined significance
Adenocarcinoma
Other epithelial malignant neoplasm

---

high-risk related HPV types, whereas high-grade CIN is associated with predominantly high and intermediate risk types.[20] The majority of invasive lesions are positive for high-risk HPV types. Evidence further implicating the high-risk HPV types is a markedly increased risk for progression of low-grade CIN to high-grade CIN when these virus types are present.[25] In addition, women who have negative cervical cytology but whose cervical sample tests positive for HPV (especially type 16 or 18) demonstrate a markedly increased risk of developing CIN II or III within 2 years.[26] Applying Koch's postulate for disease causation to viruses such as HPV, which will not grow in cell culture, is problematic. Histologic and molecular transformation has been demonstrated after transfection of a keratinocyte cell culture with HPV 16 DNA.[27]

Although there is strong evidence to support the etiologic role of certain HPV types, it appears that other factors or circumstances must also be at work for cervical neoplasia to occur, since a large percentage of women test positive for the virus and yet only a small percentage develop cervical neoplasia.[28]

SCREENING
Papanicolaou Smear

Initially using vaginal pool smears to study hormonal status, Papanicolaou and Traut[29] realized the usefulness of the technique for detecting neoplastic cervical cells and reported this in 1941. Using a modeled wooden spatula Ayre proposed direct sampling of the cervix, and this produced a much improved sample.[30] In the late 1940s to early 1950s the Pap smear came into widespread use as a screening technique for cervical precancerous conditions and cancers.

The concept of the Pap smear evolved into a technique to screen for cervical precancerous conditions, which are then histologically confirmed and treated, with the idea of preventing progression to invasive cancer.

> *In countries such as the United States and others that have implemented widespread cervical cytologic screening programs there has been a reduction in the incidence of and mortality from invasive cervical cancer.*

In lieu of a prospective randomized trial between screened and nonscreened populations, the decreasing mortality rate for cervical cancer is solid evidence that screening for this tumor is efficacious.[31,32] The resulting widespread incorporation of the Pap smear into everyday medical practice is a good demonstration that not every treatment or practice recommendation has to be supported by a prospective randomized trial. In 1980 cervical cancer remained the second most frequent neoplasm in women worldwide.[33] The extent of reduction in cervical cancer mortality is in proportion to the number of women being screened, with no decrease in incidence or mortality noted in unscreened populations.

It is an unfortunate misconception that the Pap smear is highly accurate and that errors in sampling or interpretation are unacceptable. The test involves cytologic interpretation of a smear of cells taken from the cervix and is subject to error at a number of levels.[34] The false negative rate of the Pap smear is not exactly known, but according to some estimates is around 10% to 20%.[35-39] In the presence of invasive cancer the false negative rate actually appears to be much higher, probably because of obscuring inflammation,[36,40,41] resulting in a delay in diagnosis and a reduced chance for survival. The false positive rate of the Pap smear is also unknown but may be substantial.[38,39,42] This leads to different problems, such as anxiety on the part of the patient, expense associated with a futile investigation, and in some cases unnecessary treatment.

The Pap smear technique is illustrated in Figure 3-1. A woman scheduled for a Pap smear should not douche or have intercourse for at least 24 hours before the examination and should not be menstruating. A speculum is carefully placed to expose the cervix, lubricated only with water or a specialized lubricant. Using an Ayer spatula the entire circumference of the external cervical os area is gently scraped, with the aim being to harvest cells from the area of the transformation zone. The specimen is quickly but gently and evenly spread on a glass slide. An additional sample may be taken from the vaginal pool or posterior vaginal fornix, but it is important to obtain an adequate sample from the endocervical canal. This is best done with an endocervical brush.[43] In certain populations, such as postmenopausal women, it is especially important to obtain a good endocervical sample.[44,45] Also important is rapid fixation of the specimen with cytofixative to avoid an air-drying artifact. An adequate history must also accompany the smear, including information such as the date of the last menstrual period, hormonal medications, prior genital tract neoplasia, and treatment.

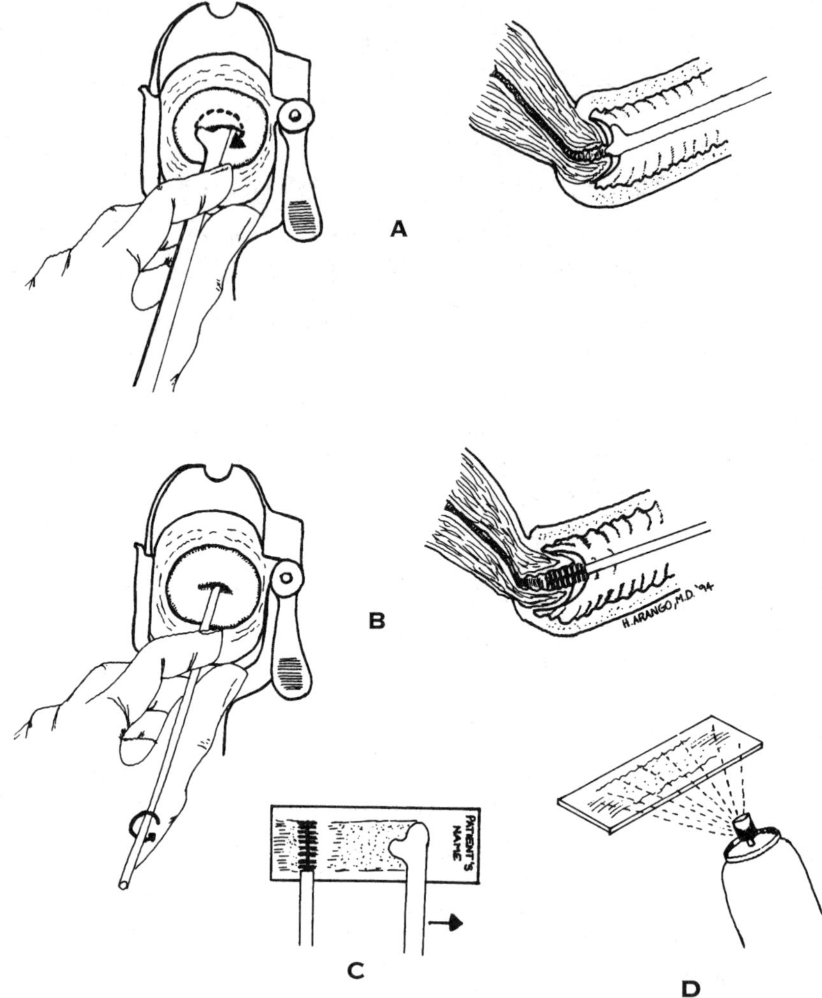

Figure 3-1   Taking a Papanicolaou smear.

Women should begin Pap smear screening once they have become sexually active or reach age 18. The optimal screening interval thereafter is a subject of much controversy. In 1988 a consensus statement from the American College of Obstetricians and Gynecologists and the American Cancer Society was published and accepted by other organizations. It reads as follows[46,47]:

All women who are or who have been sexually active, or who have reached age 18, should undergo an annual Pap test and pelvic examination. After a woman has had three or more consecutive, satisfactory annual examinations with normal findings, the Pap smear may be performed less frequently at the discretion of her physician.

The false negative rate of the Pap smear, the frequent difficulty in determining the risk status of an individual patient, recent evidence that the transit time from CIN to invasive cancer in some patients is quite short, and the opportunity to screen for other medical conditions including other malignancies have led most obstetrician-gynecologists in the United States to recommend annual screening.[48]

Despite the limitations just mentioned, a well-taken, well-fixed, well-stained, and well-read Pap smear is the best method of screening for cervical cancer.

Other Screening Methods

Recognizing the inherent false negative rate of the Pap smear, a few alternative or adjunctive methods of cervical screening have been reported.

Colposcopy

Colposcopy is the usual method of evaluating a cervix following the report of an abnormal Pap smear. For satisfactory colposcopy the entire transformation zone (squamocolumnar junction) must be visualized because most cervical cancers begin in this area. The colposcope magnifies the cervix 10 to 20 times, and special attention is paid to the transformation zone, usually with the aid of 3% to 5% acetic acid. This removes mucus, dehydrates the cells, and accentuates abnormalities such as mosaicism, punctation, and white epithelium. The vascular pattern is brought out using a green filter, and all abnormal areas are biopsied. In nonpregnant women an endocervical curettage is performed. Prior studies have demonstrated some improvement in screening sensitivity by combining the Pap smear and colposcopy.[49-52] The use of the colposcope in a screening setting is not really practical, however, because of the cost and need for expertise in colposcopy.

Cervicography

Originally described by Adolf Stafl in 1981, cervicography is basically a picture of what is seen through the colposcope.[53] The picture may be sent to an expert for interpretation. There are several reports on the use of this technique as a screening method.[54-59] However, the results are varied, with some showing high false positive and false negative rates. The technique also involves significantly more expense as an initial screening method than the Pap smear alone.

Schiller's Test

Schiller's test consists of applying Lugol's iodine to the cervix. Normal ectocervical tissue contains glycogen and turns a mahogany brown. Pale areas are positive and should be biopsied. False positive tests are too frequent to make this useful for screening.

Acetic Acid Test

Three prior studies have evaluated the use of acetic acid application alone to determine whether this would improve detection of CIN missed by the Pap smear.[60-62] The test does appear to detect a few patients with CIN who have a normal Pap smear, but false positive and false negative rates are high.

HPV DNA Test

HPV DNA testing has also been studied as a screening tool for cervical cancer.[26,58,63] As previously discussed, a large percentage of patients who test positive for HPV have no current evidence of cervical neoplasia, and the expense of routine testing would be prohibitive. In certain populations where screening can be done only infrequently and especially when the patients are at high risk, the addition of this technique and colposcopy may be appropriate. If colposcopy is performed, a good plan of management is essential.

PREVENTION OF INVASIVE CERVICAL CANCER
Patient Education and Access to Care

> *Cancer of the cervix still accounts for more cancer deaths than any other cancer in third-world countries.*

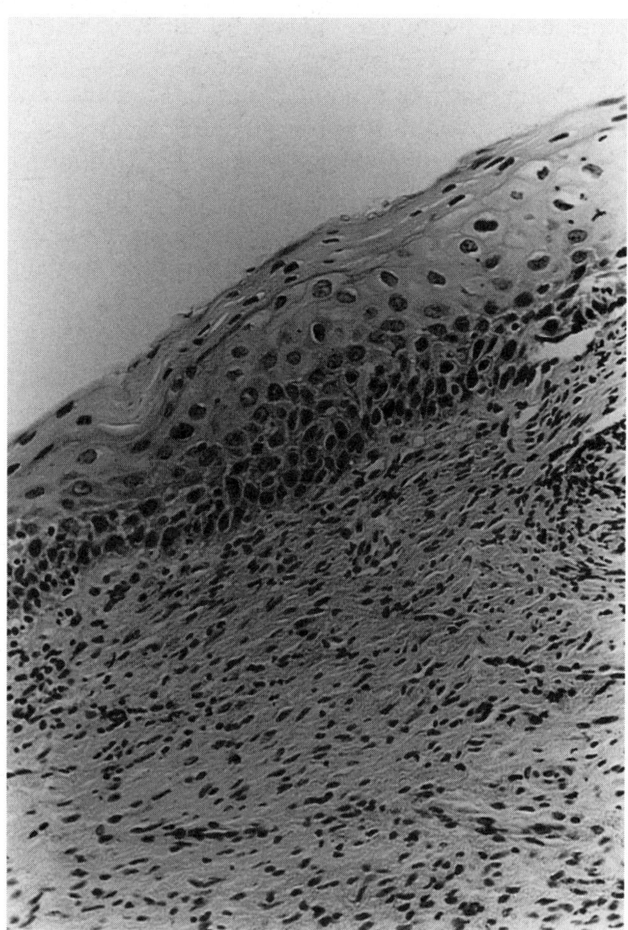

Figure 3-2   Cervical intraepithelial neoplasia (CIN) I (mild dysplasia). Cytologic changes characteristic of malignancy are present in the lower half of the epithelium. (From Cavanagh D, Ruffolo EH, Marsden DE: *Gynecologic cancer—a clinicopathologic approach,* Norwalk, Conn, 1985, Appleton-Century-Crofts.)

This is largely attributed to the lack of widespread programs for cervical cytologic screening in these areas. However, to a lesser degree significant segments of the minority population in countries such as the United States still do not get the benefit of routine Pap smear screening.[48] Socioeconomic factors are undoubtedly the major reason for this deficiency. Studies have shown that in many instances, however, reasons for not being screened have much to do with lack of educational awareness of the importance of this aspect of preventive care. Allocation of resources and widespread educational programs directed particularly toward African-American, Hispanic, and poor white women are needed to improve this situation and reduce the death rate from squamous carcinoma of the cervix. With adequate cytologic screening programs it is within our grasp to make this a largely preventable disease in the United States.

Treatment of Precancerous Conditions

The reasons for reduction in cervical cancer mortality in screened populations are not entirely clear. Identification of invasive cancer at an earlier and

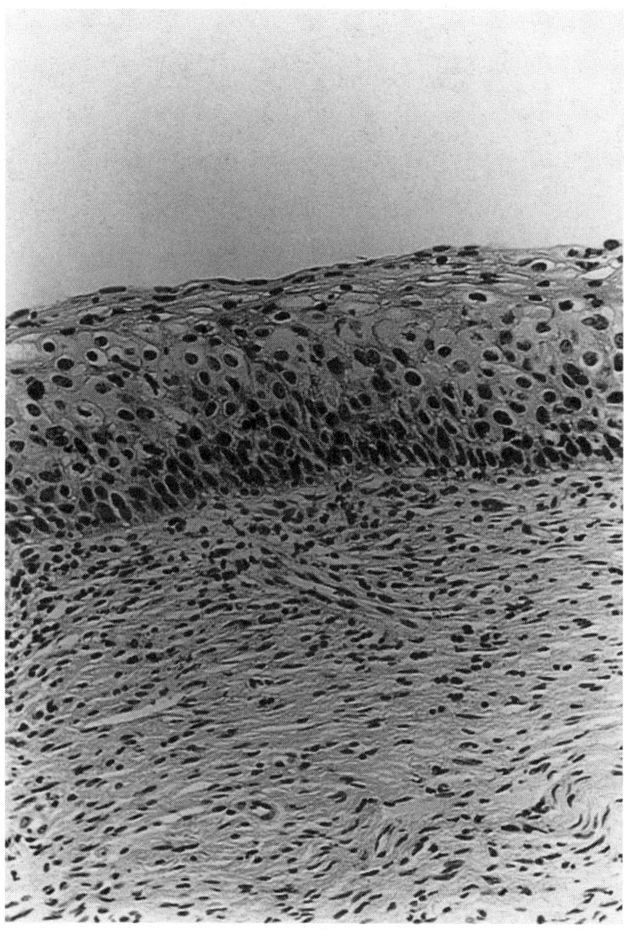

Figure 3-3 Cervical intraepithelial neoplasia (CIN) II (moderate dysplasia). Cytologic changes characteristic of malignancy extend between half and three fourths of the thickness of the epithelium. (From Cavanagh D, Ruffolo EH, Marsden DE: *Gynecologic cancer—a clinicopathologic approach,* Norwalk, Conn, 1985, Appleton-Century-Crofts.)

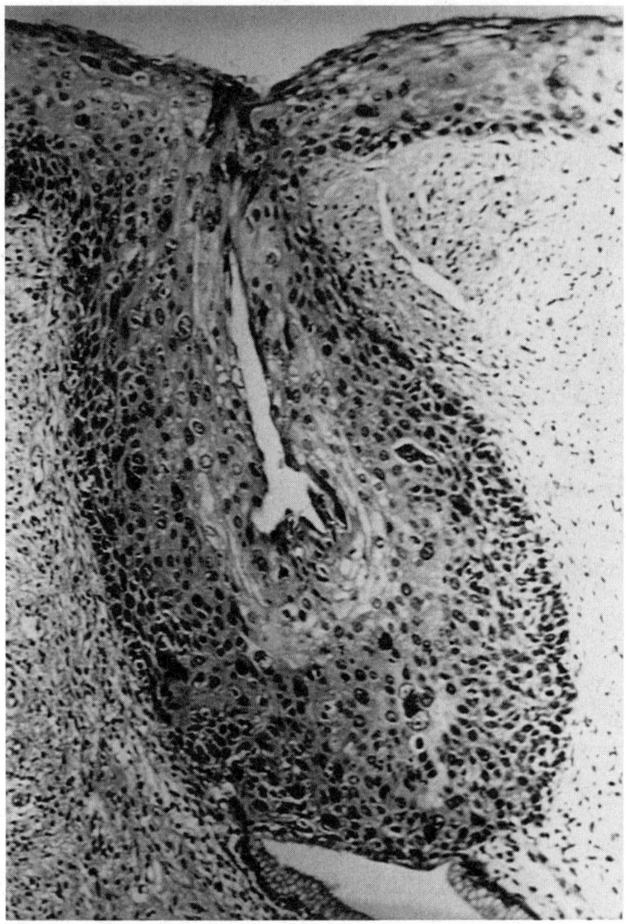

Figure 3-4   Cervical intraepithelial neoplasia (CIN) III (severe dysplasia). Cytologic changes characteristic of malignancy extend into the upper fourth of thickness of the epithelium. In this example the lesion extends into an endocervical gland. (From Cavanagh D, Ruffolo EH, Marsden DE: *Gynecologic cancer—a clinicopathologic approach,* Norwalk, Conn, 1985, Appleton-Century-Crofts.)

more curable stage certainly contributes. Much of the benefit is thought to be through identification and treatment of precancerous cervical lesions and thus prevention of invasive disease. As many as 600,000 women could be diagnosed with CIN each year in the United States.[64] There are several relatively simple and highly effective local treatments that eradicate these CIN lesions. The progressive nature of CIN I to III is illustrated in Figures 3-2 to 3-5. Severe dysplasia and carcinoma in situ have the same prognosis, so both are graded as CIN III.

When a woman is found to have an abnormal Pap smear suggestive of cervical neoplasia and the cervix is grossly normal, the next step in evaluation is colposcopy. The colposcope allows the physician to evaluate the extent and direct a biopsy of dysplastic or neoplastic appearing areas. Depending on the results of this evaluation, the plan of management for CIN lesions may vary widely, from observation only to hysterectomy. A large percentage of patients with a significant CIN lesion (CIN II or III) are treated by

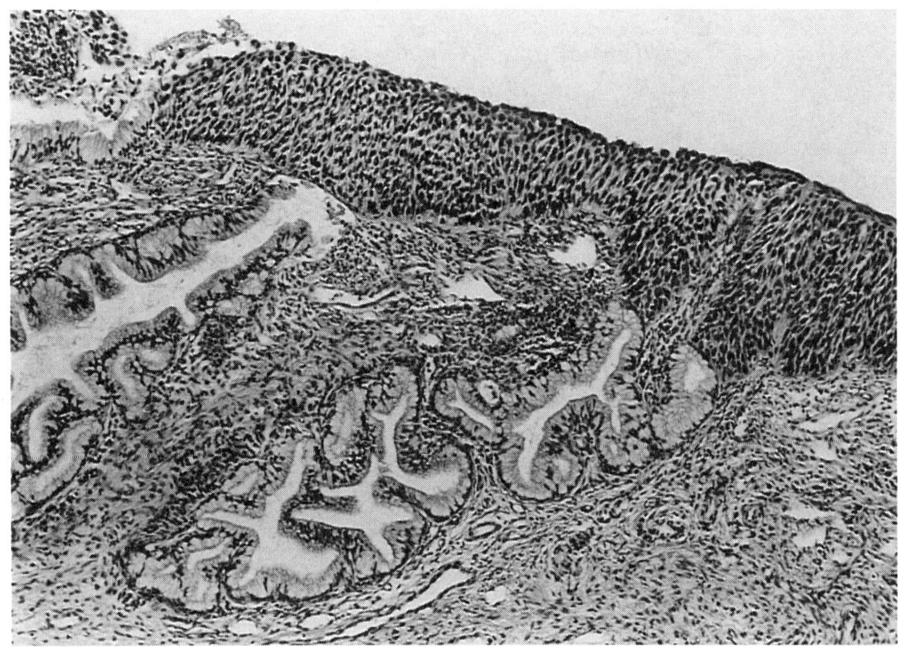

Figure 3-5 Cervical intraepithelial neoplasia (CIN) III (carcinoma in situ). The full thickness of the epithelium exhibits the cellular changes characteristic of malignancy. (From Cavanagh D, Ruffolo EH, Marsden DE: *Gynecologic cancer—a clinicopathologic approach,* Norwalk, Conn, 1985, Appleton-Century-Crofts.)

a locally ablative method (cryotherapy or laser) or local excision by cone biopsy or large loop excision of the transformation zone (LLETZ). On long-term follow-up few patients so managed develop invasive cancer.[65-67] Hysterectomy should be offered to healthy women with CIN III who do not intend to have any more children.

FUTURE DIRECTIONS

It had been anticipated that through widespread implementation of screening programs and treatment of cervical precancerous conditions, invasive cervical cancer could largely be eliminated. As previously discussed, large segments of the population do not undergo regular screening, and this group accounts for most of the patients with invasive cancer in the United States and worldwide. Even in screened populations, however, invasive squamous cervical cancers do develop and adenocarcinoma of the cervix, although only accounting for 20% of cases in the United States, is on the rise. Thus it is unlikely, given present methods, that invasive cervical cancer is an entirely preventable disease. The screening-prevention system for cervical neoplasia is prone to several sources of error. This includes the false negative rate of the Pap smear, precancerous conditions and cancers arising high in the endocervical canal that may escape sampling, a rapid transit from a preinvasive to an invasive lesion in some cases, and de novo development of invasive cancers without a preliminary preinvasive state.

> *Future directions in cervical screening will include efforts at inclusion of the entire population at risk and improvements in screening methodology.*

As stated, reaching out to currently unscreened segments of the population will be a matter of resource allocation and education. Currently, the greatest area of need for improvement in screening is to find methods that will reduce the false negative and false positive rates to more acceptable levels. Obviously there are biochemical changes in the cervix before the development of the earliest histopathologic change, but so far a test based on biochemical indicators such as pentose shunt enzymes has eluded investigators.

REFERENCES

1. Boring CC et al: Cancer statistics, 1994, *CA Cancer J Clin* 44:7, 1994.
2. *Cancer facts and figures, 1984,* New York, 1984, American Cancer Society.
3. Brinton LA et al: Risk factors for cervical cancer by histology, *Gynecol Oncol* 51:301, 1993.
4. Benda JA: Pathology of cervical carcinoma and its prognostic implications, *Semin Oncol* 21:3, 1994.
5. Nasiell K, Roger V, Nasiell M: Behavior of mild cervical dysplasia during long-term follow-up, *Obstet Gynecol* 67:665, 1986.
6. Nasiell K, Nasiell M, Vaclavinkova V: Behavior of moderate cervical dysplasia during long-term follow-up, *Obstet Gynecol* 61:609, 1983.
7. Peterson O: Spontaneous course of cervical precancerous conditions, *Am J Obstet Gynecol* 72:1063, 1956.
8. McIndoe WA et al: The invasive potential of carcinoma in situ of the cervix, *Obstet Gynecol* 64:451, 1984.
9. Koss LG, Stewart FW, Foote FW: Some histological aspects of behavior of epidermoid carcinoma in situ and related lesions of the uterine cervix, *Cancer* 16:1160, 1963.
10. Qizilbash AH: In situ and microinvasive adenocarcinoma of the cervix, *Am J Clin Pathol* 64:155, 1975.
11. Ostor AG et al: Adenocarcinoma in situ of the cervix, *Int J Gynecol Pathol* 3:179, 1984.
12. Bertrand M, Lickrish GM, Colgan TJ: The anatomic distribution of cervical adenocarcinoma in situ: implications for treatment, *Am J Obstet Gynecol* 157:21, 1987.
13. Hopkins MP, Roberts JA, Schmidt RW: Cervical adenocarcinoma in situ, *Obstet Gynecol* 71:842, 1988.
14. Anderson ES, Arffmann E: Adenocarcinoma in situ of the uterine cervix: a clinico-pathologic study of 36 cases, *Gynecol Oncol* 35:1, 1989.
15. Muntz HG et al: Adenocarcinoma in situ of the uterine cervix, *Obstet Gynecol* 80:935, 1992.
16. Poynor EA et al: Management and follow-up of patients with adenocarcinoma in situ of the uterine cervix, *Gynecol Oncol* 57:158, 1995.
17. Fujimoto I et al: Epidemiologic study of carcinoma in situ of the cervix, *J Reprod Med* 30:535, 1985.
18. Parazzini F et al: Risk factors for cervical intraepithelial neoplasia, *Cancer* 69:2276, 1992.
19. Vonka V et al: Prospective study on the relationship between cervical neoplasia and herpes simplex virus II: herpes simplex type II antibodies present in serum taken at enrollment, *Int J Cancer* 33:61, 1984.

20. Lorincz AT et al: Human papillomavirus infection of the cervix: relative risk associations of 15 common anogenital types, *Obstet Gynecol* 79:328, 1992.

21. Richart RM, Wright TC Jr: Controversies in the management of low-grade cervical intraepithelial neoplasia, *Cancer* 71:1413, 1993.

22. Kurman RJ et al: From Papanicolaou to Bethesda: the rationale for a new cervical cytologic classification, *Obstet Gynecol* 77:779, 1991.

23. Richart RM, Jones HW III, Reid R: Classification and interpretation of Pap smears, *Am Coll Obstet Gynecol* Update 18(10):1, 1993.

24. Durst M et al: The physical state of human papillomavirus type 16 DNA in benign and malignant genital tumours, *J Gen Virol* 66:1515, 1985.

25. Campion MJ et al: Progressive potential of mild cervical atypia: prospective cytological, colposcopic and virological study, *Lancet* 2:237, 1986.

26. Kovtsky LA et al: A cohort study of the risk of cervical intraepithelial neoplasia grade 2 or 3 in relation to papillomavirus infection, *N Engl J Med* 327:1272, 1992.

27. McCance DJ et al: Human papillomavirus type 16 alters human epithelial cell differentiation in vitro, *Proc Natl Acad Sci USA* 85:7169, 1988.

28. Schiffman MH: Recent progress in defining the epidemiology of human papillomavirus infection and cervical neoplasia, *J Natl Cancer Inst* 84:394, 1992.

29. Papanicolaou GN, Traut HF: The diagnostic value of vaginal smears in carcinoma of the uterus, *Am J Obstet Gynecol* 42:193, 1941.

30. Ayre JE: Selective cytology smear for diagnosis of cancer, *Am J Obstet Gynecol* 53:609, 1947.

31. Bocciolone L et al: Trends in uterine cancer mortality in the Americas, 1955-1988, *Gynecol Oncol* 51:335, 1993.

32. Adami HO et al: Survival trend after invasive cervical cancer diagnosis in Sweden before and after cytologic screening, *Cancer* 73:140, 1994.

33. Parkin DM, Laara E, Muir CS: Estimates of the worldwide frequency of sixteen major cancers in 1980, *Int J Cancer* 41:184, 1988.

34. Koss LG: Cervical (Pap) smear: new directions, *Cancer* 71:1406, 1993.

35. Gay JD, Donaldson LD, Goellner JR: False-negative results in cervical cytologic studies, *Acta Cytol* 29:1043, 1985.

36. Van der Graaf Y et al: Screening errors in cervical cytology screening, *Acta Cytol* 31:434, 1987.

37. Melamed MR: Quality control in the cytology laboratory, *Acta Cytol* 20:203, 1976.

38. DiBonito L et al: Cervical cytopathology: an evaluation of its accuracy based on cytohistologic comparison, *Cancer* 72:3002, 1993.

39. Yobs AR, Swanson RA, Lamotte LC Jr: Laboratory reliability of the Papanicolaou smear, *Obstet Gynecol* 65:235, 1985.

40. Wain GV, Farnsworth A, Hacker NF: Cervical carcinoma after negative Pap smears: evidence against rapid-onset cancers, *Int J Gynecol Cancer* 2:318, 1992.

41. Stanbridge CM et al: A cervical smear review in women developing cervical carcinoma with particular reference to age, false-negative cytology and the histologic type of the carcinoma, *Int J Gynecol Cancer* 2:92, 1992.

42. Pearlstone AC, Grigsby PW, Mutch DG: High rates of atypical cervical cytology: occurrence and clinical significance, *Obstet Gynecol* 80:191, 1992.

43. Hoffman MS et al: Comparing the yield of the standard Papanicolaou and endocervical brush smears, *J Reprod Med* 36:267, 1991.

44. Hoffman MS et al: Use of the cytobrush in postmenopausal women, *J Gynecol Surg* 7:23, 1991.

45. Hoffman MS, Gordy LW, Cavanagh D: Use of the cytobrush for cervical sampling after cryotherapy, *Acta Cytol* 35:79, 1991.

46. American College of Obstetricians and Gynecologists: *Report of the task force on routine cancer screening,* Washington, DC, 1989, The College.

47. Fink DJ: Change in American Cancer Society guidelines for detection of cervical cancer, *CA Cancer J Clin* 38:127, 1988.

48. DiSaia PJ, Creasman WT: Preinvasive disease of the cervix. In Disaia PJ, Creasman WT, editors: *Clinical gynecologic oncology*, ed 4, St Louis, 1993, Mosby.

49. Giles JA et al: Colposcopic assessment of the accuracy of cervical cytology screening, *Br Med J* 296:1099, 1988.

50. Navratil E et al: Simultaneous colposcopy and cytology used in the screening for carcinoma of the cervix, *Am J Obstet Gynecol* 75:1292, 1297, 1958.

51. Limburg H: Comparison between cytology and colposcopy in the diagnosis of early cervical carcinoma, *Am J Obstet Gynecol* 75:1298, 1958.

52. Olatunbosun OA, Okonofua FE, Ayangade SO: Screening for cervical neoplasia in an African population: simultaneous use of cytology and colposcopy, *Int J Gynecol Obstet* 36:39, 1991.

53. Stafl A: Cervicography: a new method for cervical cancer detection, *Am J Obstet Gynecol* 139:815, 1981.

54. Blythe JG: Cervicography: a preliminary report, *Am J Obstet Gynecol* 152:192, 1985.

55. Hall JB et al: Evaluation of the cerviscope as a screening instrument, *Gynecol Oncol* 20:17, 1985.

56. Tawa K et al: A comparison of the Papanicolaou smear and the cervigram: sensitivity, specificity, and cost analysis, *Obstet Gynecol* 71:229, 1988.

57. Szarewski A et al: The use of cervicography in a primary screening service, *Br J Obstet Gynecol* 98:313, 1991.

58. Reid R et al: Should cervical cytologic testing be augmented by cervicography or human papillomavirus deoxyribonucleic acid detection? *Am J Obstet Gynecol* 164:1461, 1991.

59. Kesic VI et al: A comparison of cytology and cervicography in cervical screening, *Int J Gynecol Cancer* 3:395, 1993.

60. Ottaviano M, LaTorre P: Examination of the cervix with the naked eye using acetic acid test, *Am J Obstet Gynecol* 143:139, 1982.

61. Fiscor G et al: Enhancing cervical cancer detection using nucleic acid hybridization and acetic acid tests, *Nurse Pract* 15:326, 1990.

62. Van Le L et al: Acetic acid visualization of the cervix to detect cervical dysplasia, *Obstet Gynecol* 891:293, 1993.

63. Bauer HM et al: Genital human papillomavirus infection in female university students as determined by a PCR-based method, *JAMA* 265:472, 1991.

64. Sadeghi SB, Sadeghi A, Robboy SJ: Prevalence of dysplasia and cancer of the cervix in a nationwide Planned Parenthood population, *Cancer* 61:2359, 1988.

65. Draeby-Kristiansen J et al: Ten years after cryosurgical treatment of cervical intraepithelial neoplasia, *Am J Obstet Gynecol* 165:43, 1991.

66. Andersen ES, Husth M: Cryosurgery for cervical intraepithelial neoplasia: 10-year follow-up, *Gynecol Oncol* 45:240, 1992.

67. Boyes DA, Worth AS, Fidler HK: The results of treatment of 4389 cases of preclinical squamous carcinoma, *J Obstet Gynaecol Br Commonw* 77:769, 1970.

COLON AND RECTAL CANCER

4

Jack S. Mandel

Observational studies of screening flexible sigmoidoscopy
Conclusions

OTHER SCREENING PROCEDURES

RECOMMENDATIONS FOR PRACTICE AND FUTURE RESEARCH

INCIDENCE

Cancers of the colon and rectum occur throughout the world.[1] The incidence rate varies widely from about 2 per 100,000 population in India to 30 per 100,000 population in U.S. whites.[2] The highest rates (>20) occur in developed countries, including those in North America, western Europe, and Australia; the lowest rates (<10) occur in eastern Europe, the Philippines, and India. Between 1960 and 1985 worldwide incidence generally increased.[3] Mortality increased somewhat, although notable decreases of about 6% to 9% every 5 years occurred in Canada, the United States, Sweden, and western Europe. This decline in mortality has been greater among women than men.

> *In 1995 it is estimated that 138,200 new cases and 55,300 deaths will occur in the United States from cancer of the colon and rectum. These cancers account for about 12% of all incident cancers and 10% of all cancer deaths.*

TABLE 4-1

AGE-ADJUSTED INCIDENCE AND MORTALITY RATES AND 5-YEAR RELATIVE SURVIVAL RATES FOR COLORECTAL CANCER BY GENDER AND RACE

	Incidence*	Mortality*	Survival (%)
Whites			
Men	59.8	23.8	59.9
Women	40.9	16.0	58.7
TOTAL	48.8	19.2	59.3
African-Americans			
Men	60.1	28.0	46.6
Women	46.8	20.6	48.9
TOTAL	52.2	23.5	47.8

From Miller BA et al, editors: *Seer Cancer Statistics Review 1973-1990,* National Cancer Institute, NIH Pub No 93-2789, Bethesda, Md, 1993, US Government Printing Office.
*Rates per 100,000 population adjusted to 1970 U.S. population.

Colorectal cancer deaths account for 758,000 person-years of life lost, an average of 13.3 years per person dying of colorectal cancer.[4]

The age-adjusted incidence rate in the United States is 49 per 100,000 population.[5] As shown in Table 4-1, the age-adjusted incidence rate is about 50% higher in men than women. The rates are about equal for African-American and white men; African-American women, however, have a 14% higher rate than white women.

Between 1973 and 1985 the incidence rates increased for white men and women and then began to decline (Figure 4-1). For African-Americans incidence increased from 42.6 per 100,000 population in 1973 to 59 per 100,000 population in 1990 for men and from 41.1 per 100,000 population in 1973 to 48.8 per 100,000 population in 1990 for women. African-Americans have higher colorectal cancer mortality than whites (23.5 versus 19.2 per 100,000 population). Five-year survival rates are 59.3% for whites and 47.8% for African-Americans.

Between 1973 and 1990, age-adjusted mortality decreased for whites (10% for men and 22% for women) and increased for African-Americans (26.4% for men and 3.2% for women) (Figure 4-2).

It has been suggested recently that the declining colorectal cancer mortality in the late 1980s for whites, the steady declines in distant (late-stage) disease incidence rates, the increases in regional disease incidence rates in the early 1980s followed by declines in the late 1980s, and the increases in localized (early-stage) disease incidence rates in the mid-1980s may reflect improved early detection and changes in lifestyle factors associated with the disease.[6]

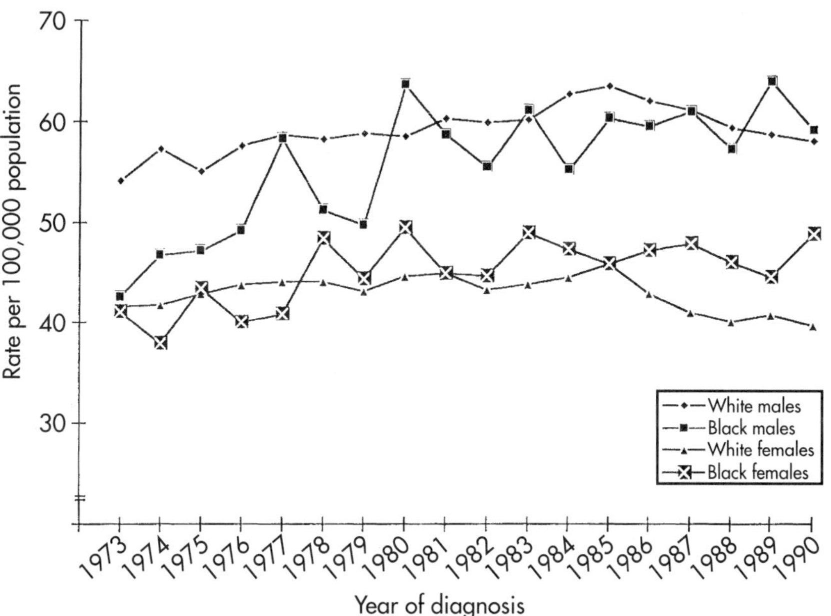

Figure 4-1   Age-adjusted incidence rates (per 100,000 population adjusted to U.S. population) for colorectal cancers by gender and race, 1973-1990. (From Miller BA et al, editors: *Seer Cancer Statistics Review 1973-1990,* National Cancer Institute, NIH Pub No 93-2789, Bethesda, Md, 1993, US Government Printing Office.)

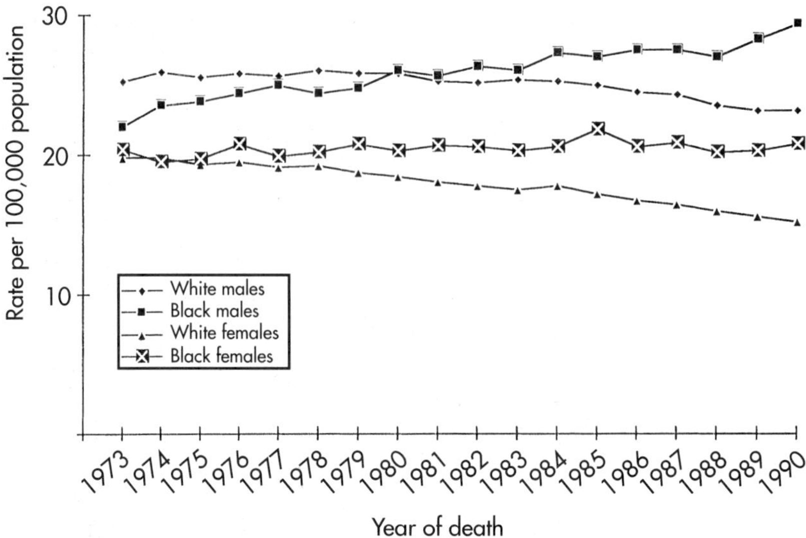

Figure 4-2   Age-adjusted mortality rates (per 100,000 population adjusted to U.S. population) for colorectal cancers by gender and race, 1973-1990. (From Miller BA et al, editors: *Seer Cancer Statistics Review 1973-1990,* National Cancer Institute, NIH Pub No 93-2789, Bethesda, Md, 1993, US Government Printing Office.)

ETIOLOGY AND PREVENTION

Little is known about the etiology of colorectal cancer. A recent review of the literature offers a few factors that are positively or negatively associated with the disease.[7] Those positively associated include a diet high in fat, meat, and protein, a family history of colorectal cancer, exposure to asbestos, and ulcerative colitis. Those negatively associated or protective include a diet high in vegetables, fruits, and fibers, physical activity, and the use of nonsteroidal antiinflammatory drugs. The available data suggest that colorectal cancer incidence might be lowered over time if the population consumed less fat, meat, and protein and more fruits and vegetables, although definitive evidence from randomized trials is not yet available.

> *Screening average risk asymptomatic people over the age of 50 with Hemoccult will reduce colorectal cancer mortality.[8]*

Other guaiac, immunochemical, and heme-porphyrin tests, as well as procedures such as flexible sigmoidoscopy and colonoscopy, have been suggested for screening, but there are insufficient data to support the widespread use of any of these except in further clinical trials.

FECAL OCCULT BLOOD TESTS

The development of a fecal occult blood test (FOBT) for home use to screen for colorectal cancer was stimulated by Greegor[9] in 1967. Since then, there has been considerable debate about the effectiveness of FOBTs as a screening method for colorectal cancer. Despite the absence of adequate data from randomized controlled trials or well-designed observational studies, the FOBT was recommended for screening,[10-12] yet agreement was not universal.[13,14] In 1993 results from the first randomized controlled trial helped focus the debate on the relative merits of an FOBT.[8] The concurrent publication of results from a prospective study and two case-control studies added further to the evidence in support of FOBTs.[16-18]

Types

The three principal types of FOBTs are guaiac, immunochemical, and hemeporphyrin assays. The guaiac tests, which detect heme in any form provided that the iron has not been removed from the porphyrin ring, react to any peroxidase. Guaiac tests have been studied more than the other FOBTs. A more detailed review of these tests is presented later in this chapter.

Immunochemical tests are the most selective in that they detect only hemoglobin and globin and perhaps early degradation products of globin. A variety of immunochemical tests are available, including the enzyme-linked immunosorbent assay (ELISA), FECA-EIA (Labsystems, Oy), the radial immunodiffusion test Detectacol (IMVS, Adelaide); the latex agglutination tests Hemolex (Orion) and OC Hemodia (Eiken); and the hemagglutination test HemSp (Fujirebio), marketed in North America and Europe as HemeSelect (SmithKline Diagnostics, Inc.). These are predominantly qualitative tests, utilizing antibodies directed against the intact globin moiety of human hemoglobin and possibly also against large fragments of globin.[19]

A number of studies have evaluated immunochemical tests. Turunen et al.[20] found that combining them with a guaiac test (Fecatwin [S]ensitive) was most effective in detecting neoplastic lesions. They recommended the use of the combined Fecatwin S and FECA-EIA kit.

Armitage et al.[21] used the ELISA (Feca-EIA) combined with a guaiac test, Fecatwin Sensitive/Feca EIA, to screen an asymptomatic population and compared it with the unhydrated Hemoccult. They concluded that Feca EIA increased the yield of neoplastic disease detection over the Hemoccult test; however, the high false positive rate made the test unsuitable for population screening.

Songster et al.[22] reported on an immunochemical screening test (Fecal Smear Punch-Disc Test), which employed high-titer monospecific antisera to intact human hemoglobin in a radial immunodiffusion assay. They found that immunochemical screening for occult blood loss provided a higher rate of detection of colon cancer than Hemoccult.

HemeSelect, a hemagglutination test with an intermediate threshold of sensitivity for hemoglobin, uses formalin-fixed chicken erythrocytes coated with anti–human hemoglobin AO blood group antibodies. It has been evaluated in studies comparing four fecal occult blood tests for the detection of colorectal neoplasia.

St. John et al.[23] compared Hemoccult II (nonrehydrated), Hemoccult-SENSA (a more sensitive guaiac test), HemeSelect, and HemoQuant (a hemeporphyrin assay). HemeSelect and HemoccultSENSA had significantly higher sensitivity for colorectal cancer (97% and 94%, respectively) than Hemoccult II (89%)

and HemoQuant (71%). There were no significant differences in sensitivity among the four tests for cancers proximal to the splenic flexure. In contrast, the sensitivity for HemoQuant (65%) was considerably lower than the other three tests for distal cancer (89% for Hemoccult II, 94% for HemoccultSENSA, and 96% for HemeSelect). The sensitivity rate for HemoQuant was also significantly lower for distal cancers (65%) than for proximal cancers (89%).

HemeSelect had the highest sensitivity for all adenomas combined (58% versus 31% for Hemoccult II, 44% for HemoccultSENSA, and 37% for HemaQuant). For large (>1 cm) adenomas, the sensitivity for HemeSelect was the highest (76%). In comparison, the sensitivity was 60% for HemoccultSENSA and 42% for both Hemoccult and HemoQuant. For small (<1 cm) adenomas, sensitivity ranged from a high of 36% for HemeSelect to a low of 17% for Hemoccult II.

Castiglione et al.[24] compared the specificity and positive predictivity of four fecal occult blood tests, for both 1-day and 3-day testing using rehydrated Hemoccult II, HemoccultSENSA, OC-Hemodia, and HemeSelect, which were 4.8%, 5.6%, 8.4%, and 11.2%, respectively. The immunochemical tests were generally less predictive than the guaiac tests in all subgroups of neoplastic disease, but especially for adenomas. The specificity of rehydrated Hemoccult II, HemoccultSENSA, OC Hemodia, and HemeSelect in the overall series was 96.1%, 96.0%, 93.8% and 91.2%, respectively. The differences in specificity between guaiac and immunochemical tests were statistically significant; the only exception was HemoccultSENSA as compared with OC Hemodia in asymptomatic patients. No significant difference was evident between the two guaiac tests, whereas OC Hemodia was significantly more specific than HemeSelect, particularly in asymptomatic subjects. None of the differences between tests was statistically significant in the group of symptomatic subjects. Values of specificity as determined on the first fecal sample only in the overall series were 98%, 98%, 96%, and 95% for Hemoccult II, HemoccultSENSA, OC Hemodia, and HemeSelect, respectively. No significant difference in specificity was evident when 3-day guaiac tests were compared to 1-day immunochemical tests. The authors concluded that 1-day immunochemical testing with HemeSelect might be an alternative to classic 3-day guaiac testing.

The heme-porphyrin tests detect the broadest range of blood derivatives, namely deironed hemes (heme-derived porphyrins) as well as intact heme in any form (free or as hemoprotein). HemoQuant is a biochemical method for the assay of fecal heme and its degradation products in stool. This test showed promise early[25-27]; however, more recent studies have shown that this test is probably less sensitive and specific than Hemoccult.[23,28,29]

The performance of any given type of FOBT in a screening program is likely to depend on the nature of blood derivatives present in the feces in a given clinical situation.[30] Only the guaiac tests (namely Hemoccult) have been sufficiently studied so that enough data are available on which to base a recommendation for screening.

Blood in Stool

Heme is an iron compound of protoporphyrin that constitutes the pigment portion or protein-free part of the hemoglobin molecule. Its fate in the gut is not well understood.

> *Fecal excretion of heme can be an indicator of gastrointestinal mucosal pathology.[31]*

The amount excreted depends on the balance between the amount delivered to the lumen, including that which is present in the diet as myoglobin and hemoglobin, and its loss from the lumen.[32]

In the stomach heme is rapidly released from the binding protein and precipitated. In the small intestine it is solubilized, and about 5% to 15% is absorbed.[31] Globin (a protein from hemoglobin) is rapidly digested in the stomach and small intestine. The majority of heme presenting to the upper gut is passed to the colon.[30] Heme in the colonic lumen may be derived from the small intestine as heme or from colonic bleeding or desquamation as hemoprotein. Hemoglobin, which enters the large intestine from bleeding in the upper gastrointestinal tract, either remains whole and is excreted as intact hemoglobin in the feces or undergoes proteolytic digestion of the globin to become heme.[30]

Protoheme—heme coming from the ileum or from hemoglobin—is either excreted in the feces as intact heme or converted by bacteria to a range of heme-derived porphyrins lacking iron.[30] This conversion is a slow and incomplete process, and the amount converted in this way depends on colonic transit rate, site of bleeding, and amount of luminal heme.[32] In addition to the removal of iron, bacterial activity can cause modifications of the vinyl side chains of heme to produce various iron-porphyrin derivatives, which are excreted in the feces.[30] As a consequence, feces contain variable proportions of heme and heme-derived porphyrins.[32]

From in vivo and in vitro studies it is possible to predict the nature of hemoglobin derivatives likely to be found in feces, based on the site of bleeding.[30] The more proximal the bleeding, the more likely are heme-derived porphyrins to be the principal products. The more distal the bleeding, the more likely it is that intact hemoglobin will be present in the feces.

> *Many conditions can result in blood in stool. These include cancer, polyps, peptic ulcers, hemorrhoids, and diverticulitis.*

The bleeding tends to be intermittent,[33] and the blood is not distributed equally throughout the stool.[34] These factors affect the sensitivity and specificity of all types of FOBTs.[30]

Blood Loss from Colorectal Cancers and Adenomas

Data on daily blood loss have been obtained from radiochromium blood loss studies and more recently from heme-porphyrin assays.[34a,35] The validity of using the ^{51}Cr label method for measurement of blood loss rests on evidence that the isotopic label is neither secreted into nor reabsorbed from the gastrointestinal tract.[36]

There have been a number of studies on fecal blood loss from colorectal cancers and polyps. Turunen et al.[20] collected a total of 30 48-hour fecal samples from 19 colorectal cancer patients and 11 controls for quantitative determination of fecal blood loss using the ^{51}Cr method. The tests were performed after administration of a peroxidase-free diet. The geometric mean level of daily gastrointestinal blood loss in the controls (12 samples) was 0.4 ml/day. The mean level of blood loss was 18.4 ml/day for cancers in the right colon and 2.8 ml/day for cancers in the left colon and rectum. There was a significant correlation between Dukes stage and blood loss. The geometric mean levels of blood loss were considerably higher in patients with Dukes C or D cancers than in patients with Dukes A or B cancers.

Macrae and St. John[37] measured ^{51}Cr-labeled blood loss for an average of 9.1 days in 46 patients with colorectal cancer and 28 patients with adenomas at the Royal Melbourne Hospital in Australia. The patients were placed on a strict low-peroxidase diet before surgery. Daily stool collections were begun at least 2 days after intravenous injection of ^{51}Cr-labeled blood and continued for a minimum of 5 days.

The mean level of blood loss was 9.3 ml/day in the right colon and 1.5 ml/day, 1.9 ml/day, and 1.8 ml/day for transverse and descending colon, sigmoid colon, and rectum, respectively. The relationship between daily blood loss and anatomic location was significant ($P < .05$), but Dukes stage and degree of differentiation were unrelated to amount of blood loss.

Ahlquist et al.[38-40] conducted a retrospective study of fecal blood levels in colorectal adenocarcinoma patients identified from the surgical pathology tissue registry at the Mayo Clinic. Records were reviewed from 160 consecutive primary colorectal adenocarcinoma patients diagnosed in 1985 or 1986 and for whom a prediagnosis fecal blood test (HemoQuant) had been reported. Of these, 71% had suggestive colorectal symptoms (particularly stool changes, overt bleeding, and abdominal pain) or anemia at presentation, and 29% were asymptomatic. Restrictions on diet and medication use were not consistently followed. Results for only one fecal sample were reported for over 95% of the patients. Although contamination from toilet water was avoided with the use of a stool collection device, the timing of stool collection followed bowel purgation in about half of the patients, and this was associated with lower fecal blood levels. For the entire study population the mean fecal blood level was 6.6 ± 11 mg of hemoglobin per gram of stool (median, 2.7 mg/g; range, 0.1 to 69 mg/g).

Fecal blood levels were significantly higher in patients with advanced-stage cancers, with larger tumors, with proximal lesion sites, and with stools collected before any bowel purgation. Patient age, gender, tumor grade, and manner of presentation (symptoms or anemia versus asymptomatic) did not affect fecal blood level distributions.

Herzog et al.[41] determined fecal daily blood loss after intravenous administration of ^{51}Cr-labeled erythrocytes in 44 patients with colonic polyps over 15 mm in diameter who were referred for endoscopic polypectomy and 11 controls without gastrointestinal bleeding over 2 weeks. Both patients and controls were instructed to follow their customary diets without restrictions. Eighteen of the 34 patients with polyps in the descending colon and rectosigmoid and 1 of the 10 patients with polyps in the ascending colon and transverse colon had previously noticed blood in their stools, which had prompted them to seek medical care. The absence of a bleeding lesion was diagnostically confirmed in each control subject. The mean fecal daily blood loss was significantly different between polyp patients and controls (1.36 ± 0.14 ml/day for left colon, 1.28 ± 0.31 ml/day for right colon, and 0.62 ± 0.07 ml/day for controls).

Macrae and St. John[37] found geometric mean levels of blood loss from cancers were 9.3 ml/day for the cecum and ascending colon, 1.5 ml/day for the transverse and descending colon, 1.9 ml/day for the sigmoid colon, and 1.8 ml/day for the rectum. Blood loss in 28 patients with adenomas was over 2 ml/day only when adenomas exceeded 2 cm in diameter. Because only two adenomas were in the right side of the colon, no analysis could be made of the relationship between the anatomic site of adenomas and the degree of blood loss.

> *The data suggest that cancers bleed more from right-sided than left-sided lesions and more from late- than early-stage cancers. Blood loss from polyps, although considerably less than from cancers is probably greater in larger (>2 cm) than in smaller polyps.*

Characteristics of Hemoccult Tests

Sensitivity is the ability of the test to detect the disease of interest—colorectal cancer, adenomatous polyps, or both. A number of studies have reported on the sensitivity of Hemoccult and other FOBTs. Results for Hemoccult varied from 26% to 92% for colorectal cancer.[29,37,42-45] Most of the studies have shown sensitivity values of 65 percent or greater for colorectal cancer. Studies using rehydrated slides have reported sensitivities between 83 and 92 percent. Test sensitivity for adenomatous polyps is lower, ranging from 15% to 30% for all polyps but higher for larger polyps.[23,25,43]

The wide range in sensitivity values reported is not surprising. Hemoccult is a test for blood in the stool. It is not a direct test for cancer or polyps. The rationale for its use as a screening test for colorectal neoplasms is based on the fact that many, perhaps most and eventually all, cancers bleed. Some polyps bleed, particularly those which are larger. Bleeding is intermittent and not evenly distributed throughout stool.

> *A test for blood in stool should effectively identify most cancers and some polyps if it is applied repeatedly with multiple samples to overcome the intermittent bleeding and the unequal distribution of blood in stool.*

Thus the rationale for Greegor's original recommendation for multiple sampling is evident.[46]

Most of the studies of Hemoccult sensitivity have not evaluated the test on an average risk asymptomatic population using multiple tests from multiple stools. The use of different study populations (for example, asymptomatic, clinical) and different stool sampling methods may account for the wide variation in test sensitivity. For example, in the clinical study by St. John et al.[23,25] Hemoccult II tests were obtained from 124 patients with newly diagnosed colorectal cancer and 86 patients with adenoma after excluding dietary hemes and peroxidase-rich foods. Test sensitivity for colorectal cancer at all sites was 89.5%. The sensitivity was 30.2% for the 86 patients with adenomas. Sensitivity was significantly better for adenomas 1 cm or more in diameter (41.7%) than for adenomas less than 1 cm in diameter (15.8%).

Ahlquist et al.[29] compared the sensitivity of Hemoccult II (not rehydrated) and HemoQuant for colorectal neoplasia. Two groups were studied: (1) 1217 patients at least 18 years old undergoing routine structural surveillance evaluations following curative resection of a colorectal cancer and (2) 12,312 first-degree relatives, at least 50 years old, of colorectal cancer patients.

Subjects were instructed to refrain from eating red meat and taking nonsteroidal antiinflammatory drugs, iron supplements, and vitamin C for 5 days before and during stool collections. Subjects were directed to scoop a marble-sized stool sample from each end of three consecutive stools with a small spatula and seal it into an air-tight plastic tube. Stools were tested by both HemoQuant and Hemoccult. The median delay from stool collection to stool testing was 7 days (range, 5 to 21 days). In the postresection group, stools were collected and tested before routine annual endoscopic or radiographic surveillance evaluations for the first 3 postoperative years. The postresection group of 1217 patients returned 2946 test kits. Overall, 2.3% of all stool samples returned were Hemoccult positive. Hemoccult screens were positive for 12 of 46 colorectal cancers found on surveillance, yielding a sensitivity of 26%. The sensitivity of 255 adenomatous polyps was 8.6% for Hemoccult.

Since patients were screened after curative resection of the colon, the study was evaluating the tests' ability to detect only very early lesions. This is an interesting question, but is largely irrelevant to the issue of whether regular (for example, annual) screening of an average risk asymptomatic population with FOBT results in a significant reduction of colorectal cancer.

Hemoccult sensitivity for colorectal cancer was also determined for the group of relatives. However, only those with positive FOBTs underwent diagnostic tests. Test sensitivities were determined by estimating missed cancers based on a telephone follow-up of a small sample of test negatives.

The Minnesota study applied the Hemoccult test in the prescribed manner to average risk asymptomatic individuals annually.[15] The high sensitivity for colorectal cancer in the study (80% for nonrehydrated Hemoccults and 92% for rehydrated Hemoccult) is not surprising, given the frequent application of the test and the population screened. Cancer screening tests are generally considered for repeated (such as annual) application. The transition from normal mucosa to invasive carcinoma takes many years.

Repeat screening increases the likelihood of detecting a lesion and the probability of detecting it early enough to intervene and reduce mortality.

Specificity refers to the ability of the test to identify those without the disease of interest (true negatives). False positives are costly because of the unnecessary diagnostic procedures. The specificity of Hemoccult for colorectal cancer is 97% to 98%. It is lower for rehydrated slides.[42-44] Although the false positive rate of the test is low, it represents a large number of people because in a screening program most people do not have colorectal cancer. The lifetime prevalence of colorectal cancer is only about 5 percent.[47]

Influence of Diet

Dietary recommendations for FOBTs vary from no restriction to exclusion of all types of meat or red meat plus uncooked fruit and vegetables.[42,48,49]

The reliability of Hemoccult under both normal and restricted diets was studied in patients undergoing a ^{51}Cr fecal blood loss study for suspected gastrointestinal bleeding or iron-deficiency anemia.[50] Forty patients were advised to eat a normal diet during the test period, and 20 were placed on a restricted diet 48 hours before Hemoccult testing and for the duration of the study. The diet excluded red meat, dark fish, raw vegetables, and raw fruits except fresh oranges and strawberries. High-fiber foods were encouraged.

A single Hemoccult test was performed on each sample. Less than 1.5 ml hemoglobin per gram of feces (equivalent to less than 1.6 ml blood/day) was taken as normal fecal loss and not evidence of significant gastrointestinal bleeding. Thirteen (11%) Hemoccult tests were falsely positive on a normal diet and two (2%) on the restricted diet. This difference was statistically significant. Ten of the 40 patients on a normal diet gave false positive reactions, whereas one of 20 patients on the restricted diet gave a false positive reaction. This difference was not significant.

Macrae et al.[49] studied the influence of diets of differing peroxidase content on nonrehydrated and rehydrated Hemoccult II tests in 156 healthy young subjects under 40 years of age who did not have a history of bleeding hemorrhoids or other significant gastrointestinal disease. In a crossover design each subject followed one diet for 6 days and then a second diet for a further 6 days. Foods were selected for their high or low peroxidase content as determined by measurement of peroxidase activity.[51] The four diets used in the study were (1) full-challenge diet of rare red meat and fresh fruit and vegetables, (2) rare red meat but no fresh fruit or vegetables, (3) fresh fruit and vegetables but no red meat, and (4) strict low-peroxidase diet.

Duplicate sets of Hemoccult II slides were prepared on the last 3 days of each 6-day dietary period for testing with and without rehydration. All 52 subjects in group 1 (hospital staff members) provided additional stool samples on the last 3 days of each dietary period for quantitative measurement of fecal peroxidase activity.

When the Hemoccult slides were developed without rehydration, only seven (0.4%) of 1856 slides were positive. The positive results occurred with challenge diets containing 250 g of rare red meat. With rehydration 53 (5.7%) of 926 slides were positive in 26 of the 156 subjects on a challenge diet that included rare red meat and uncooked fruit and vegetables. Well-cooked red meat also gave positive tests.

With rehydrated tests, significantly more Hemoccults were positive ($P <$ .001) on the full-challenge diet (4.2%), compared with the strict low-peroxidase diet (0.6%) in group 1. When fresh fruit and vegetables were omitted from the challenge diet (group 2), the proportion of positives remained unchanged (6.3% for the full-challenge diet and 6.6% for the comparison diet). Exclusion of red meat from the challenge diet (group 3) led to a significant fall in Hemoccult positivity from 6.6% on the full-challenge diet to 1.6% on the comparison diet.

Direct assay of stools showed no detectable peroxidase activity in 154 of 155 stool samples from the 52 subjects following the strict low-peroxidase diet. In this study well-motivated healthy young subjects were used because they were unlikely to have occult gastrointestinal bleeding. However, there was no confirmation of Hemoccult results with colonoscopy, barium enema, or ^{51}Cr-labeled blood loss tests.

St. John and Young[52] directly compared test positivity rates and the dietary restriction for three fecal occult blood tests: Hemoccult II, Hemoccult-SENSA, and HemeSelect. Healthy volunteers participated in a randomly administered crossover study in which all three tests were performed in parallel on three serial stools in each dietary arm of the study. In one arm the volunteers followed a low-heme, low-peroxidase exclusion diet; in the other arm they were instructed to consume their usual diet and to complete a food diary.

The findings indicated that a special diet appeared to be less important with Hemoccult II, but that may have depended on the usual level of consumption of red meat in the population to be screened.

In a study to determine the duration of FOBT false positivity induced by eating red meat, 46 healthy asymptomatic medical students consumed 350 to 450 g of cooked red meat (beef, pork, lamb, or veal) per day for the first 3 days of the study.[53] From the fourth day to the tenth day they abstained from red meat. Vitamin C, horseradish, melons, and antiinflammatory medications were avoided before and during the study.

The positivity rates for rehydrated Hemoccult II were 15.4%, 5.5%, and 5.5% on days 1 to 3 and 0% thereafter. All positive results were presumed to be false positives caused by eating red meat because the population comprised young, asymptomatic subjects, unlikely to have significant colorectal pathology.

The authors stated that the presence of positive results on days 1 to 3 (beginning of the red meat–free days) and the absence of positive results thereafter supported their assertion of a substantial rate of false positivity. The recommendation for Hemoccult testing as found in the Hemoccult II product insert was to abstain from red meat for 48 hours before testing. On the basis of this study the authors advised a 3-day period of abstention from red meat before testing with Hemoccult.

In the Nottingham study, a randomized controlled trial of fecal occult blood testing (Hemoccult), the dietary restrictions that were found to be an inconvenience to participants resulting in a 30% decline in compliance, were not employed in the initial screen.[54] Participants in this study, ages 50 to 74 years, were identified from general practitioner registers. After stratification by age and sex, they were randomized by household into one test group, whose members were sent fecal occult blood tests, and one control group, which did not receive the tests. The test group was sent either 3-day or 6-day Hemoccult test packs and a letter inviting them to complete and return the test. These tests were performed without dietary restrictions.

All patients with positive results were subsequently retested with dietary restrictions and proceeded to further investigation (colonoscopy and, if necessary, double-contrast barium enema) only if they remained positive. However, because of intermittent bleeding from tumors, a second test was performed on those with negative results 3 months later. This test incorporated dietary restrictions.

During the test period 18,925 people participated in the study. After the initial Hemoccult tests without dietary restrictions 647 (3.4%) were positive. On retesting with dietary restrictions 251 (39%) remained positive and were referred for further investigation. Thirty-five (14%) carcinomas and 169 adenomas in 129 (51%) patients were identified. Of the 396 individuals with FOBT negatives, 317 (80.1%) completed and returned the test 3 months later. Thirty-one (9.8%) were positive and 286 (90.2%) were negative. Investigation of the positives revealed four (13%) carcinomas and 20 colonic polyps in 15 (48%) patients. It is interesting to note that the positive predictive values for both cancers and polyps were the same.

The authors concluded that retesting with dietary restriction reduced the false positive rate, thus reducing the need for unnecessary diagnostic investigations. Because there was a substantial yield of significant disease from rescreening, they advocated additional rescreening for this group 3 months later.

In another study subjects from the test group were sent a letter and three or six Hemoccult cards (randomly allocated), which they were invited to complete and return while eating a normal diet.[55] The Hemoccult card had two test squares, each to be smeared with a small fecal sample taken at separate sites from the stool and completed over 3 or 6 days, resulting in a total of six or 12 fecal smears. All subjects with at least one positive test during stool sampling while eating a normal diet were asked to complete a further test over 6 days with appropriate dietary restriction. If results were negative, further diet-restricted retesting over 6 days after a 3-month interval was offered. Any subject with a positive retest was advised to undergo colonoscopy.

At the initial screen 376 subjects had a positive test while on a normal diet. Of these, 165 (43.9%) remained positive on retesting and were advised to undergo colonoscopy. The proportion of subjects whose retest was positive increased with the number of positive Hemoccult squares. In all, 113 (35.6%) of 317 subjects whose initial test result was less than five squares positive and 52 (88.1%) of 59 with at least five squares positive remained positive. This difference was statistically significant. Considering only those who were investigated diagnostically following a positive retest, there was no significant difference in the predictive value of the initial test results for either carcinoma or adenoma of 1 cm or more. The data suggested that, if five or more test squares were positive, then dietary interference is unlikely to have accounted for the positive test result. But, where dietary interference had been eliminated as a cause for the positive result in those with fewer positive squares (that is, those whose retests were also positive), there appeared to be little predictive value associated with the number of initially positive squares obtained when eating a normal diet.

The authors concluded that, if dietary restriction retesting is practiced, individuals with strongly positive tests should undergo diagnostic evaluation without retesting.

> *Overall, the results from the studies of diet indicate that foods can interfere with the test, and therefore dietary restriction just before and during the testing period should be recommended.*

Randomized Controlled Trials

Randomized controlled trials of a screening test provide the most persuasive evidence of the test's effectiveness. The only FOBT that has been evaluated in a randomized controlled trial is Hemoccult, in four trials: (1) Minnesota, (2) Funen, Denmark, (3) Göteborg, Sweden, and (4) Nottingham, England. The Minnesota trial has concluded and published results. The other three are in progress, and final results are expected within the next 3 years.

Minnesota Trial

The first randomized controlled trial was initiated in Minnesota in 1975.[15,56] A total of 46,551 participants ages 50 to 80 years were recruited between 1975 and 1977 and randomly assigned to annual screening, biannual screening, or a control group. Participants in the annual and biannual groups submitted six guaiac-impregnated paper slides (Hemoccult), prepared by two smears from each of three consecutive stools. Participants were instructed to abstain from red meat, poultry, fish, and certain vegetables and fruits and to discontinue the use of vitamin C tablets and aspirin for at least 24 hours before and during the collection of the samples. Slide processing was modified early in the trial to incorporate rehydration with a drop of deionized water to restore the sensitivity that was reduced because of drying. Participants with one or more positive test slides in the set of six were invited to the University of Minnesota for a diagnostic evaluation, which included colonoscopy.

Participants in all three study groups received a questionnaire by mail each year. The purpose of this questionnaire was to ascertain (1) vital status, (2) the occurrence of colorectal cancer and polyps in the control group, and (3) colorectal lesions discovered in members of the screened groups either as a result of a diagnostic procedure unrelated to a study positive screening test or in persons who were unwilling or unable to submit the slides.

Deaths were reviewed by a deaths review committee to determine the underlying cause of death. In addition, a nosologist independently coded the death certificates according to the Eighth Revision of the International Classification of Diseases.

Follow-up for vital status through year 14 was 100%. The cumulative colorectal cancer (CRC) mortality per 1000 population was 34%, significantly lower in the annual screened group compared to the control group. The CRC mortality for the biannual group was 10% lower than for the control group. The relatively small mortality reduction in the biannual group was due, in part, to an increase in the number of deaths in the early years of the study, which was consistent with chance. When the data were analyzed with the follow-up beginning at year 6, there was a 30% CRC mortality reduction in the biannual group compared to the control group. For the annual group the reduction increased from 34% to 40%.

In support of the observed mortality reduction, survival was greatest in the annual screen group and poorest in the control group (Figure 4-3). The biannual group was intermediate. An evaluation of survival by mode of detection revealed that the screen-detected cases in both screening groups had the highest survival rate, whereas the survival for the nonscreen-detected cases was considerably lower and similar to survival for the control group.

There was a 48% and 35% reduction in Dukes D cancer in the annual and biannual groups, respectively, relative to the control group. This was particularly noteworthy, since these late-stage cancers contributed substantially to mortality because of their poor prognosis. Five-year survival for Dukes D cancers was only 2.5%.

> *Evaluating the stage data by mode of detection revealed a substantial shift to earlier stage cancers among the screen-detected cases.*

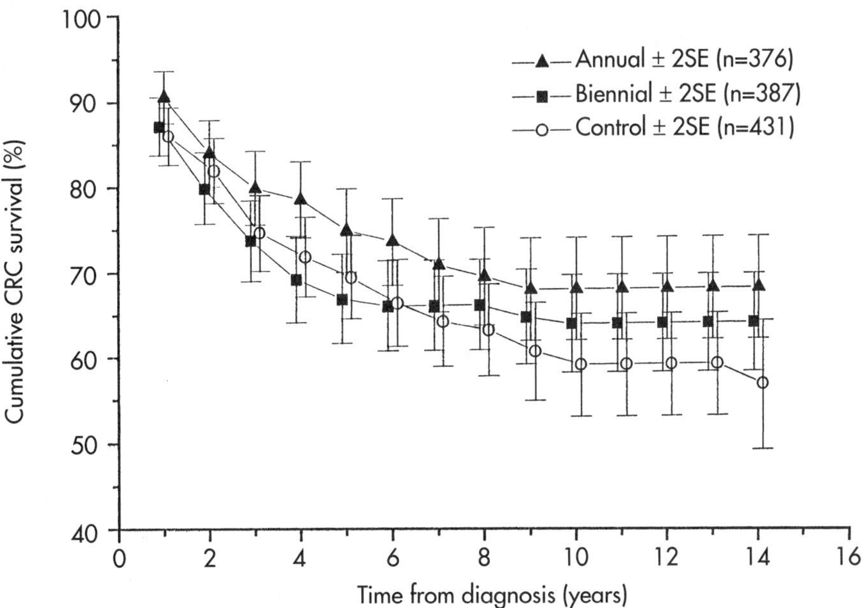

Figure 4-3 Cumulative colorectal cancer survival by study group.

A total of 75% and 66% of the annual and biannual screen-detected cases, respectively, were Dukes A or B, compared to 59% in the control group. The percent of Dukes A or B among interval-detected cases (59% and 55%) was more similar to the control group than to the screen-detected cases.

The observed 34% mortality reduction in the annual group is probably an underestimate of the true reduction, since only 46% of the participants in the annual group completed all of the screens, 10% did not do any screens, there was a 3-year period during which there was no screening, and 83% of the tests were rehydrated. In addition, some members of the control group received screening tests through their regular physicians. These factors dilute the observed difference.

Because Hemoccult is a test for blood, not for cancer, and the positivity rate was high (10%), the question was raised as to the independent contribution of colonoscopy in detecting nonbleeding cancers among false positives.[15] A number of analyses suggested that FOBT contributed substantially to the mortality reduction. These included the sensitivity of the test (92%) and the increasing positive predictive value for cancer and large polyps ($\geq$ 1 cm) with the number of Hemoccult tests positive out of the set of six. There was no such trend for all polyps, regardless of size. Since cancers and larger polyps are more likely to bleed, then the trends observed in the positive predictive value were as expected if the Hemoccult test has predictive power. A particularly compelling argument favoring the contribution of FOBT to the observed mortality reduction was the cumulative colorectal cancer incidence among those positive or negative on the first screen and among the control group. If the observed CRC mortality reduction was due to randomly performing colonoscopy, then the cumulative CRC incidence would eventually be similar among those positive or negative on the first screen. In fact, there was a highly significant fivefold difference in cumulative CRC incidence between these groups. In addition, the cumulative CRC incidence was significantly lower among those negative on the first screen than among those in the control group. This evidence strongly supports the effectiveness of FOBT in reducing CRC mortality.

Lang and Ransohoff[57] presented a model based on estimated data from the Minnesota trial which suggested that colonoscopy accounted for 33% to 50% of the mortality reduction. However, using actual rather than estimated data resulted in a substantial reduction in their estimate of the colonoscopy contribution to the observed mortality reduction.[58]

Göteborg Trial

All 68,308 inhabitants of Göteborg born between 1918 and 1931 were enrolled and randomly allocated to a control or a screen group.[45,58a-60] Three Hemoccult II guaiac-impregnated paper tests were mailed to screen group participants, who prepared two samples from each of three consecutive stools and mailed them back immediately after the last test. They were asked to avoid peroxidase-rich vegetables, food containing blood, and vitamin C and iron supplements for 2 days before and during the stool collection. One rescreen was conducted 16 to 24 months (mean = 20 months) after the initial screen. Approximately half the slides from the first screen and all the slides from the second screen were rehydrated. Because of the large number of positive tests and the subsequent increase in diagnostic examinations, participants in the last cohort recruited (birth years 1923 to 1931) who had a positive screening test at either the initial or second screen were reinvestigated with Hemoccult II, and only those positive on this test were examined. The examination conducted at the hospital included a digital rectal examination, proctoscopy, rectosigmoidoscopy (60 cm), and a double-contrast barium enema. All neoplasms were removed either endoscopically or surgically.

Of the randomized subjects, 63% participated in the first screen and 60% participated in the second screen. As in the Minnesota trial, the positivity rate was higher for rehydrated than nonrehydrated tests (6% versus 1.9%). The sensitivity for rehydrated tests was 83% higher than for nonrehydrated slides.

From the start of the first screening to the end of the rescreening there were 117 colorectal cancers and 419 adenomas diagnosed among screen group participants and 44 cancers and 51 adenomas among control group participants. The distribution of cancers according to Dukes classification was significantly better for the screen group than for the control groups. Significantly more Dukes A cancers and significantly fewer Dukes D cancers were diagnosed in the screen group during this period. In the follow-up period after screening ended fewer cancers and adenomas were diagnosed in the screen group. There were no differences in the Dukes distribution for screen and control group cancers diagnosed during the follow-up period. To date, no reduction in CRC mortality has been observed.

Nottingham Trial

The Nottingham Colorectal Cancer Screening trial, which started in 1984, was designed to enroll 156,000 asymptomatic men and women, ages 50 to 74, and randomly allocate them to a control or screen group.[61-64] Study participants, identified from general practitioner records, were sorted by household (those living at the same address), and then households were stratified by number of eligible members, gender, and by average age of eligible members in 5-year age groups, before being randomly assigned to screen or control groups. Patients with known bowel disease or a previous history of cancer and those deemed to be unsuitable by the general practitioner were excluded from the study.

Compliers with the initial screen were rescreened every 2 years with FOBT (Hemoccult, Rohm Pharma). The initial tests were carried out over 3 consecutive days without dietary restrictions and without rehydration. Since 1985, participants with a positive test were asked to repeat the test over a 6-day period while excluding red meats and vegetables high in peroxidase from their diet. Early in the study the diagnostic protocol included a digital rectal examination, proctoscopy, rigid sigmoidoscopy, a 60-cm fiberoptic sigmoidoscopy, and double-contrast barium enema. Later in the study those with a second positive test had colonoscopy, and if this was incomplete a double-contrast barium enema was administered. Subjects with a negative second test after dietary restrictions were asked to repeat the test, again with dietary restrictions, after 3 months.

The trial is still in progress, and therefore mortality data are not yet available. Among the first 71,868 participants invited to participate, 53% complied. The positivity rate was 2%. Those with negative Haemoccult tests were offered rescreening at 2-year intervals. Compliance was 77% and 84% for the first and second rescreens, respectively. Positivity rates for these rescreens were 1.3% and 0.6%.

The proportion of Dukes A cancers was significantly lower in the control group (14%) than in the screen-detected cases (47%) or in the entire screened group (28%). The proportion of Dukes D cancers was significantly higher in the control group (21%) than in the screen-detected group (6%) but similar in the entire screened group.

The sensitivity of the test for cancer was 67.6% but was higher when tests were completed over 6 rather than 3 days (74% versus 65%).[65] This might be expected, since cancers bleed intermittently and blood is not evenly distributed throughout stool. Thus the chances for detecting a bleeding cancer may have increased with the increased number of tests, as shown in the Minnesota trial.

Funen Trial

In 1985, 30,970 residents of Funen ages 45 to 75 were randomly assigned to biannual screening with Hemoccult, and 30,968 were randomly assigned to serve as controls.[66-70]

Study participants were obtained from the Central Person Register and the Patient File of the County of Funen. The latter file was used to exclude patients with known colorectal cancer, adenoma, and distant spread from all types of cancer. However, two equal samples were randomly selected from among these exclusions to compare prevalent figures for the whole population.

Six Hemoccult II slides were obtained from three consecutive stools while participants maintained a restricted diet consisting of no red meat or fresh fruit and abstained from using iron supplements, vitamin C, aspirin, or other nonsteroid antirheumatics during the 3-day testing period.

Three screenings were conducted between 1985 and 1990 at 2-year intervals. Only those who completed the previous screening were invited for the following screening. However, to maintain the integrity of the study design, all randomized subjects should have been invited to participate in every screen. Persons with positive FOBT slides were examined by colonoscopy. A double-contrast barium enema was done when colonoscopy was incomplete or the person refused colonoscopy.

Death certificates were evaluated without knowledge of group assignment and classified according to prespecified criteria. For those deaths not readily classifiable, a death review committee evaluated the information to determine if death was caused by CRC.

The total number of deaths from all causes was approximately equal between the study groups. However, there were fewer CRC deaths among screen group participants (74) than among control group participants (91). When the deaths were divided among those which occurred in subjects screened and those in nonresponders, the disparity increased. The proportion of CRC deaths among screenees, nonresponders, and control group participants was 0.17%, 0.34%, and 0.30%, respectively.

There was a greater percentage of Dukes A cancers in the screened group than in the control group (25% versus 9%). Dukes A and B accounted for 55% and 45% of the screened and control group cancers, respectively. About 25% of the classified cancers in both groups were Dukes D.

A more favorable stage distribution was found among screen-detected cancers (51% Dukes A, 6% Dukes D) than among interval-detected cancers (18%

Dukes A, 22% Dukes D), cancers in nonresponders (11% Dukes A, 41% Dukes D), and cancers among control group participants (9% Dukes A, 24% Dukes D). Interval cancers were larger than screen-detected cancers, and cancers 2 cm or larger occurred more often among those who were screen detected.

The preliminary results from this trial showed a 19% decrease in CRC mortality and a more favorable stage distribution among screen group participants compared to control group participants.

Comparison of Results

The main features of these four randomized controlled trials are shown in Table 4-2. All the trials used an FOBT with dietary restrictions. In Nottingham initial testing was done without any dietary restriction but was used on retesting of test positives. Minnesota and Göteborg rehydrated most of the slides, which resulted in an increase in positivity, higher sensitivity, lower specificity, and a lower positive predictive value. Compliance varied considerably, from 53% in Nottingham to 85% in Minnesota on the first screen. Compliance on rescreening ranged from 75% in Minnesota to 41% in Nottingham when all randomized participants are considered. Screening intervals varied as well. Minnesota screened annually and biannually. The other trials were essentially biannual intervals (Sweden was 16 to 24 months).

There was a wide variation in positivity rates (1% to 9.8%), which was due to at least two factors, the age groups tested and rehydration of the tests. The latter was the more significant contributor to the positivity rate. One other difference worth noting that would influence the outcome is the FOBT used. Although all the studies used a Hemoccult test, two used the original Hemoccult and two used Hemoccult II. Each test required two independent samples from each of three stools. However, it was unknown if three Hemoccult II tests result in two smears from each of three samples or six separate smears from six samples. The latter is more likely with Hemoccult, since each slide requires one sample.

> *The likelihood of detecting blood increases with more sampling because of the intermittence of the bleeding and the uneven distribution of blood in stool.*

Minnesota is the only study to date that has demonstrated a statistically significant mortality reduction.

> *Through 14 years of follow-up there was a statistically significant 34% reduction in CRC mortality in the annual group compared to the control group.*

The biannual group mortality reduction was 10%. A somewhat higher than expected mortality in the early years of the study, consistent with chance, contrib-

TABLE 4-2

SUMMARY OF RANDOMIZED CONTROLLED TRIALS

	Minnesota	Göteborg	Nottingham	Funen
Date started	1975	1982	1981	1985
Number of participants	46,551	68,308	144,103	61,938
Age	50-80	60-64	50-74	45-74
Screening test	Hemoccult	Hemoccult II	Hemoccult	Hemoccult II
Slides rehydrated	83	83	0	0
Diet restrictions	Yes	Yes	Yes[*]	Yes
Study groups	3	2	2	2
Frequency of screening	Annual, biannual	16-24 months	Biannual	Biannual
Number of screens	Annual (11), biannual (6)	2	3	3
Compliance with first screen (%)	85	63	53	67
Rescreening compliance (%)	75	60	77[†]	93[†]
Diagnostic examination	Colonoscopy	Double-contrast barium enema	Colonoscopy	Colonoscopy
Slides positive (%)				
Rehydrated	9.8	6	—	—
Not rehydrated	2.4	1.9	2.1	0.9
Sensitivity for colorectal cancer (%)	92[‡,§]	83[‡,‖]	68[¶]	48
Specificity for colorectal cancer (%)	90[‡]	96[‡]	98	99
Positive predictive value for colorectal cancer (%)	2.2[‡]	5.2[‡]	11.5	8.2

[*]On retesting after a positive test.
[†]Rescreening offered only to those who complied with initial screen.
[‡]Rehydrated slides.
[§]False negatives or interval cancers defined as those occurring within 1 year after a negative screen.
[‖]False negatives or interval cancers defined as those occurring 16 to 24 months after a negative screen.
[¶]False negatives or interval cancers defined as those occurring within 2 years after a negative screen. Sensitivity was 65% if tests were collected over 3 days and 74% if collected over 6 days.

uted to this relatively small cumulative 14-year mortality reduction in the biannual group.

> *A larger reduction may be observed with additional follow-up based on the stage distribution, which showed a 35% reduction in Dukes D cancers and a survival rate for screen-detected cancers; this is more similar to the reduction for the annual group than for the control group.*

The other three trials in process do not have final mortality results. However, interim results from the Funen study on CRC mortality and staging data from all three trials are consistent with a screening benefit.

Nonrandomized Controlled Studies

Burgundy Study

A study in the Burgundy area of France was initiated in 1988 and involved 91,000 participants ages 45 to 74 years.[71,72] All residents of certain towns and administrative districts of the department of Saone et Loire were offered the screening test. The controls, residents of areas of similar size and similar risk of CRC in the neighboring department of Côte d'Or, were not offered the screening test.

The first screen with Hemoccult was conducted in 1988 and 1989, the second in 1990. The third screen was scheduled to be conducted 2 years after the second. Participants were asked to complete Hemoccult tests from three consecutive stools without adhering to any dietary restrictions. However, it was suggested that vitamin C and aspirin not be used during the testing period. Those with a positive screening test were offered colonoscopy. Double-contrast barium enema was used when colonoscopy was incomplete. This study is still ongoing, and results are not yet available.

The compliance rate was 54% in the first screen and 55.5% in the rescreen. Overall, 63.7% of the screened group participants completed at least one screen. Compliance was greater in women than men. For both men and women compliance was poorest among the oldest (70 to 74) study participants. The positivity rate was 2.3%; 84% of test positives had a complete bowel examination. Compliance was considerably better when the test was proposed by the physician than when it was mailed.

Colon Project

The Colon Project, a controlled nonrandomized study conducted between 1975 and 1984 by the Memorial Sloan-Kettering Cancer Center in collaboration with the Preventive Medicine Institute (PMI)-Strang Clinic in New York, was designed to evaluate the effectiveness of FOBT as a supplement to 25-cm rigid sigmoidoscopy.[16,73]

Between 1975 and 1979, 21,756 patients over the age of 40 who came to the clinic were enrolled. Those with a prior history of colon cancer or membership in group health insurance or corporate health plans were excluded.

There were two groups of patients coming to the clinic: one group responded regularly to reminders for annual checkups, and another group came for single visits, often because of specific health concerns. The former group was designated the Regulars and the latter the First Timers.

The Regulars and First Timers were separately allocated to study and control groups. Randomization was not feasible in the context of the operation of the clinic; therefore allocation was based on enrollment date. Those assigned to a study group were sent three Hemoccult slides and instructions for completing them before their clinic visit. They were asked to adhere to a meat-free, high-bulk diet for 1 day before and 3 days during slide preparation. Slides were tested without rehydration. Participants with a positive FOBT were referred for double-contrast barium enema and full colonoscopy.

All participants underwent the standard PMI-Strang Clinic examination at enrollment, which included a 25-cm rigid proctosigmoidoscopy. Those found to have a polyp at least 3 mm in size were referred for colonoscopy.

Follow-up for vital status was completed for 97% of the cohort. Deaths were reviewed by a committee who examined death certificates, hospital records, autopsy reports, physicians' statements, and, when available, x-rays and pathology slides. There were 9277 (7168 study, 2109 control) participants enrolled as Regulars and 12,479 (5806 study, 6673 controls) as First Timers.

A greater proportion of Regulars than First Timers had a personal history of cancer or polyps, whereas a greater proportion of First Timers were symptomatic at enrollment. Study and control groups were better balanced on gender and age among First Timers than among Regulars.

Compliance with FOBT at the first screen was 80% among First Timers and 70% among Regulars. It declined in subsequent screens to 20% and 16%, respectively, at 1 and 2 years among First Timers. Positivity was higher among First Timers (2.6%) than Regulars (1.4%) and, as expected, was higher on the first (prevalence) screen than on subsequent (incidence) screens. Over 75% of test positives received a diagnostic examination within 1 year after a positive test.

The prevalence rate of CRC was higher in the study group than control groups, whereas incidence rates were approximately equal. At the prevalence screen there was a greater proportion of Dukes A cancers and a smaller proportion of Dukes D cancers in the study group compared to the control group for both Regulars and First Timers. The stage distribution was more similar for incident cancers, which was probably due to the low compliance that resulted in very few screen-detected cancers.

The significant difference in survival between the First Timers study and control group (70% versus 48%) but not the Regulars study and control group was notable. This difference is affected in part by lead time and length bias. However, there was also a 43% reduction ($P = .053$) in CRC mortality between the First Timers study and control group. This mortality reduction occurred among all age groups but was somewhat greater among those over 65 than those under 65 years of age.

Among First Timers the reduction in CRC mortality, the shift to earlier stage cancers, and the improved survival rate all provide evidence of a screening benefit.

Case-Control Studies

Case-control studies of cancer screening must be interpreted cautiously because of selection bias.[74] Nevertheless, despite the potential problem, they warrant review and consideration to evaluate whether the results generally support findings from randomized controlled trials.

Kaiser-Permanente Study

In a case-control study of FOBT screening among members of the Kaiser-Permanente Medical Care Program of Northern California, potential cases were members age 50 or over who were diagnosed with colorectal adenocarcinoma between 1981 and 1987 and who subsequently died of the disease before December 1988.[17] One control matched to each case on age, sex, and date of health plan entry was randomly selected from the Kaiser membership lists. For 96 cases with distal location of the CRC, four controls were selected for a separate analysis of screening sigmoidoscopy. Thus the study included 486 cases and 727 controls.

Outpatient medical records were reviewed for 10 years before the index date, which was defined as the date immediately before onset of the case's symptoms or before the screening test that led to the diagnosis. Potential confounders included a history of adenomatous polyps or colorectal cancer before the 10-year interval, a family history of CRC noted before the case's diagnosis, and the number of periodic health checkups in a 10-year period. Because FOBT screening was rarely done before 1979, only a 5-year screening history was considered. Two years of data were available for 79% of the case-control sets.

An adjusted-odds ratio of 0.69 (95% confidence interval [CI] = 0.52 to 0.91) was observed for exposure to at least one screening FOBT during the 5-year interval.

> *The results indicated that CRC mortality could be reduced by 31% with FOBT screening.*

Saarland Study

A population-based case-control study was conducted in the Saarland in Germany to evaluate effectiveness of FOBT screening for CRC.[18] The FOBT was introduced in the Federal Republic of Germany in 1977 and was offered to all men and women ages 45 years and over.

Cases in the study were individuals 55 to 74 years of age who had died between 1983 and 1986 and who had been initially diagnosed with CRC between 1979 and 1985. The cause of death and the screening history were obtained from the decedent's physicians.

Up to five age-matched controls were identified from the files of the physician of the corresponding case. Information on the controls had to be available for at least 3 years before diagnosis of the matched case, since FOBT screening for both cases and controls was ascertained for this period. Information was abstracted on whether the FOBT was conducted on a symptomatic or asymptomatic person. The study included 429 cases (220 men, 209 women) and 3412 controls (694 men, 2718 women).

Six to 36 months before diagnosis 13% of male cases and 14% of male controls had at least one asymptomatic FOBT (odds ratio = 0.92; 95% CI = 0.54 to 1.57). For the same prediagnostic period 16% of female cases and 29% of female controls had at least one asymptomatic FOBT (odds ratio = 0.43; 95% CI = 0.27 to 0.68). For the period 12 to 36 months before diagnosis the corresponding odds ratios were 0.73 (95% CI = 0.40 to 1.32) for men and 0.40 (95% CI = 0.25 to 0.65) for women. Thus for men in whom screening participation rates were very low, there was a 27% nonsignificant benefit, but for women in whom participation rates were considerably higher, a significant 60% benefit from screening was observed.

Marshfield Study

In a third case-control study the medical records of 66 members of the Greater Marshfield Community Health Plan who died of CRC from 1979 to 1988, and 196 members matched on gender, age, and enrollment duration were reviewed for a history of screening for CRC.[75] Only screening tests done in the absence of symptoms were considered.

FOBT screening was not associated with a lower CRC mortality (odds ratio = 1.15; 95% CI = 0.93 to 1.44). However, the study cannot be considered as providing evidence for or against FOBT screening because only 21% of the cases and 16% of the controls received multiple-slide evaluation of stool. Most screening was done on a single sample obtained during a digital rectal examination.

Puget Sound Study

In this case-control study cases were members of an HMO who were diagnosed with and subsequently died of colorectal adenocarcinoma.[76] Controls were randomly selected from the HMO membership lists and matched to the cases based on their year of birth, gender, and year of enrollment. The odds ratio for those who were ever screened with FOBT was 0.71 (95% CI = 0.50 to 1.00) for home use of FOBT and 0.95 (95% CI = 0.67 to 1.36) for office use of FOBT. A statistically significant reduced odds ratio of 0.65 (95% CI = 0.44 to 0.97) was found for those who were screened before age 75 but not for those who were screened after age 75 (odds ratio = 0.98; 95% CI = 0.49 to 1.96).

Conclusions

Of the many FOBTs, only Hemoccult has been adequately studied. Hemoccult is a test for blood in stool, not for cancer or polyps. However, most cancers and some polyps do bleed. The bleeding is intermittent and the blood is not uniformly distributed throughout the stool. The test is sensitive for cancer, but not for polyps, although it is somewhat better for larger than smaller polyps.

It is a fairly inexpensive test and is generally acceptable to the general population. Compliance in the randomized trials ranged from 53% to 75%.

> *There is now evidence from a randomized controlled clinical trial, a prospective nonrandomized study, and three case-control studies that screening for FOBT with Hemoccult can reduce CRC mortality from about 30% to 60%.*

The Marshfield study is the only completed study that did not find a benefit from FOBT. As mentioned earlier, the FOBTs were primarily single tests done as a part of a digital rectal examination.

It is clear, therefore, that the weight of evidence supports a recommendation for screening with FOBT. Although there are preliminary data that FOBTs other than Hemoccult may be more sensitive and specific, only Hemoccult has been properly evaluated to date.

FLEXIBLE SIGMOIDOSCOPY

Screening with a 60-cm flexible sigmoidoscopy has received considerable attention recently.[77-79] The rationale for using this procedure relates to the direct visualization and subsequent removal of neoplastic lesions to prevent the development of cancer (in the case of polyp removal) or to prevent the progression of cancer (in the case of cancer removal). The underlying assumption to support this approach is the following:

> *Most, and perhaps all, cancers arise from polyps, and therefore removal of polyps with continued surveillance to identify and remove new or recurrent polyps will prevent cancer.*

The data in support of this hypothesis are speculative but reasonably persuasive.

Adenoma-Carcinoma Sequence

The idea that the majority of CRCs evolve from benign adenomas has been discussed in the literature for more than 50 years and is widely accepted.[80-82] Dukes[83] was among the first to comment, in 1925, on the malignant potential of villous and adenomatous polyps. Even though the evidence is indirect, most investigators[84-90] believe that the majority of colorectal cancers arise from polyps (Figure 4-4).

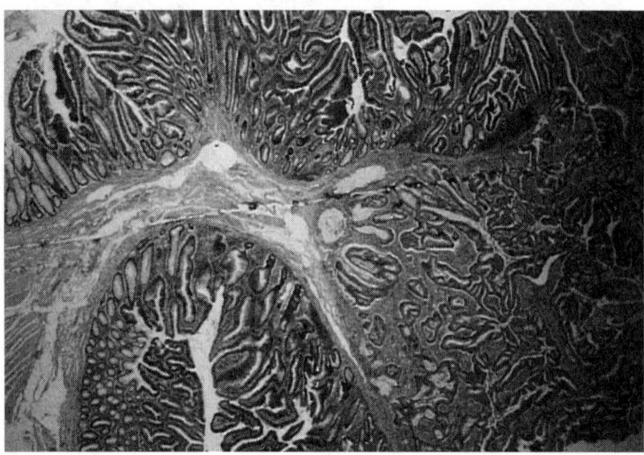

Figure 4-4   Photomicrograph depicting a well-differentiated adenocarcinoma occurring in a previous polyp.

CRC probably develops through a sequence of stages beginning with environmental carcinogens acting on a genetically susceptible mucosa and resulting in a hyperproliferative state, followed by a series of oncogene mutations and chromosome deletions.[81,91] This leads to a precursor adenoma, successive stages of dysplasia, and then invasive cancer.

It must be stressed that the evidence implicating adenomas as precursors of carcinomas is indirect, since these lesions are generally resected when discovered rather than left intact and observed to determine their natural history.[90] The present belief that all polyps should be removed makes it impossible to design a randomized trial to better understand the physiologic process.

The de novo origin of cancer has received more attention in recent years as an alternative pathway in some cases of CRC.[88] Some carcinomas appear to have arisen out of flat mucosa and in the absence of adenomatous tissue.[92-94]

The term *de novo carcinoma* has been applied to small ulcerating or non-ulcerating carcinomas in which no residual adenomatous tissue can be identified.[84] Microscopically, these tumors present as a firm, pale button 5 to 15 mm in diameter with a depressed center, although histologically there may be no ulceration. These lesions are rare, particularly found within the rectum and sigmoid colon, but it is conceivable that many escape endoscopic detection or evolve rapidly into invasive malignancy. Therefore it does appear that a proportion of large bowel cancers do not develop within a conventional polypoid adenoma. The size and hence clinical importance of this group are unknown.[87]

There may be two alternative pathways in the development of CRC, one in which the patient develops malignancy through a stage of benign polypoid growth (the adenoma-carcinoma sequence) and one in which the patient develops dysplastic epithelium that has the property of growing invasively directly from flat mucosa (de novo).[88]

Adenoma prevalence was first assessed in 1947 with a study of 1460 consecutive autopsies in which the entire bowel was examined.[95] Since this landmark study, similar autopsy surveys have been conducted. In most of these studies the prevalence of adenomas increased with age, and in some older age groups the prevalence rate exceeded 50%. These observations parallel those for CRCs, lending credence to the adenoma-carcinoma theory.[90]

Further evidence has been provided by studies of the prevalence of colorectal adenoma at autopsy, which were conducted in populations with differing risks of large bowel cancer.[81,84,88-90] In general, there was a correlation between the prevalence of adenoma and the incidence of CRC. The correlation coefficient was 0.73 for men, 0.43 for women, and 0.67 for men and women combined. These observations were offered as evidence to support the hypothesis that adenomas are an intermediate step in colon carcinogenesis.

The time required for the evolution from a clean colon to adenoma to CRC was recently studied in the U.S. National Polyp Study.[96,97] The temporal sequence was derived from single time point observations of mean ages of subsets of the cohort.

> *Age frequency distributions indicated a 10-year interval from clean colon to invasive cancer with a 5-year interval from clean colon to adenomas.*

The interval was shorter for patients with a single adenoma, and there was a larger interval from clean colon to patients having multiple adenomas, adenomas with infiltrating cancer, or significant dysplasia, all of which fell in the same general time frame.

The natural history of 5 to 10 years for the adenoma-carcinoma sequence was suggested earlier by several studies.[98-100]

The frequently repeated demonstration of foci of invasive cancer in adenomas provides additional evidence of the premalignant nature of adenomas.[88,101,102] Pathologically it is extremely rare to find a small focus of cancer in normal mucosa, whereas this is common in adenomas.[89]

Remnants of adenomas have been found in 14% to 23% of all colorectal carcinomas.[85,87,101,103,104] Adenomatous remnants were more frequently present in carcinomas only infiltrating the submucosa (57%) than in those extending beyond the muscularis propria (8%). The implication is that, as carcinomas grow and infiltrate, they destroy preexisting adenomatous tissue.

In one study 90% of early cancers in a series contained remnants of adenomas.[105] The high proportion of adenomatous remnants in carcinomas in a very early stage of the disease has been taken to indicate that most CRC develops through a stage of benign disease.[88] Residual adenomatous tissue adjacent to a carcinoma provides only circumstantial evidence for the adenoma-carcinoma concept.[84]

Lev[85] concluded that the most convincing evidence of the adenoma-carcinoma sequence has been the histologic demonstration of varying grades of dysplasia and of invasive carcinoma in the same polyp, and the demonstration of adenomatous remnants in early carcinomas.

The natural history of familial polyposis coli strongly argues in favor of an adenoma-carcinoma sequence.[86] Familial polyposis is an inherited disease with a mendelian autosomal dominant pattern and a high degree of penetration. The trait first becomes manifest with the appearance of colonic adenoma shortly after puberty. The average age of the onset of symptoms is about 20 years.[106]

Many of the basic data on familial polyposis coli have been supplied from the Polyposis Register of over 300 families at St. Mark's Hospital in London.[107] In a series of patients with familial polyposis, the colons that were removed contained between 157 and 3676 polyps, with an average of 981. The average age of patients at the time of diagnosis of CRC was 35 years. The average age of death of patients with familial polyposis was 40 years. The uniform sequence of first having large numbers of polyps develop followed by the development of carcinoma of the colon and rectum 15 to 20 years later would support the adenoma-carcinoma theory.[86]

The WHO Collaborating Centre for the Prevention of Colorectal Cancer also concluded in 1990 that support for the adenoma-carcinoma sequence was found in inherited CRC syndromes, both familial polyposis and the cancer family syndrome.[81]

The biologic changes observed in the development of neoplasia generally reflect alterations in cell proliferation or the regulation of cell proliferation.[90] Many such changes associated with CRC also have been found in adenomas. Abnormal activation of small *ras* oncogenes has been demonstrated in the early stages of carcinogenesis in CRC and also occurred in colorectal adenomas.[108]

Familial adenomatous polyposis patients have been shown to have deletion of part of chromosome 5, reducing production of a tumor suppressor (or antioncogene).[109] Recent studies have shown similar deletions of chromosome 17 (reducing production of the p53 suppressor protein) and chromosome 18 (reducing the deleted in colorectal cancer (DCC) gene, which affects cell surface interactions.[110] Vogelstein et al.[91] showed (1) *ras* gene mutations in many adenomas over 1 cm in size and in carcinomas and (2) deletions in certain gene sequences in chromosomes 5, 17, and 18 in substantial numbers of adenomas or carcinomas. Specifically, they showed that the frequency of genetic defects increases with increasing size and dysplasia of colorectal adenomas up to a maximum of 75% chromosome 17 and 18 gene deletions in carcinomas.

Fearon and Vogelstein[111] developed a hypothesis of colorectal carcinogenesis.

> *The model postulated a sequence of genetic alteration involving the mutational activation of an oncogene coupled with the loss of several genes that normally suppress tumorigenesis. Initially there is a chromosome 5 and ras oncogene mutation, then chromosome 18 loss resulting in severe dysplasia in adenomas, and finally chromosome 17 loss before progression to invasive carcinoma.*

Other genetic defects may be involved in tumor progression and metastasis. Although this schema of molecular events is presented in a sequential manner, the chronology of alterations is not absolute, that is, an early adenoma may already exhibit a 17p deletion.[89,112] Two points are most important in this context. First, it is the accumulation of genetic alterations, rather than the exact order, that was associated with colonic tumorigenesis. Second, these genetic studies have convincingly shown that cancer cells arising within an adenoma exhibited the identical molecular alterations as the adenoma cells but also acquired mutations that were presumably critical for the malignant phenotype.[113] This latter point is one of the stronger arguments that colon carcinomas derive from preexisting adenomas.

Histochemical abnormalities have been studied in both CRC and adenomas. Tierney et al.[86] concluded that, even though adenomas of the colon and rectum lack the capacity of invasion or metastatic characteristics of a malignant lesion, sufficient evidence suggested that adenomas shared, to various degrees, the anaplastic characteristics of carcinoma. The loss of cellular control mechanisms in both adenomas and carcinomas is reflected by abnormalities in DNA ploidy, enzymatic activities, expression of carcinoembryonic antigen, and composition of mucin. Neugut et al.[90] concluded there was some evidence for the following abnormalities in both adenoma and carcinoma: DNA aneuploidy, cell kinetics, enzyme activity and expression, carcinoembryonic antigen expression, and presence of abnormal blood group antigens on cancer cell surfaces.

Adenomas are considerably more common than carcinomas. Only a small proportion (about 10%) of adenomas give rise to carcinomas.[88,104] Results are available from two recent adenoma follow-up studies, which have identified factors of importance for risk of new adenomas and thereby possibly increased risk of carcinoma.[114] High-grade dysplasia represents the extreme end of the spectrum of abnormal histologic changes, short of invasive carcinoma, encountered in CRCs.[115] Considerable evidence supports the view that high-grade dysplasia, as defined in the National Polyp Study, is a valid marker of the potential for malignant transformation.[116]

Risk of Cancer Following Polypectomy

National Polyp Study

Evidence that removal of polyps and ongoing colonoscopy surveillance reduce the incidence of CRC has been provided by the National Polyp Study (NPS), the Funen Adenoma Follow-up Study, and the St. Mark's Hospital Study.

The NPS is a multicenter prospective randomized trial designed to evaluate follow-up surveillance strategies in patients who have undergone polypectomy for the control of large bowel cancer.[96,97,117] The NPS was designed as a multicenter study to establish a cohort that was representative geographically rather than that of a single institution. Also, multiple centers allowed the inclusion of several types of practice. These included a Veterans Administration center, a cancer center, university medical centers, community hospitals, and private office practices.

All 9112 patients referred to the seven participating centers for initial colonoscopy or polypectomy between November 1980 and February 1990 who did not have a family or personal history of familial polyposis, inflammatory bowel disease, history of polypectomy, or history of CRC were evaluated for enrollment in the study.

After colonoscopy, patients were excluded if they had no polyps, nonadenomatous polyps, malignant polyps, a sessile adenoma larger than 3 cm in diameter, or CRC. Eligible patients had at least one histologically documented adenoma of the colon or rectum and had undergone a complete colonoscopy during which all identified polyps were removed. Of the 9112 referred patients, 6480 became ineligible at this stage. The remaining 2632 patients had one or more adenomas.

The study cohort consisted of the 1418 patients who were randomly assigned to more frequent follow-up (1 and 3 years after initial polypectomy) or less frequent follow-up (3 years) with colonoscopy and barium enema. The patients were also offered a follow-up examination at 6 years. All patients completed a questionnaire, had FOBT, and were contacted annually by a study coordinator. All endoscopic, pathologic, and surgical findings from other institutions were reviewed. Data on the patients in both treatment arms of the study were pooled for the analysis of the incidence of CRC. Death certificates were obtained for all patients who died, and patients' records, pathology reports, slides, and x-ray films were reviewed by a death review committee. All pathology slides were reviewed by a pathology review committee.

Three reference groups were used to determine the expected incidence rates of CRC in the study cohort. The first reference group was a retrospective cohort of 226 patients studied at the Mayo Clinic in Rochester, Minnesota, between 1965 and 1970 who had polyps 1 cm or larger in diameter that were above the reach of a rigid sigmoidoscope and were detected by barium enema. These patients had declined surgical polypectomy. Patients presenting with CRC were excluded. The cumulative incidence of colon cancer was 4% at 5 years and 14% at 10 years.

The second reference group was a cohort of 1618 patients who underwent excision of rectal adenomas between 1957 and 1980 at St. Mark's Hospital in London. Patients who had CRC or were diagnosed with CRC within 2 years after the excision of adenomas were excluded.

The age- and sex-specific rates of CRC for 1983 to 1987 from the Surveillance, Epidemiology, and End Results (SEER) Program of the National Cancer Institute were used for the third reference group, since this period represented the midpoint of accrual and follow-up for the cohort in the National Polyp Study. The mean age of the 1418 patients who entered the study was 61 ± 10 years (range 22 to 88); 70% were men and 30% were women. Of these patients, 1210 (85%) were followed until the end of the study, and 169 (12%) were followed until death, for a total of 8401 person-years at risk (average, 5.9). Only 39 (3%) patients were lost to follow-up during the study; 80% returned for one or more of their scheduled colonoscopies. About 92% (1310) had been referred for colonoscopy because of symptoms or positive results on screening or a diagnostic test. As a result, five asymptomatic CRCs (malignant polyps) were detected in NPS at follow-up colonoscopy in five patients, none of whom had rectal bleeding or a change in bowel habits. No patient had a symptomatic cancer or died of CRC.

The expected numbers of CRCs in the study cohort, based on the Mayo Clinic, St. Mark's, and SEER rates, were 48.3, 43.4, and 20.7, respectively. In each case the observed incidence of CRC in the study cohort (5) was significantly lower ($P < .001$) than the expected incidence. The standardized incidence ratio was 0.10 (95% CI = 0.03 to 0.24) for the Mayo Clinic group, 0.12 (95% CI = 0.04 to 0.27) for the St. Mark's group, and 0.24 (95% CI = 0.08 to 0.56) for the SEER group. Therefore the incidence of CRC in the NPS cohort was significantly lower (90%) than expected on the basis of the rate in the Mayo Clinic group, the St. Mark's cohort (88%), and the SEER group (76%).

> *The authors concluded that the significantly reduced incidence of CRC provided evidence of the progression of adenoma to adenocarcinoma and of the effectiveness of the current practice of searching for and removing adenomatous polyps in the colon.*

A multiple logistic model was used in the NPS to assess the independent risk factors of patient and polyp characteristics associated with high-grade dysplasia in adenomas.[115] The data, based on the results of the initial colonoscopic examination, included 3371 adenomas from 1867 patients. Of the total adenomas, 206 (6.2%) showed high- grade dysplasia, a category composed of features of either severe dysplasia or carcinoma in situ. Severe dysplasia was present in 2.5% and carcinoma in situ in 3.7% of adenomas. Adenoma size and the extent of the villous component were found to be the major independent polyp risk factors associated with high-grade dysplasia. They were statistically significant and independent but not interactive effects. The adjusted odds ratios were 3.3 for medium-size adenomas and 7.7 for large adenomas relative to small adenomas, and 2.7 for villous A adenomas, 3.4 for villous B adenomas, and 8.1 for villous C and D adenomas relative to tubular adenomas.

Increased frequency of high-grade dysplasia in adenomas located distal to the splenic flexure was attributable mainly to increased size and villous component rather than to location per se. The adjusted odds ratio was 1.4 for left-sided location, which was not statistically significant. An evaluation of the association of patient variables with the presence of high-grade dysplasia in adenomas was also done. Increasing age was associated with risk for high-grade dysplasia in patients, and this effect was independent of the effect of adenoma size and histologic type. The adjusted odds ratio was 1.8 ($P < .0016$) for ages 60 years and older. Gender was not associated with high-grade dysplasia; an adenoma removed from a male was no more likely to show high-grade dysplasia than a comparable adenoma in a female. Multiplicity of adenomas affected the risk for high-grade dysplasia in patients but depended on adenoma size and villous component and was not an independent factor.

The odds ratio for the combined effects of size and histology from the logistic model was the product of the individual adjusted odds ratios. The odds ratio for high-grade dysplasia increased to 62.7 for large and villous C and D adenomas relative to small and tubular adenomas.

Funen Adenoma Study

The goal of The Funen Adenoma Follow-up Study was to reduce the incidence of CRC in adenoma patients and thereby reduce mortality.[118] By identifying factors associated with high risk of subsequent neoplasia, the study hoped to establish appropriate follow-up intervals and thereby reduce the incidence of carcinoma.

Between 1978 and 1992 a total of 1042 patients (606 males and 436 females) with colorectal adenomas were allocated to different follow-up intervals ranging from 6 to 48 months. The median age at intake was 62 years (range 25 to 77 years). There were 841 patients referred because of colorectal symptoms (symptomatic population), and 201 were referred from an ongoing screening study evaluating Hemoccult II (screened population), which began in 1985. All persons in the screening study with positive Hemoccult II were offered colonoscopy, and persons with one or more adenomas and no carcinoma were transferred to the adenoma follow-up study. A clean colon was ensured by total colonoscopy in 1013 of the patients. Double-contrast barium enema was performed if colonoscopy was not completed. The pathologic classification of all adenomas was performed by one pathologist who was unaware of the group in which the patient belonged.

The size of the largest adenoma and the structure of the most villous adenoma were found to be independent predictors of severe dysplasia. No independent associations were found between patient characteristics of age, sex, multiplicity of adenomas, study subpopulation (symptomatic or screening), and the risk of severe dysplasia, and no interactions were found.

Anatomic location was not an independent risk factor in the NPS, whereas it was in the Funen Adenoma Follow-up Study. An association between age and severe dysplasia would have been expected in accordance with the adenoma-carcinoma sequence but was not found in the Funen Study, in contrast to the NPS. A possible explanation may be that no upper age limit was used for inclusion in the NPS.

Between 1978 and 1992 a total of 1689 colorectal adenomas were removed in 1042 patients with no history of previous colorectal neoplasms. Dysplasia was graded as mild, moderate, or severe in accordance with Konishi and Morson.[119] Adenomas with so-called intraepithelial carcinoma or intramucosal carcinoma were graded as severe dysplasia; 118 patients had severe dysplasia in one or more adenomas. Of 1689 adenomas 122 showed severe dysplasia. A multiple logistic model was used to assess the independent risk factors associated with severe dysplasia in all 1689 colorectal adenomas. Size, structure, and anatomic location were controlled for independent effects on risk of severe dysplasia in the logistic model, and all were found to be independent risk factors.

The adjusted odds ratio was 9.3 for adenomas of 10 to 19 mm and 25.2 for adenomas 20 mm or greater relative to small adenomas. Adjusted odds ratios were 1.9 (95% CI = 1.2 to 3.0) for tubulovillous adenomas and 2.3 (95% CI = 0.7 to 7.3) for villous adenomas relative to tubular adenomas. Distal location of adenomas was independent of size and extent of villous component associated with severe dysplasia. The adjusted odds ratios for anatomic location were 0.7 (95% CI = 0.4 to 1.0) for the sigmoid colon, 0.4 (95% CI = 0.1 to 1.6) for the descending colon, and 0.2 (95% CI = 0.1 to 0.7) for the right colon relative to the rectum.

St. Mark's Hospital Study

This study evaluated the subsequent risk of CRC after removal of rectosigmoid adenomas.[120] Over 2000 symptomatic patients who underwent excision of one or more rectosigmoid adenomas were followed for up to 30 years to determine their incidence of CRC. The incidence of rectal cancer overall was similar to that in the general population (standardized incidence rate = 1.2; 95% CI = 0.7 to 2.1); however, those with a rectosigmoid adenoma that was tubulovillous, villous, or over 1 cm had 3.6 times (95% CI = 2.4 to 5.0) the risk of developing colon cancer. Those with multiple rectosigmoid adenomas had 6.6 times (95% CI = 3.3 to 11.8) the risk of developing colon cancer. Those with only small tubular adenomas (43% of the case group) had no increased risk of CRC.

Observational Studies of Screening Flexible Sigmoidoscopy

Given that there is an arguable basis for the adenoma-carcinoma sequence and that removal of adenomas might prevent colorectal cancers, the question then becomes how best to accomplish this. FOBT is not a sensitive enough test for adenomas because most do not bleed.

Flexible sigmoidoscopy (60 cm) has been proposed. It has the obvious advantage of direct visualization of adenomas but the disadvantage of examining only the distal portion of the colon. There has not been a randomized controlled clinical trial to demonstrate its effectiveness as a screening procedure, yet it is recommended based on observational (mainly case-control) studies[78] despite the biases with these types of studies.[74,121,122] Atkin et al.[123] suggested that a one-time flexible sigmoidoscopy at about age 55 could reduce CRC mortality by about 45%. They propose a randomized trial to evaluate their hypothesis. Such a trial is necessary to provide definitive evidence of the effectiveness of flexible sigmoidoscopy screening. Circumstantial evidence is available from observational studies, although these studies must be interpreted cautiously because of biases inherent in the design.

Gilbertsen reported on 113,800 proctosigmoidoscopies of 21,140 adults attending a cancer detection center at the University of Minnesota.[124,125] Follow-up of patients with diagnosed and removed adenomas failed to find a single death from rectal cancer. This widely cited finding has been used to argue the case for screening sigmoidoscopy; however, in an insightful analysis of the Gilbertsen studies, Miller[47] presented persuasive evidence that these studies were inappropriately conducted and subsequently misinterpreted.

The Multiphasic Checkup Evaluation Study, a randomized trial to test the effectiveness of periodic multiphasic health checkups in preventing or postponing illness, disability, and death, was initiated in 1964 as part of the Kaiser-Permanente Medical Care Program.[126] The study group, 5156 persons ages 35 to 54 years, was contacted annually and urged to attend a comprehensive screening examination, which consisted of a blood pressure measurement, electrocardiogram, audiogram, visual acuity measurement, tonometry, spirometry, chest x-ray, mammography for women ages 40 and older, urinalysis, and blood tests, including hematology and serum chemistry panels. Sigmoidoscopy using a 25-cm rigid sigmoidoscope was a recommended but optional addition for men and women ages 40 and older.

A group of 5557 persons assigned to the control group was not urged to take any of the tests but was free to do so as part of the Kaiser program.

Deaths among the study and control members were ascertained through 1982 by follow-up through the Kaiser records and by matching names of subjects who left the plan against California vital records.

Early in the study a lower CRC mortality was observed in the study group.[127] By the seventh year (1971) of follow-up there were two CRC deaths in the study group and 10 in the control group ($P < .05$). By the sixteenth year (1980) the number of CRC deaths increased to 12 and 29 in the study and control groups, respectively.[128] This mortality difference was accompanied by a stage shift toward earlier cancers in the study group. Although more 25-cm rigid sigmoidoscopies were performed on the study group members than control group members (8.1% versus 5.2%), there was no difference in the frequency with which polyps were removed. The authors concluded that, if sigmoidoscopy screening accounted for the mortality reduction, it was due to early detection of cancer rather than to the removal of premalignant adenomas.

Selby et al.[129] attempted to clarify the mechanisms that could account for the significant reduction in CRC mortality. By reexamining 8891 medical charts to reconstruct relevant histories that had been erased from computer tapes, they found the following: (1) that sigmoidoscopy did not account for the reduction in study group CRC incidence because there was no group difference in the rate of detection or removal of polyps; (2) that the incidence of CRC was similar to expected based on general population data; (3) that the mortality difference could be related to small differences in screen-detected cancers, which could be explained by chance, lead time, or length bias; (4) that most tumors in both study and control groups were detected because of symptoms rather than by screening of asymptomatic individuals; (5) that the slight improvement of stage distribution in the study group was not related to screening sigmoidoscopy; and (6) that particularly noteworthy was the absence of a substantial difference in exposure to sigmoidoscopy between the two groups. As suggested by Miller,[47] the apparent benefit to the study group may have been due to a chance difference between the groups in the prevalence of risk factors for CRC and the probability of the development of, and thus death from, CRC in the two groups.

Two recent case-control studies concluded that a single screening sigmoidoscopy could reduce mortality from cancers of the rectum and distal colon by between 59% and 79%.[75,130]

At Kaiser-Permanente Medical Care Program of Northern California, cases were plan members 45 years of age or older diagnosed with adenocarcinoma of the colon or rectum between 1971 and 1987, and who died of the cancer by the end of 1988.[130] Cases were identified from the SEER Registry, which collects information on incident cancer cases diagnosed among residents of the study area. Deaths were ascertained from registry information or by linking the case file to the California vital records. This system of case ascertainment would miss eligible cases who were health plan members and who left the area before their cancer was diagnosed, deaths among ascertained cases that occurred outside of California, and deceased cases who did not match the California vital statistics records because of an error in matching variables. It has been estimated that the Kaiser system of matching cases to vital records missed between 8% and 18% of deaths.[128]

After reviewing 1712 patient records, it was determined that there were 261 deaths from adenocarcinomas that could have been detected by rigid sigmoidoscopy, that is, cancers of the rectum or rectosigmoid and cancers of the sigmoid colon that were visualized by rigid sigmoidoscopy or described as within 20 cm of the anus in pathologic or surgical reports. A random sample of 268 fatal cancers that were above 20 cm was selected from the remaining cases for separate analysis.

Four matched (age, sex, date of entry into the health plan) controls per case were selected from membership lists. One control was selected for each of the 268 patients with cancer above 20 cm. Controls had to be alive and a member of the health plan when the matched cases died. However, it was not apparent if cases had to be members of the health plan until the time of their death. If not, a bias may have been introduced.

The analyses considered the 10-year period immediately before the onset of symptoms or the screening test that led to the diagnosis of fatal CRC. The same 10-year period was examined for the matched controls. A reviewer, blinded to the subject's case-control status, reviewed outpatient medical records and abstracted all instances of screening tests with sigmoidoscopy, digital rectal examination, FOBTs, barium enema examination, and colonoscopy.

Several possible confounding factors were considered based on their availability in the medical records. No attempt was made to systematically obtain data on these confounders for all study subjects, nor was there any attempt to obtain data on potential confounders not readily available in the charts.

A history of CRC or adenomatous polyps before the 10-year observation period and a family history of CRC were noted more frequently among cases than controls. Thus their risk of CRC was greater.

Significantly fewer cases than controls had one or more screening rigid sigmoidoscopies during the 10-year period (adjusted odds ratio = 0.41; 95% CI = 0.25 to 0.69). The optimum screening interval could not be determined, since the small numbers of cases resulted in wide confidence intervals. There was no evidence of screening efficacy for the 268 cases with cancer beyond the reach of the rigid sigmoidoscopy (adjusted odds ratio = 0.96; 95% CI = 0.61 to 1.50).

This study showed that screening with rigid sigmoidoscopy could reduce mortality from cancers within 20 cm of the bowel by 59%. This result must be interpreted in the context of the study design, a design likely to overestimate the benefit of screening. Furthermore, extrapolation of the finding to 60 cm of the colon suggests that overall CRC mortality could be reduced by at most 30%, assuming that 50% of the CRCs and adenomatous polyps arise within 60 cm of the large bowel and that screening with 60-cm flexible sigmoidoscopy will reduce deaths from distal cancers by 59%.

Newcomb et al.[75] conducted a case-control study of 66 cases who were members of the Greater Marshfield Community Health Plan, who died of cancer of the colon or rectum between 1979 and 1988, and who were enrolled in the health plan at least 12 months before diagnosis. Controls were 196 randomly selected Marshfield members of the same gender, similar age, and enrollment duration.

Information was collected from records on dates, signs and symptoms, and results of screening tests (FOBT, digital rectal examination, and sigmoidoscopy) done in the absence of symptoms. Additional information abstracted from records included personal history of polyps or digestive disease, familial history of colon cancer, and limited demographic data. No attempt was made to systematically collect these data from all subjects or to obtain information on other potential confounding factors. A total of 29.1% of controls and 10.6% of cases had at least one screening sigmoidoscopy. Both rigid and flexible sigmoidoscopy were used; however, a majority of the examinations were flexible sigmoidoscopies. A greater proportion of cases than controls had a family history of CRC and a history of polyps. Controls had a somewhat longer affiliation with the health plan than cases.

The risk for death from CRC was reduced among individuals having had a single screening sigmoidoscopy (odds ratio = 0.21; 95% CI = 0.08 to 0.52). The reduction in cancer mortality risk appeared to be limited to cancer of the rectum and distal colon.

The authors noted a number of limitations to their study, including the reliance on medical records for screening histories, the limited ability to identify potential confounders, and their reliance on judgment as to whether symptoms plausibly related to the cancer were present at the time the tests were performed.

Conclusions

Flexible sigmoidoscopy screening has considerable appeal, but there is insufficient evidence to recommend it for mass screening. The observational studies suggest that sigmoidoscopy screening may reduce CRC mortality; however, these studies are not adequate proof of effectiveness. The two case-control studies could well have overstated the benefit because of selection bias. For example, in the Selby study the odds ratio increased from 0.30 to 0.41 by adjusting for three known confounders. Additional adjustment for other potential confounders could further increase the odds ratio, thus reducing the apparent screening benefit. Further research is needed, preferably a randomized controlled trial to obtain definitive evidence of the potential benefit of screening with flexible sigmoidoscopy. Consideration must also be given to compliance and cost.

OTHER SCREENING PROCEDURES

> *Colonoscopy has been suggested as a one-time screen during the sixth decade of life.*

The appeal is apparent: visualizing the entire colon could lead to the identification of 95% of the patients with larger adenomatous polyps or cancers. Follow-up examinations would depend on the findings from the baseline colonoscopy. Lieberman[131] proposed no follow-up if no polyps or hyperplastic polyps are found, 10-year follow-up for tubular adenomas, a 1-year then 5-year follow-up for adenomas greater than 1 cm or villous adenomas, and a 1-year, then 3- to 5-year follow-up for carcinomas. His theoretical cost-effectiveness analysis showed that colonoscopy screening was more cost-effective than flexible sigmoidoscopy or FOBT screening.

This idea warrants further exploration. Two issues to consider, in addition to cost and effectiveness, are compliance and risk. There are no data on colonoscopy compliance of an asymptomatic average risk population. Additional studies are needed to provide data on effectiveness and compliance before considering colonoscopy as a screening procedure.

RECOMMENDATIONS FOR PRACTICE AND FUTURE RESEARCH

The only test that has proven to be effective in reducing CRC mortality is Hemoccult applied annually to a population over the age of 50. Other FOBTs, such as HemoccultSENSA, show promise, but there is insufficient evidence to recommend their use.

Problems with the Hemoccult include low sensitivity for adenomas, a large number of false positives, and therefore relatively high cost. If the ongoing randomized trials demonstrate a significant benefit from biannual screening, as has been demonstrated for annual screening, then the screening cost will be substantially reduced by screening half as often.

Observational studies show a benefit from flexible sigmoidoscopy screening. If these studies are correct, CRC mortality could be reduced by about 30% to 40%. However, a recommendation for flexible sigmoidoscopy screening is premature because there has not been a definitive study of flexible sigmoidoscopy screening, observational studies may overestimate the benefit, compliance is unknown but likely to be lower than with FOBT, and cost-effectiveness cannot be determined because effectiveness is not known.

REFERENCES

1. Parkin DM, Laara E, Muir CS: Estimates of the worldwide frequency of 16 major cancers in 1980, *Int J Cancer* 41:184, 1988.
2. Whelan SL, Parkin DM, Masuyer E, editors: *Patterns of cancer in five continents,* Pub No 102, Lyon, France, 1990, International Agency for Research on Cancer.
3. Coleman MP et al: *Trends in cancer incidence and mortality,* Pub No 121, Lyon, France, 1993, International Agency for Research on Cancer.
4. Wingo PA, Tong T, Bolden S: Cancer statistics, 1995, *CA Cancer J Clin* 45:8, 1995.
5. Miller BA et al, editors: *Seer Cancer Statistics Review 1973-1990,* National Cancer Institute, NIH Pub No 93-2789, Bethesda, Md, 1993, US Government Printing Office.
6. Chu KC et al: Temporal patterns in colorectal cancer incidence, survival, and mortality through 1990, *J Natl Cancer Inst* 86:997, 1994.
7. Potter JD et al: Colon cancer: a review of the literature, *Epidemiol Rev* 15:499, 1993.
8. Mandel JS et al: Reducing mortality from colorectal cancer by screening for fecal occult blood, *N Engl J Med* 328:1365, 1993.
9. Greegor DH: Diagnosis of large-bowel cancer in the asymptomatic patient, *JAMA* 201:943, 1967.
10. Levin B, Murphy GP: Revision in American Cancer Society recommendations for the early detection of colorectal cancer, *Cancer* 42:296, 1992.
11. Mettlin C et al: Defining and updating the American Cancer Society Guidelines for the cancer-related checkup, *Cancer* 43:42, 1993.
12. Ferruci JT: Screening for colon cancer: programs of the American College of Radiology, *Am J Radiol* 160:999, 1993.
13. Canadian Task Force on the Periodic Health Examination: The periodic health examination. 2. 1989 update, *Can Med Assoc J* 141:4, 1989.

14. Knight KK, Fielding JE, Battista RN: Occult blood screening for colorectal cancer, *JAMA* 261:587, 1989.

15. Reference deleted in proofs.

16. Winawer SJ et al: Screening for colorectal cancer with fecal occult blood testing and sigmoidoscopy, *J Natl Cancer Inst* 85:1311, 1993.

17. Selby JV et al: Effects of fecal occult blood testing on mortality from colorectal cancer: a case-control study, *Ann Intern Med* 118:1, 1993.

18. Wahrendorf J et al: Effectiveness of colorectal cancer screening: results from a population-based case-control evaluation in Saarland, Germany, *Eur J Cancer Prev* 2:221, 1993.

19. St. John DJB: Faecal occult blood tests: a critical review. In Hardcastle JD, editor: *Screening for colorectal cancer,* Englewood, NJ, 1990, Normed Verlag.

20. Turunen MJ et al: Immunological detection of faecal occult blood in colorectal cancer, *Br J Cancer* 49:141, 1948.

21. Armitage N et al: A comparison of an immunological faecal occult blood test Fecatwin sensitive/FECA EIA with Haemoccult in population screening for colorectal cancer, *Br J Cancer* 51:799, 1985.

22. Songster CL, Barrows GH, Jarrett DD: Immunochemical detection of fecal occult blood. The fecal smear punch-disc test: a new noninvasive screening test for colorectal cancer, *Cancer* 45:1099, 1980.

23. St. John DJB et al: Evaluation of new occult blood tests for detection of colorectal neoplasia, *Gastroenterology* 104:1661, 1993.

24. Castiglione G, Grazzini G, Ciatto S: Guaiac and immunochemical tests for faecal occult blood in colorectal cancer screening, *Br J Cancer* 65:942, 1992.

25. Schwartz S et al: The HemoQuant test: a specific and quantitative determination of heme (hemoglobin) in feces and other materials, *Clin Chem* 29:2061, 1983.

26. Schwartz S, Ellefson M: Fecal recovery of hemoproteins from blood, meat, and fish ingested by normal volunteers: the HemoQuant assay, *Gastroenterology* 84:1302, 1983.

27. Ahlquist DA et al: Fecal blood levels in health and disease: a study using HemoQuant, *N Engl J Med* 312:1422, 1985.

28. St. John DJB et al: Comparison of the specificity and sensitivity of Hemoccult and Hemo-Quant in screening for colorectal neoplasia, *Ann Intern Med* 117:376, 1992.

29. Ahlquist DA et al: Accuracy of fecal occult blood screening for colorectal neoplasia: a prospective study of Hemoccult and HemoQuant tests, *JAMA* 269:1262, 1993.

30. Young GP, St John DJB: Selecting an occult blood test for use as a screening tool for large bowel cancer. In Rozen P, Reich CB, Winawer SJ, editors: *Large bowel cancer: policy, prevention, research and treatment, Gastrointest,* Basel, Switzerland, 1991, Karger.

31. Young GP, Rose IS, St John DJB: Haem in the gut. I. Fate of haemoproteins and the absorption of haem, *J Gastroenterol Hepatol* 4:537, 1989.

32. Young GP et al: Haem in the gut. II. Faecal excretion of haem and haem-derived porphyrins and their detection, *J Gastroenterol Hepatol* 5:194, 1990.

33. Farrands PA, Hardcastle JD: Accuracy of occult blood tests over a six-day period, *Clin Oncol* 9:217, 1983.

34. Rosenfield RE et al: Nonuniform distribution of occult blood in feces, *Am J Clin Pathol* 71:204, 1979.

34a. Tameron AD: Gastrointestinal blood loss measured by radioactive chromium, *Gut* 1:177, 1960.

35. St. John DJB: Screening tests for colorectal neoplasia, *J Gastroenterol Hepatol* 6:538, 1991.

36. Roche M et al: Study of urinary and fecal excretion of radioactive chromium Cr in man: its use in the measurement of intestinal blood loss associated with hookworm infection, *J Clin Invest* 36:1183, 1957.

37. Macrae FA, St. John DJB: Relationship between patterns of bleeding and Hemoccult sensitivity in patients with colorectal cancers or adenomas, *Gastroenterology* 82:891, 1982.

38. Ahlquist DA et al: Patterns of occult bleeding in asymptomatic colorectal cancer, *Cancer* 63:1826, 1989.

39. Ahlquist DA et al: Colorectal cancer detection in the practice setting: impact of fecal occult blood testing, *Arch Intern Med* 150:1041, 1990.

40. Ahlquist DA et al: A stool collection device: the first step in occult blood testing, *Ann Intern Med* 108:609, 1988.

41. Herzog P et al: Fecal blood loss in patients with colonic polyps: a comparison of measurements with chromium-labeled erythrocytes and with the Haemoccult test, *Gastroenterology* 83:957, 1982.

42. Simon JB: Occult blood screening for colorectal carcinoma: a critical review, *Gastroenterology* 88:820, 1985.

43. Simon JB: The pros and cons of fecal occult blood testing for colorectal neoplasms, *Cancer Metastasis Rev* 6:397, 1987.

44. Mandel JS et al: Sensitivity, specificity and positive predictivity of the Hemoccult test in screening for colorectal cancers, *Gastroenterology* 97:597, 1989.

45. Kewenter J et al: Follow-up after screening for colorectal neoplasms with fecal occult blood testing in a controlled trial, *Dis Colon Rectum* 37:115, 1994.

46. Greegor DH: Detection of silent colon cancer in routine examination, *Cancer* 19:330, 1969.

47. Miller AB: Review of sigmoidoscopy screening for colorectal cancer. In Chamberlain J, Miller AB, editors: *Screening for gastrointestinal cancer,* Toronto, 1988, Hans Huber.

48. Illingworth DG: Influence of diet on occult blood tests, *Gut* 6:595, 1965.

49. Macrae FA et al: Optimal dietary conditions for Hemoccult testing, *Gastroenterology* 82:899, 1982.

50. Bassett ML, Goulston KJ: False positive and negative Hemoccult reactions on a normal diet and effect of diet restriction, *Aust N Z J Med* 10:1, 1980.

51. Caligiore P et al: Peroxidase levels in food: relevance to colorectal cancer screening, *Am J Clin Nutr* 35:1487, 1982.

52. St. John DJB, Young GP: Is there a need to restrict diet in occult blood screening for colorectal cancer? *Gastroenterology* 102:A402, 1992.

53. Feinberg EJ et al: How long to abstain from eating red meat before fecal occult blood tests, *Ann Intern Med* 113:403, 1990.

54. Thomas WM et al: Role of dietary restriction in Haemoccult screening for colorectal cancer, *Br J Surg* 76:976, 1989.

55. Robinson MHE et al: Is dietary restriction always necessary in Haemoccult screening for colorectal neoplasia? *Eur J Surg Oncol* 19:539, 1993.

56. Gilbertsen VA et al: The design of a study to assess occult blood screening for colon cancer, *J Chron Dis* 33:107, 1980.

57. Lang CA, Ransohoff D: Fecal occult blood screening for colorectal cancer, *JAMA* 271:1011, 1994.

58. Mandel JM et al: Letter to the editor, *JAMA* 272:1090, 1994.

58a. Kewenter J et al: Screening and rescreening for colorectal cancer, *Cancer* 62:645, 1988.

59. Kewenter J et al: A randomized trial of faecal occult blood testing for early detection of colorectal cancer: results of screening and rescreening of 51,325 subjects. In Miller AB et al, editors: *Cancer screening,* Cambridge, England, 1991, Cambridge University Press.

60. Kewenter J et al: Results of screening, rescreening and follow-up in a prospective randomized study for detection of colorectal cancer by fecal occult blood testing: results for 68,308 subjects, *Scand J Gastroenterol* 29:468, 1994.

61. Hardcastle JD et al: Controlled trial of faecal occult blood testing in the detection of colorectal cancer, *Lancet* 2:1, 1983.

62. Hardcastle JD et al: Randomized, controlled trial of faecal occult blood screening for colorectal cancer: results for first 107,349 subjects, *Lancet* 1:1160, 1989.

63. Hardcastle JD: Randomized control trial of faecal occult blood screening for colorectal cancer: results for the first 144,103 patients, *Eur J Cancer Prev* 1:21, 1991.

64. Thomas WM, Hardcastle JD: An update on the Nottingham trial of fecal occult blood screening for colorectal cancer. In Miller AB et al, editors: *Cancer screening,* Cambridge, England, 1991, Cambridge University Press.

65. Thomas WM et al: Screening for colorectal carcinoma: an analysis of the sensitivity of Haemoccult, *Br J Surg* 79:833, 1992.

66. Klaaborg K et al: Participation in mass screening for colorectal cancer with fecal occult blood test, *Scand J Gastroenterol* 21:1180, 1986.

67. Krönborg O et al: Initial mass screening for colorectal cancer with fecal occult blood test: a prospective randomized study at Funen in Denmark, *Scand J Gastroenterol* 22:677, 1987.

68. Krönborg O et al: Repeated screening for colorectal cancer with fecal occult blood test: a prospective randomized study at Funen, Denmark, *Scand J Gastroenterol* 24:599, 1989.

69. Krönborg O et al: Causes of death during the first 5 years of a randomized trial of mass screening for colorectal cancer with fecal occult blood test, *Scand J Gastroenterol* 27:47, 1992.

70. Jensen BM, Krönborg O, Fenger C: Interval cancers in screening with fecal occult blood test for colorectal cancer, *Scand J Gastroenterol* 27:779, 1992.

71. Faivre J et al: Participation in mass screening for colorectal cancer: results of screening and rescreening from the Burgundy study, *Eur J Cancer Prev* 1:49, 1991.

72. Arveux P et al: Views of a general population on mass screening of colorectal cancer: the Burgundy study, *Prev Med* 21:574, 1992.

73. Winawer SJ, Schottenfeld D, Flehinger BJ: Colorectal cancer screening, *J Natl Cancer Inst* 83:243, 1991.

74. Moss SM: Case-control studies of screening, *Int J Cancer* 20:1, 1991.

75. Newcomb PA et al: Screening sigmoidoscopy and colorectal cancer mortality, *J Natl Cancer Inst* 84:1572, 1992.

76. Lazovich D: A case-control study to evaluate efficacy of screening for faecal occult blood, *J Med Screening* 2:84, 1995.

77. Shapiro S: Case-control studies of colorectal cancer mortality: is the case made for screening sigmoidoscopy, *J Natl Cancer Inst* 84:1546, 1992.

78. Ransohoff DF, Lang CA: Sigmoidoscopy screening in the 1990s, *JAMA* 269:1278, 1993.

79. Lieberman D: Colon cancer screening: beyond efficacy, *Gastroenterology* 106:803, 1994.

80. Morson BC: Evolution of cancer of the colon and rectum, *Cancer* 34:845, 1974.

81. Winawer SJ et al: Risk and surveillance of individuals with colorectal polyps, *Bull World Health Organ* 68:789, 1990.

82. Bronner MP, Haggitt RC: The polyp-cancer sequence: do all cancers arise from benign adenomas? In Sivak MV, editor: *Gastrointestinal endoscopy,* Philadelphia, 1993, WB Saunders.

83. Dukes CE: Simple tumors of the large intestine and their relationship to cancer, *Br J Surg* 13:720, 1925.

84. Jass JR: Do all colorectal carcinomas arise in preexisting adenomas? *World J Surg* 13:45, 1989.

85. Lev R: *Adenomatous polyps of the colon: pathobiological and clinical features,* New York, 1990, Springer-Verlag.

86. Tierney RP, Ballantyne GH, Modlin IM: The adenoma to carcinoma sequence, *Surg Gynecol Obstet* 171:81, 1990.

87. Williams CB, Bedenne L: Management of colorectal polyps: is all the effort worthwhile? *J Gastroenterol Hepatol* (suppl 1):144, 1990.

88. Eide TJ: Natural history of adenomas, *World J Surg* 15:3, 1991.

89. Itzkowitz SH: The adenomatous polyp, *Semin Gastrointest Dis* 3(1):3, 1992.

90. Neugut AI, Jacobson JS, DeVivo I: Epidemiology of colorectal adenomatous polyps, *Cancer Epidemiol Biomarkers Prev* 2:159, 1993.

91. Vogelstein B et al: Genetic alterations during colorectal-tumor development, *N Engl J Med* 319:525, 1988.

92. Kuramoto S, Oohara T: Minute cancers arising de novo in the human large intestine, *Cancer* 61:829, 1988.

93. Shimoda T et al: Early colorectal carcinoma with special reference to its development de novo, *Cancer* 64:1138, 1989.

94. Bedenne L et al: Adenoma-carcinoma sequence or "de novo" carcinogenesis? A study of adenomatous remnants in a population-based series of large bowel cancers, *Cancer* 69:883, 1992.

95. Helwig EB: The evolution of adenomas of the large intestine and their relation to carcinoma, *Surg Gynecol Obstet* 84:36, 1947.

96. Winawer SJ et al: The National Polyp Study: design, methods, and characteristics of patients with newly diagnosed polyps, *Cancer* 70:1236, 1992.

97. Winawer SJ et al: Prevention of colorectal cancer by colonoscopic polypectomy, *N Engl J Med* 329:1977, 1993.

98. Wolff WI, Shinya H: Polypectomy via the fiberoptic colonoscope: removal of neoplasms beyond the reach of the sigmoidoscope, *N Engl J Med* 288:329, 1973.

99. Kozuka S et al: Premalignancy of the mucosal polyp in the large intestine. II. Estimation of the periods required for malignant transformation of mucosal polyps, *Dis Colon Rectum* 18:494, 1975.

100. Morson BC: The evolution of colorectal carcinoma, *Clin Radiol* 35:425, 1984.

101. Muto T, Bussey HJR, Morson BC: The evolution of cancer of the colon and rectum, *Cancer* 36:2251, 1975.

102. Shinya H, Wolff WI: Morphology, anatomic distribution and cancer potential of colonic polyps: an analysis of 7,000 polyps endoscopically removed, *Ann Surg* 190:679, 1979.

103. Eide TJ: Remnants of adenomas in colorectal carcinomas, *Cancer* 51:1866, 1983.

104. Eide TJ: Risk of colorectal cancer in adenoma-bearing individuals within a defined population, *Int J Cancer* 38:173, 1986.

105. Hermanek P: Dysplasia-carcinoma sequence, types of adenomas and early colorectal carcinoma, *Eur J Surg Oncol* 13:141, 1987.

106. Dukes CE: Familial intestinal polyposis, *Ann R Coll Surg Engl* 10:293, 1952.

107. Bussey HJR: *Familial polyposis coli: family studies, histopathology, differential diagnosis, and results of treatment,* Baltimore, 1975, Johns Hopkins University Press.

108. Meltzer SJ et al: Protooncogene abnormalities in colon cancers and adenomatous polyps, *Gastroenterology* 92:1174, 1987.

109. Bodmer WF et al: Localization of the gene for familial adenomatous polyposis on chromosome 5, *Nature* 328:614, 1987.

110. Stanbridge EJ: Identifying tumor suppressor genes in human colorectal cancer, *Science* 247:12, 1990.

111. Fearon ER, Vogelstein B: A genetic model for colorectal tumorigenesis, *Cell* 61:759, 1990.

112. Bishop DT, Burt RW: Genetic epidemiology and molecular genetics of colorectal adenomas and cancer. In Rozen P, Reich CB, Winawer SJ, editors: *Large bowel cancer: policy, prevention, research and treatment,* Basel, Switzerland, 1991, Karger.

113. Baker SJ et al: p53 gene mutations occur in combination with 17p allelic deletions as late events in colorectal tumorigenesis, *Cancer Res* 50:7717, 1990.

114. Krönborg O: Colorectal polyps: introduction, *World J Surg* 15:1, 1991 (editorial).

115. O'Brien MJ et al: The National Polyp Study: patient and polyp characteristics associated with high-grade dysplasia in colorectal adenomas, *Gastroenterology* 98:371, 1990.

116. Day DW, Morson BC: Pathology of adenomas in the pathogenesis of colorectal cancer. In Morson BC, editor: *Major problems in pathology,* Philadelphia, 1978, WB Saunders.

117. Winawer SJ, Zauber A, Diaz B: The National Polyp Study: temporal sequence of evolving colorectal cancer from the normal colon, *Gastrointest Endosc* 33:167, 1987.

118. Jorgensen OD, Krönborg O, Fenger C: The Funen adenoma follow-up study: characteristics of patients and initial adenomas in relation to severe dysplasia, *Scand J Gastroenterol* 28:239, 1993.

119. Konishi F, Morson BC: Pathology of colorectal adenomas: a colonoscopic survey, *J Clin Pathol* 35:830, 1982.

120. Atkin WS, Morson BC, Cuzick J: Long-term risk of colorectal cancer after excision of rectosigmoid adenomas, *N Engl J Med* 326:658, 1992.

121. Connor RJ, Prorok PA, Weed DL: The case-control design and the assessment of the efficacy of cancer screening, *J Clin Epidemiol* 44:1215, 1991.

122. Weiss NS, McKnight B, Stevens NG: Approaches to the analysis of case-control studies of the efficacy of cancer screening, *Am J Epidemiol* 135:817, 1992.

123. Atkin WS et al: Prevention of cancer by once-only sigmoidoscopy, *Lancet* 341:736, 1993.

124. Gilbertsen VA: Proctosigmoidoscopy and polypectomy in reducing the incidence of rectal cancer, *Cancer* 34:936, 1994.

125. Gilbertsen VA, Nelms JM: The prevention of invasive cancer of the rectum, *Cancer* 41:1137, 1978.

126. Cutler JL et al: Multiphasic checkup evaluation study. I. Methods, *Prev Med* 2:197, 1973.

127. Dales LG et al: Multiphasic checkup evaluation study. Outpatient clinic utilization, hospitalization and mortality experience after seven years, *Prev Med* 2:221, 1973.

128. Friedman GD, Collen MF, Fireman BH: Multiphasic health checkup evaluation: a 16-year follow-up, *J Chron Dis* 39:453, 1986.

129. Selby JV, Friedman GD, Collen MF: Sigmoidoscopy and mortality from colorectal cancer: the Kaiser Permanente multiphasic evaluation study, *J Clin Epidemiol* 41:427, 1988.

130. Selby JV et al: A case-control study of screening sigmoidoscopy and mortality from colorectal cancer, *N Engl J Med* 326:653, 1992.

131. Lieberman D: Screening colonoscopy: has the time come? In Swak MV, editor: *Gastrointestinal endoscopy clinics of America*, Philadelphia, 1993, WB Saunders.

PROSTATE CANCER

5

William J. Catalona

Mortality and morbidity benefits of PSA screening
Cost effectiveness of PSA screening

RECOMMENDATIONS ABOUT SCREENING

PROSTATE CANCER SCREENING DEBATE

Screening for prostate cancer is controversial. The controversy is about whether screening will improve patient outcomes and what the costs will be in terms of money, anxiety, and the morbidity and mortality caused by the screening tests and by the treatment of the cancers detected.[1-8] To prove that screening is worthwhile, it is not sufficient merely to show that screening detects more cancers or even that it detects them earlier.

> *It must be shown that screening reduces the morbidity and mortality rates of prostate cancer, preferably in a cost-effective manner.*

Some physicians, notably epidemiologists and family practitioners, have questioned the value of screening and treatment for localized prostate cancer.

> *This movement has been based largely on misleading studies that have left the general public and much of the medical community with the erroneous impression that deferred treatment is as effective as active therapy for all men with clinically localized prostate cancer.*

This specious conclusion has been advanced to challenge the ethics of screening and treatment for early prostate cancer. Recently even the ethics of performing screening trials have been questioned. Some authors who believe that screening and early treatment for prostate cancer may do more harm than good have called for a moratorium on prostate cancer screening until the results of a prospective clinical trial are available to resolve these issues.

This debate has carried over to professional societies. On one side, the American Urological Association, the Canadian Urological Association, the American Cancer Society, and the American College of Radiology all have recommended routine annual prostate-specific antigen (PSA) screening for prostate cancer. On the other side, the U.S. Preventive Services Task Force and the Canadian Task Force on the Periodic Health Examination have not recommended PSA screening. The National Cancer Institute, which recommends the routine performance of digital rectal examination (DRE), does not recommend using PSA for screening until more information is available. In general, physicians who are directly responsible for diagnosing and treating prostate cancer patients, such as urologists and radiation oncologists, favor screening, whereas those who do not have direct patient responsibility, such as epidemiologists, do not favor screening.

> *Some of the technical arguments advanced against screening relate to inherent biases that may produce the false impression that screening is useful.*

Lead time bias, an apparent increase in survival when the total length of life is *not* prolonged, and length time bias, the tendency to detect preferentially the slowly growing cancers through screening because they remain in the population longer, may create the false impression that early detection leads to prolonged survival.[1,7,9] Because of the comparatively slow growth rate of many prostate cancers and the usual advanced age at the time of diagnosis, prostate cancer is especially prone to lead time and length time bias.[1,9] Some authors have also criticized existing screening trials for selection bias, that is, studying only men who volunteer to be studied, because they may not be representative of the general population.[10] This criticism is less valid because, in practice, the results of screening are relevant only to men who have submitted to being screened.

It is indisputable that prostate cancer is an increasingly common cause of cancer deaths in American men, and to a considerable extent the high prostate cancer mortality rate is caused by late detection. Early-stage cancers have favorable outcomes with treatment, whereas advanced cancers have unfavorable outcomes.[11]

> *It is reasonable to expect that earlier detection will benefit individuals in at least some subsets, and therefore overall prostate cancer morbidity and mortality rates will be reduced by screening.*

This is the case in other similar cancers.[12,13]

> *The only current practical means for reducing the morbidity and mortality rates of prostate cancer are through early detection and treatment of curable disease.*

The National Cancer Institute is sponsoring the prospective, Prostate, Lung, Colorectal, Ovarian (PLCO) Trial to determine whether screening reduces the prostate cancer death rate.[1,14] This trial will take 15 years to complete, and it is estimated that half a million men will die of prostate cancer during that interval. There are further concerns about the PLCO trial. First, most test subjects and controls previously will have undergone screening with PSA testing and DRE. Second, the age range selected for screening in the PLCO trial (60 to 74 years) is too high and will not give screening a fair trial. In this regard, since screening is most likely to be beneficial for men ages 50 to 65, it is unrealistic to expect a demonstrable benefit from screening men age 74. Third, the number of screenings planned (four) is insufficient to evaluate the benefits of measuring PSA rate of change in the early detection of prostate cancer. Fourth, not all persons diagnosed with cancer will receive effective treatment; some will opt for expectant management or one of the experimental treatments such as cryoablation or interstitial radiation therapy.

> *Therefore, it is likely that after 15 years we still will lack valid data to resolve the screening controversy.*

BASIS FOR SCREENING WITH SERUM PSA MEASUREMENTS

Serum PSA concentrations are lower than 4 ng/ml in virtually all normal men without prostatic disease and also in about 25% of men with palpable prostate cancer.[4] Elevated PSA concentrations (higher than 4 ng/ml) are observed not only in men with prostate cancer, but also in some men with benign prostatic hyperplasia (BPH), urinary tract infection, prostatitis, and in men who recently have undergone prostatic manipulation, such as prostatic biopsy or urethral instrumentation.[15] False elevations of serum PSA concentrations in men with infections and in those who have undergone urinary tract manipulation can be excluded readily, leaving those with BPH and prostate cancer to be distinguished from each other. Approximately 25% of men with clinical BPH have elevated serum PSA concentrations, which are generally higher in patients with larger prostate glands.[15] It has been estimated that BPH tissue contributes 0.3 ng/ml per gram of tissue to the serum PSA concentration; in contrast, prostate cancer tissue contributes about tenfold more PSA to the serum concentration (3 ng/ml per gram of tissue). Autopsy studies suggest that approximately 30% of men older than 50 years of age have occult prostate cancer, but only about 10% to 20% who undergo prostatectomy for BPH are found to have cancer in the resected specimen.[16]

WASHINGTON UNIVERSITY PSA SCREENING STUDIES

For the past 5 years prostate cancer screening trials at Washington University in St. Louis have involved more than 27,000 men.[4,9,17] The author has participated in a multiinstitutional trial involving more than 6000 men enrolled at six medical centers to evaluate PSA in conjunction with rectal examination and prostatic transrectal ultrasonography (TRUS) as screening tests.[4] These trials have provided useful insights about PSA-based screening and are used extensively in this chapter to illustrate the performance characteristics of prostate cancer screening. The most current results are summarized below.

There are currently two prostate cancer screening studies at our institution, PSA-1 and PSA-2. Volunteers have been recruited for PSA-1 and PSA-2 through press releases asking healthy men to participate in a study of serum antigen (PSA) measurement as a screening test for prostate cancer. Exclusion criteria for both studies include age under 50, history of prostate cancer, and active prostatitis.

PSA-1 Study Protocol

In our PSA-1 study protocol[9,17] men whose initial PSA concentrations were 4 ng/ml or less were not evaluated further. Rather, their PSA levels were measured again at 6-month intervals for the duration of the study unless the PSA level increased to over 4 ng/ml (Figure 5-1).

If the PSA value was over 4 ng/ml, another blood sample was collected within 1 to 2 weeks to verify the elevation. Men who had two serum PSA values over 4 ng/ml within that period underwent both DRE and prostatic TRUS. If either or both of these procedures revealed abnormal or suspicious findings, we performed a needle biopsy under ultrasound guidance of the areas involved. If the PSA concentration was over 4 ng/ml but the rectal and ultrasound examinations were normal, no biopsy was performed.

Men whose biopsies were negative for cancer had serum PSA measurements at 6-month intervals. Repeat DRE, TRUS, and biopsy, if indicated, were recommended for men whose PSA levels were again over 4 ng/ml at a later evaluation.

We measured serum PSA concentrations using an immunoenzymetric assay (Tandem-E PSA, Hybritech, Inc.) and used the normal range recommended by the manufacturer (0 to 4 ng/ml), considering PSA values over 4 ng/ml as grounds for suspecting prostate cancer.

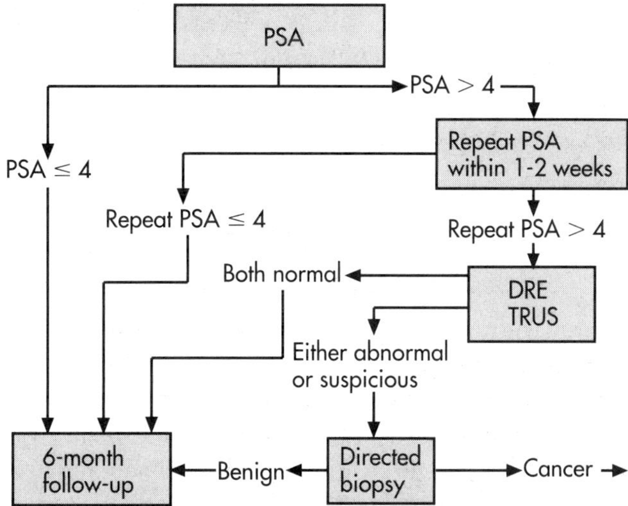

Figure 5-1 Prostate-specific antigen (PSA)-1 study protocol. *DRE,* Digital rectal examination; *TRUS,* transrectal ultrasonography.

The following data were recorded:

1. Findings on DRE, which were categorized as normal, abnormal but benign (including enlargement), or suspicious for cancer (including induration, asymmetry, irregularity)
2. TRUS findings, categorized as normal, abnormal but benign (including enlargement, asymmetry, calculi, transition zone hypoechoic areas), or suspicious for cancer (hypoechoic area in the posterior peripheral zone)
3. PSA level in serum drawn before each DRE, ultrasonographic examination, or biopsy
4. Results of biopsy
5. Clinical and pathologic tumor stage

From June 1989 through September 1991, 10,249 men were enrolled in the PSA-1 study. PSA-1 volunteers have been screened at 6-month intervals for the past 5 years, and the study is projected to continue for an additional 3 years. Since recruitment of new participants ended in September 1991, all PSA-1 volunteers have been enrolled for at least 30 months.

> *Data for the first 30 months of the PSA-1 study show a consistently high compliance rate for twice yearly PSA screening. At 30 months 86% of the men without cancer detected on a previous visit returned for PSA testing.*

The compliance rate for further evaluation (that is, DRE and TRUS following an elevated PSA level) was very good at entry (95%) but decreased substantially at 30 months (46% of men with elevated PSA at 30 months complied with recommendation for DRE and TRUS). However, the group of men with elevated PSA who refused further evaluation at 30 months had a median number of three previous negative biopsies.

Compliance with recommendation for prostatic biopsy following an abnormal or suspicious DRE or TRUS remained consistently high throughout the 30-month interval, ranging from 92% at entry to 96% at 30 months.

PSA-2 Study Protocol

The study protocol for PSA-2 differs from the PSA-1 protocol in that all men were initially screened with *both* PSA and DRE.[4] Blood samples were obtained before DRE, or at least 1 week after (Figure 5-2).

Within the PSA-2 study protocol, men with normal PSA levels (0 to 4 ng/ml) and normal DRE findings, or DRE findings that were abnormal but benign, were not further evaluated. Rather, PSA measurements and DRE were repeated at 6-month intervals for the duration of the study unless the PSA level became elevated (>4 ng/ml) or the DRE became suspicious for cancer. If either test was suspicious for cancer, the subject underwent four (quadrant) TRUS-guided needle biopsies (two apex, two base). Ultrasound findings were recorded, but TRUS results were not used to determine whether a biopsy was performed. All four quadrants were biopsied even if no suspicious areas on DRE or TRUS

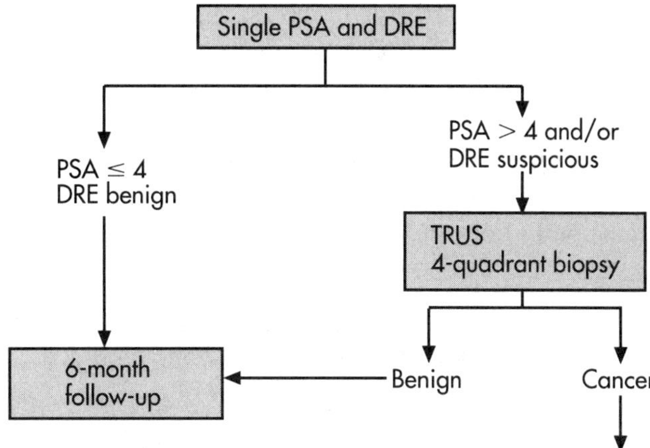

Figure 5-2   Prostate-specific antigen (PSA)-2 study protocol. *DRE,* Digital rectal examination; *TRUS,* transrectal ultrasonography.

were present. According to standard medical practice, we performed additional biopsies directed at palpable abnormalities and hypoechoic areas. Men whose biopsies were negative continued with serum PSA measurements and DRE at 6-month intervals.

Results

From May 1991 through March 1994, 15,314 men were enrolled in the PSA-2 study. Unlike PSA-1, enrollment is still ongoing. PSA-2 originated as one of six centers included in the Hybritech, Inc., multicenter trial of PSA and DRE combined screening.[4] The protocol for the multicenter study involved a once-only screen with both PSA and DRE. However, we are in the process of converting PSA-2 to a serial screening study, that is, screening men with both PSA and DRE every 6 months.

To date, 81% of the men with elevated PSA or suspicious DRE upon initial screening have complied with recommendations for TRUS and prostatic biopsy. Compliance is somewhat higher for the subset of men with *both* elevated PSA and suspicious DRE (89% of this group have undergone TRUS and prostatic biopsy).

Age and Race of PSA Screening Volunteers

The majority of the volunteers for both PSA-1 and PSA-2 studies were below the age of 70. More specifically, 36% of PSA-1 volunteers were between the ages of 50 and 59, 49% were between 60 and 69, 19% were between 70 and 79, and 1% were 80 years of age or older. Overall, the mean age for PSA-1 volunteers was 63 (SD = ±7, range = 50 to 90).

The men enrolled in PSA-2 were somewhat younger (mean age = 60, SD ±8, range = 50 to 95). More specifically, 50% were between the ages of 50 and 59, 37% were between 60 and 69, 12% were between 70 and 79, and 1% were 80 years of age or older.

The vast majority of screening volunteers in both studies were white (99% white in PSA-1 and 95% white in PSA-2). However, we have initiated community outreach efforts to increase enrollment of African-American men. The increased number of African-American men enrolled in the PSA-2 study represents the result of these efforts.

Initial Screening Results

Upon initial screening the distribution of PSA levels was approximately the same in both PSA-1 and PSA-2.

> *Approximately 10% of the men who volunteered for PSA screening or PSA and DRE screening combined had PSA levels of more than 4 ng/ml. Similarly, 11% of the PSA-2 volunteers were found to have suspicious DRE upon initial screening.*

Prostatic ultrasonography yielded abnormalities in the majority of PSA-1 and PSA-2 volunteers. However, all the men who underwent TRUS were preselected on the basis of elevated PSA or suspicious findings on DRE.

Within PSA-1 only 6% of the men with elevated PSA levels upon initial screening had both normal DRE and TRUS and therefore were not recommended for biopsy according to the study protocol. The vast majority of men with elevated PSA concentration upon initial screening underwent prostatic biopsy.

Biopsy Rate and Overall Cancer Detection Rate

Upon initial screening 8% of PSA-1 volunteers and 15% of PSA-2 volunteers underwent prostatic biopsy. The cancer detection rate was identical for both study groups (3%).

To date 10% of the PSA-1 volunteers and 6% of the PSA-2 volunteers have undergone at least one biopsy after initial screening. As expected from the longer duration of PSA study 1, the cancer detection rate for serial screening is slightly higher in the PSA-1 study group (3%) than in the PSA-2 study group (1%).

Cancer Detection Rate Stratified by PSA Level

> *Upon initial screening 34% of the men who had biopsies in accordance with the PSA-1 study protocol were diagnosed with cancer. In contrast, 23% of the men who had biopsies in accordance with the PSA-2 study protocol were diagnosed with cancer.*

The low yield from biopsy in men with suspicious findings on DRE whose PSA concentrations were 4 ng/ml or less accounts for the lower rate of cancer detection in PSA-2. Not surprisingly, PSA levels of 10 ng/ml or less at initial screening were associated with a higher cancer detection rate in both studies.

For the men who through serial screening underwent at least one biopsy after initial screening, 29% of the PSA-1 volunteers were diagnosed with cancer as compared with 16% of the PSA-2 volunteers. In contrast to the results for initial screening, with *serial* screening a PSA concentration of 10 ng/ml or greater immediately preceding the most recent biopsy was not associated with a higher rate of cancer detection in either PSA-1 or PSA-2.

Positive Predictive Value for PSA, DRE, and TRUS

Based on the initial PSA-2 screening results, we calculated positive predictive value (PPV) for cancer on the basis of PSA over 4 ng/ml, suspicious DRE, or suspicious TRUS. PPV was calculated as the proportion of cancers detected in men with positive screens.

> *The PPV for PSA (34%) was greater than that for DRE (21%) or TRUS (25%).*

It should be noted that the PPV for TRUS applies only to prescreened men who also had elevated PSA and/or suspicious DRE.

Clinical Staging of Cancers Detected

About 98% of the tumors detected through the PSA-1 study protocol (including both initial and serial screening) and 92% of the tumors detected through the PSA-2 study protocol (including both initial and serial screening) were clinically staged. Clinical staging consisted of DRE, determination of serum acid phosphatase levels, and radioisotope bone scanning with confirmatory imaging studies or bone biopsies, if necessary.

We originally used a modification of the Jewett-Whitmore staging system[18]; however, to facilitate comparisons with other studies, we have attempted retrospectively to translate it into the 1992 tumor-nodes-metastases (TNM) staging system.[19] Individuals were classified as having stage T_{1c} disease if they had a clinically localized nonpalpable tumor detected through PSA testing. Based on the pathologic report from the biopsy, we classified T_{1c} tumors as minimal if they were described in the pathology report as being microscopically focal and well differentiated (Gleason sum 2 to 4). Individuals were classified as having clinical stage T_{2a} disease if they had palpable carcinoma involving less than half of a lobe of the prostate and judged to be confined within the prostatic capsule. Stage T_{2b} disease denoted palpable tumors involving more than half of a lobe and judged to be confined within the prostatic capsule. The men were classified as having clinical stage T_3 disease if they had palpable extracapsular tumor extension, as D_0 disease if there was evidence of persistently elevated acid phosphatase (no analog exists in the TNM system for this category), and M_1 disease if there was radiographic or histologic evidence of distant metastases.

> *Combining clinical staging results for both PSA-1 and PSA-2, approximately 98% of the tumors detected through initial or serial screening were clinically confined to the prostate.*

Pathologic Staging of Cancers Detected

About 73% of the tumors detected through the PSA-1 study protocol (including both initial and serial screening) and 66% of the tumors detected through the PSA-2 study protocol (including both initial and serial screening) were pathologically staged.

For this analysis cancer confined to the prostate with clear margins was categorized as pathologic stage pT_1 or pT_2. Pathologic stage pT_{1c} denoted clinical stage T_{1c} tumors that were pathologically organ confined. As with clinical staging, we also subclassified pT_{1c} tumors as minimal if they were microscopically focal and well differentiated. Pathologic staging of stage pT_2 tumors was identical to clinical staging, except that the extent of the cancer was documented histologically. Men with microscopic periprostatic cancer extension, or those in whom the resected prostatic tissue contained cancer at the margins, were categorized as having pathologic stage pT_{3a} disease; those with seminal vesicle invasion were categorized as having stage pT_{3b}; and those with lymph node metastases were categorized as having N_1 disease.

Combining pathologic staging results for both PSA-1 and PSA-2, approximately 71% of the tumors detected through initial or serial screening were pathologically confined to the prostate. This indicates that, through PSA-based screening, more than 70% of cancers were potentially curable at diagnosis.

> *This represents a nearly twofold increase in the proportion of tumors pathologically organ confined and therefore curable when compared with staging results in the era before PSA was widely used for cancer detection.*

For example, both the American College of Surgeons and Surveillance Epidemiology End Results (SEER) have reported approximately 30% of tumors to be pathologically organ confined at the time of diagnosis.[11,20,21]

Possibly Unimportant Tumors: Clinical and Pathologic Staging

A common criticism of PSA-based screening is the unfounded concern that a large number of medically unimportant cancers will be detected.[1,3,7] Although the definition of unimportant cancers may vary widely, our data show the following[4,17]:

> *The vast majority of tumors detected through PSA-based screening have clinical and pathologic features traditionally associated with medically important tumors (palpable tumor mass, multifocal or diffuse involvement, and moderately or poorly differentiated histology).*

Combining clinical staging results for PSA-1 and PSA-2, only 15% to 17% of tumors were categorized as clinical stage A_1/T_{1c}–minimal (that is, microscopically focal, well-differentiated [Gleason sum 2 to 4], clinically localized nonpalpable tumors).

> *Similarly, only 2% to 4% of surgically staged tumors detected through our screening protocols could be defined as medically unimportant (pathologic stage A_1/pT_{1c}–minimal).*

PSA SCREENING ISSUES

> *Screening for prostate cancer with serum PSA measurements identifies in healthy populations of men a small subset (about 10% to 15%) of individuals who are at high risk for prostate cancer (25% to 70%).*

With prostate cancer, by the time the cancer produces symptoms, it usually is already too late for cure. The lifetime risk of having clinically significant prostate cancer is so high—about one in eight men—that, if screening is to be recommended, it should be recommended for the general population.

Prevalence of Suspicious Screening Tests

Previous studies have demonstrated that screening with DRE alone fails to increase the proportion of pathologically organ-confined cancers detected.[22] The incidence of suspicious DRE findings or elevated serum PSA concentrations is only 10% to 15% in men age 50 and rises to about 50% at age 80. This may seem to suggest that the yield is too low to justify screening men at age 50. However, younger men are more likely to have organ-confined cancers and also have a longer life expectancy.[17,23]

Therefore, if the screening tests are simple, not too expensive, and have reasonable performance characteristics, men are likely to benefit from prostate cancer screening.

Candidates for Screening

Familial prostate cancer has an earlier age of onset,[24] and focal prostate cancers are found at autopsy in a significant proportion of young African-American men.

> *Therefore beginning screening at an even earlier age may be appropriate in high-risk men such as African-Americans and men with an affected primary relative (a father or brother).*

Screening Tests to be Used: Pros and Cons

> *PSA and DRE should be the primary screening tests; ultra-sonography and systematic biopsy should be reserved for men with suspicious findings on either of these two tests.*

PSA measurements and DRE are complementary tests. For example, in our studies, DRE alone would have missed about 40% of the cancers and PSA alone would have missed about 25%. The addition of PSA to DRE increased the prostate cancer detection rate by 78%.[4] PSA also detected more organ-confined cancers.

> *In our studies, when we added PSA to the DRE, we detected nearly 80% more organ-confined cancers.[4]*

Effects of Screening on Stage of Cancers Detected

Our first study of PSA-based screening showed that, if the serum PSA concentration was elevated in the 4- to 10-ng range, about 25% of men had prostate cancer detected on the first biopsy. If the level was over 10 ng/ml, nearly 60% had cancer detected.[17]

Men who passed the first screening test were serially screened at 6-month intervals. With a follow-up ranging to 5 years, 2.6% had prostate cancer detected on subsequent screening.

> *This indicates that, in men with suspicious screening results, prostatic biopsies have a substantial sampling error and that serial screening in men with initially normal results is useful in detecting both initially missed and emerging cancers.*

The most recent tabulation our data show is that, if the initial PSA concentration was 0 to 4 ng/ml, 1.7% had cancer detected when evaluated within 5 years for a subsequently elevated PSA concentration. If the initial PSA concentration was 4 to 10 ng/ml, 36% had cancer detected within 5 years, and if the PSA concentration was over 10, 70% had cancer detected during the subsequent 5 years.

Serial Screening

Serial screening with the blood test alone also may be successful. Our data suggest that by using serial PSA screening the results may not be seriously compromised. For example, in our first study of PSA as the first-line screening test in men who were screened at 6-month intervals over 5 years, the overall cancer detection rate was 5.4%.

> *This rate was similar to the 5% detection rate achieved through initial screening with both DRE and PSA in our second screening study as well as in the multiinstitutional trial.*

Screening in African-Americans

In the African-American community there is a 31% higher incidence rate and a 117% higher mortality associated with prostate cancer.[25] Traditionally this community has a low participation rate in cancer screening programs. This may be reflected in the percentage of African-American patients with metastatic cancer at the time of diagnosis, which is twice as high as in whites. [26] In recent years the disparity in prostate cancer incidence rates between African-Americans and whites has decreased, probably because of more screening in whites. However, at the same time the disparity in age-adjusted mortality has increased.[25]

In our studies DRE findings were suspicious for cancer in 8.4% of African-Americans and 10.6% of whites (difference not significant). Significantly more African-Americans (13.2%) than whites (9.2%) had elevated PSA levels. As in clinical studies, African-Americans had a significantly higher prostate cancer detection rate (5.5% versus 3.3% in whites). Based on the screening test results, prostatic biopsies were recommended to 19.6% of African-Americans and 17.6% of whites. African-Americans living in low-income areas were less likely to comply with the recommendation for biopsy than comparable whites; however, the compliance rates were nearly identical for members of both populations who lived in higher income areas. African-American men had a significantly higher proportion with *clinically* advanced disease (9% versus 1% for white men), but there was no racial difference in the proportion with pathologically advanced or those with either clinically or pathologically advanced disease. There was also no significant racial difference in the distribution of tumor grades. African-American men with clinically localized disease were less likely than white men to select radical prostatectomy for treatment.

> *Our results suggest that the stage disparity between African-Americans and whites may be reduced or eliminated through screening.*

Follow-up studies of these patients will provide important information on the effect of screening on cancer-specific morbidity and mortality rates.

These results underscore the potential importance of screening in African-American populations. To the extent that their poor treatment outcomes are caused by late detection, earlier diagnosis through screening along with the implementation of effective treatment may reduce their excessive prostate cancer mortality and morbidity rates.

Significance of Symptoms in Screening Populations

Some authors have claimed that the results of most screening studies reported to date are suspect because they have not measured the accuracy of PSA screening in men without signs or symptoms of prostatic disease.[10] The reasoning is that, because at least some prostatic symptoms are due to prostate cancer, the prevalence of cancer in a symptomatic group of men would be higher than in an asymptomatic group. A substantial proportion of symptomatic men in a screening group would be expected to inflate calculations of the predictive value of an early detection test. In reality, PSA-based screening has been extensively studied in the target population of men who would participate in screening programs.[4]

> *Results in our multicenter screening population revealed that symptoms did not correlate with an increased risk for prostate cancer.*

In our studies[17] in 47 consecutive, concurrently studied, nonscreened cancer patients whose cancer was detected through the traditional approach, that is, biopsies were performed because of a suspicious DRE, 57% had clinically or pathologically advanced cancer at the time of detection. In concurrently studied screened patients whose cancer was detected through the initial PSA-based screen, only 37% had advanced disease, whereas of those with cancer detected through serial PSA-based screening, 29% had advanced cancer. In our second PSA study in which men were screened with both DRE and PSA testing, only 1% had clinically advanced cancer and only 29% who were surgically staged had pathologically advanced cancer at the time of detection. All screened groups had a significantly lower incidence of advanced cancer than the nonscreened patients.

> *Screening nearly doubled the percentage of men who have organ-confined (curable) cancers at the time of diagnosis.*

The key to reducing the high prostate cancer mortality rate is to detect and treat the cancer before the serum PSA concentration rises much above 10 ng/ml. In our studies 82% of men with PSA levels under 4 and 75% with levels between 4 to 10 ng/ml had pathologically organ-confined prostate cancer as compared with only 48% of those with PSA levels over 10 ng/ml.

Interpretation of PSA Tests

If the DRE is suspicious for cancer or if the PSA level is over 4 ng/ml, the patient should be fully evaluated, including systematic biopsies, unless he is too old or too ill for treatment. PSA, DRE, and ultrasonography all have false positive and false negative results. PSA is the most accurate single test, with a positive predictive value of 30% to 35% on the initial biopsy, using a cutoff of 4 ng/ml.

> *In fact, the PPV of PSA for prostate cancer (30% to 35%) is higher than that of mammography for predicting breast cancer (9% to 17%).*[27]

The most common reasons for false positive PSA elevations are BPH and prostatitis.

Proposed PSA Measures for Reducing False Positives

A criticism of PSA-based screening has been its false positive rate. Four alternative PSA measures have been proposed to reduce the false positives and decrease the number of unnecessary prostatic biopsies performed.

PSA Density

It has been suggested that the ratio of serum PSA level to the prostate volume—called the PSA density—may be more helpful in distinguishing BPH from prostate cancer.[28] Based on initial screening results from our PSA-2 study, the use of PSA density as a screen in men with normal DREs would result in fewer negative biopsies; however, the number of cancers detected also would substantially decrease. Most of the cancers missed would be organ confined.[29] Furthermore, estimates of prostatic volume based on ultrasonography are not highly reproducible. In our multicenter trial the use of PSA density would reduce the number of biopsies performed by more than 50%, but would also miss nearly half of the organ-confined cancers.[29]

> *Therefore, PSA density should not be used for primary prostate cancer screening.*

Age-Specific PSA Reference Ranges

Our data suggest the most practical serum PSA threshold for recommending prostatic biopsy is 4 ng/ml (Hybritech) for men of all ages. The use of lower PSA cut points for men in their 40s and 50s (2.5 or 3.5 ng/ml, respectively) and higher cut points for men in their 60s and those older than 70 (4.5 and 6.5 ng/ml, respectively) also has been proposed.[30] Our results reveal that the use of a PSA cut point of 3.5 ng/ml in men 50 to 59 years old with a normal DRE would result in a 29% to 45% increase in the number of biopsies performed with only an estimated 5% to 15% increase in cancers detected.[31,32] Use of a PSA cut point of 4.5 in men 60 to 69 years old with a normal DRE would result in a 15% to 18% reduction in the number of biopsies and a 6% to 10% reduction in the number of cancers detected (including an 8% to 13% reduction in the number of organ-confined cancers detected). Use of a PSA cut point of 6.5 ng/ml in men over 70 years of age with a normal DRE would result in a 44% to 52% reduction in number of biopsies, a 39% to 43% reduction in number of cancers detected, and a 42% to 47% reduction in number of organ-confined cancers detected.[32]

> *Because of the simultaneously increasing prevalence of both benign prostatic hyperplasia and prostate cancer with age, the PPV of PSA testing remains fairly constant across age groups. Thus, the 4 ng/ml cut point need not be altered in older men.*

Some investigators have recommended using 10 ng/ml as the cutoff in men with normal DRE and TRUS examinations. In our studies men with a PSA level of 4.1 to 10 ng/ml and a benign DRE had a higher incidence of detectable cancer (21%) than those with a suspicious DRE and a normal PSA level (11%).[4,33]

We found that more than two thirds of cancers were found in quadrants of the prostate that were not suspicious on rectal examination or ultrasonography.[34] Moreover, more than half of cancer patients whose serum PSA concentrations were higher than 10 ng/ml had extraprostatic spread of their cancer.

Thus our data support the concept that a biopsy—which is always indicated for a suspicious DRE—is also indicated for an elevated serum PSA concentration. If one waits until the PSA concentration rises higher than 10 ng/ml before recommending a biopsy, it will be too late to cure the cancer in more than half of the patients.

PSA Rate of Change

The rate of change in PSA (PSA slope) has been suggested as a more precise method for selecting men for biopsy. Based on reports from other investigators[35] and on our own serial screening results from PSA-1,[36] PSA slope has some promise in detecting cancers.

However, PSA slope measurements are most useful for men younger than 70 whose initial serum PSA concentrations are normal. The disadvantage of PSA slope is that multiple PSA measurements over time (at least 12 to 18 months) are required for slope calculations to be meaningful.

Measurement of PSA slope has been shown in a retrospective study to be helpful over intervals of 5 to 20 years.

Free and Bound PSA Forms

Although still in the early stages of development, researchers have developed assays to measure free and bound PSA forms in the serum.[37]

Preliminary reports suggest that the ratios of free to bound PSA forms may increase specificity by distinguishing PSA elevations caused by benign conditions from those caused by prostate cancer.

The proportion of free PSA is lower in patients with cancer than in those with benign hyperplasia.

Medically Unimportant Cancers Detected Through Screening

One concern about screening for prostate cancer is that it might detect low-grade, low-volume cancers which may progress so slowly that they do not pose an immediate threat to the patient. Recent studies have demonstrated that screening with DRE and serum PSA concentrations detects only a small fraction of the possibly latent prostate cancers in screened populations.[4,17,38-40]

> *The great majority of cancers detected through PSA screening have the histologic features of medically important cancers.*

Thus, although screening with PSA detects prostate cancer earlier, none of the screening tests is so sensitive that it detects many of the so-called insignificant cancers. There is a trend toward detecting more focal, well-differentiated cancers with serial screening. These results would be expected from the known relationship between serum PSA levels and tumor volume.

Mortality and Morbidity Benefits of PSA Screening

If treatment is beneficial to some patient subsets with early-stage prostate cancer—as it almost certainly is—early detection will have morbidity and mortality benefits.[41] Screening increases the proportion of organ-confined cancers from 35% using traditional methods to 70% or more.[17] Even older patients with a 10-year life expectancy benefit by avoiding death caused by prostate cancer, but younger patients benefit more from prolonged survival.

Cost Effectiveness of PSA Screening

Screening with PSA and DRE is associated with a very low morbidity rate. A cost-effectiveness analysis must weigh the costs of screening against the costs of treating advanced prostate cancer.

> *An analysis using Markov modeling showed that, because treating advanced prostate cancer is more costly than treating early disease, the total costs per prostate cancer detected and treated through screening with PSA and DRE are less than for those detected using DRE only.[42]*

Thus, based on this analysis, the choice seems to be between (1) performing screening and paying for the detection and treatment of early disease, and (2) not performing screening and paying the greater costs of treating advanced disease. Another study performing a cost-benefit analysis suggested that, after the third year of screening, the use of PSA testing in combination with DRE becomes cost-effective.[43]

RECOMMENDATIONS ABOUT SCREENING

The author believes that screening with an annual rectal examination and serum PSA measurement using the 4-ng cutoff should be encouraged. The preferred age range for maximizing the potential benefits of screening is between 50 and 70 years old. Men with a strong family history of prostate cancer and African-American men should consider beginning screening at age 40. Men over 70 who are concerned about prostate cancer should also be tested. Those with suspicious findings on either PSA testing or DRE should be further evaluated with ultrasonography and systematic prostatic biopsies.

REFERENCES

1. Kramer BS et al: Prostate cancer screening: what we know and what we need to know, *Ann Intern Med* 119:914, 1993.
2. Chodak GW et al: Results of conservative management of clinically localized prostate cancer, *N Engl J Med* 330:242, 1994.
3. Adami H-O, Baron JA, Rothman KK: Ethics of a prostate cancer screening trial, *Lancet* 343:958, 1994.
4. Catalona WJ et al: Comparison of digital rectal examination and serum prostate specific antigen in the early detection of prostate cancer: results of a multicenter clinical trial of 6,630 men, *J Urol* 151:1283, 1994.
5. Fleming C et al: A decision analysis of alternative treatment strategies for clinically localized prostate cancer, *JAMA* 269:2650, 1993.
6. Scardino PT, Beck JR, Miles BJ: Conservative management of prostate cancer, *N Engl J Med* 330:1831, 1994 (letter).
7. Chodak GW: Questioning the value of screening for prostate cancer in asymptomatic men, *Urology* 42:116, 1993.
8. Catalona WJ: Urology: Contempo 1993, *JAMA* 270:265, 1993.
9. Catalona WJ et al: Measurement of prostate-specific antigen in serum as a screening test for prostate cancer, *N Engl J Med* 324:1156, 1991.
10. Sox HC Jr: Preventive health services in adults, *N Engl J Med* 330:1589, 1994.
11. Boring CC et al: Cancer statistics, 1994, *CA Cancer J Clin* 44:7, 1994.
12. Harris JR et al: Breast cancer, *N Engl J Med* 327:319, 1992.
13. Mandel JS et al: Reducing mortality from colorectal cancer by screening for fecal occult blood, *N Engl J Med* 328:1365, 1993.
14. Walsh PC: Using prostate-specific antigen to diagnose prostate cancer: sailing in uncharted waters, *Ann Intern Med* 119:948, 1993 (editorial).
15. Stamey TA et al: Prostate-specific antigen as a serum marker for adenocarcinoma of the prostate, *N Engl J Med* 317:909, 1987.
16. Halpert B et al: Carcinoma of the prostate: a survey of 5,000 autopsies, *Cancer* 16:737, 1963.
17. Catalona WJ et al: Detection of organ-confined prostate cancer is increased through prostate-specific antigen-based screening, *JAMA* 270:948, 1993.

18. Catalona WJ, Whitmore WF Jr: New staging systems for prostate cancer, *J Urol* 142:1302, 1989.

19. Genitourinary cancers: prostate. In American Joint Committee on Cancer: *Manual for cancer staging,* ed 4, Philadelphia, 1992, JB Lippincott.

20. Mettlin C, Jones GW, Murphy GP: Trends in prostate cancer care in the United States, 1974-1990: observations from the patient care evaluation studies of the American College of Surgeons Commission on Cancer, *CA Cancer J Clin* 42:83, 1993.

21. Surveillance, epidemiology, and end results: incidence and mortality data, National Cancer Institute Monograph, section 22, Bethesda, Md, 1992.

22. Gerber GS et al: Disease-specific survival following routine prostate cancer screening by digital rectal examination, *JAMA* 269:61, 1993.

23. Richie JP et al: Effect of patient age on early detection of prostate cancer with serum prostate-specific antigen and digital rectal examination, *Urology* 42:365, 1993.

24. Carter BS et al: Hereditary prostate cancer: epidemiologic and clinical features, *J Urol* 150:797, 1993.

25. Miller BA et al, editors: Cancer statistics review: 1973-1989, NIH Pub No 92-2789, National Cancer Institute, 1992.

26. Steele GD et al: Clinical highlights from the National Cancer Data Base: 1994, *CA Cancer J Clin* 44:71, 1994.

27. Kerlikewske K et al: Positive predictive value of screening mammography by age and family history of breast cancer, *JAMA* 270:2444, 1993.

28. Benson MC et al: Prostate specific antigen density: a means of distinguishing benign prostatic hypertrophy and prostate cancer, *J Urol* 147:815, 1992.

29. Catalona WJ et al: Comparison of prostate specific antigen (PSA) concentration versus prostate specific antigen density (PSAD) in the early detection of prostate cancer: receiver operation characteristic (ROC) curves, *J Urol* 152:2031, 1994.

30. Oesterling JE et al: Serum prostate-specific antigen in a community-based population of healthy men: establishment of age-specific reference ranges, *JAMA* 270:860, 1992.

31. Colberg JW, Smith DS, Catalona WJ: Prevalence and pathologic extent of prostate cancer in men with PSA levels of 2.9 to 4.0 ng per ml, *J Urol* 149:507, 1993.

32. Catalona WJ et al: Selection of optimal prostate specific antigen (PSA) cutoffs for early detection of prostate cancer: receiver operating characteristic (ROC) curves, *J Urol* 152:2037, 1994.

33. Babaian JR et al: Diagnostic testing for prostate cancer detection: less is best, *Urology* 41:421, 1993.

34. Flanigan RC et al: Accuracy of digital rectal examination (DRE) and ultrasonography (TRUS) in localizing prostate cancer, *J Urol* (in press).

35. Carter HB et al: Longitudinal evaluation of prostate-specific antigen levels in men with and without prostate disease, *JAMA* 267:2215, 1992.

36. Smith DS, Catalona WJ: Rate of change in serum prostate specific antigen levels as a method for prostate cancer detection, *J Urol* 152:1163, 1994.

37. Stenman et al: A complex between prostate-specific antigen and α_1-antichymotrypsin is the major form of prostate-specific antigen in serum of patients with prostate cancer, *Cancer Res* 51:222, 1991.

38. Brawn PN et al: Prostate-specific antigen levels from completely sectioned, clinically benign, whole prostates, *Cancer* 68:1592, 1991.

39. Stormont TJ et al: Clinical stage Bo or T_{1c} prostate cancer: nonpalpable disease identified by an elevated serum prostate-specific antigen concentration, *Urology* 41:3, 1993.

40. Epstein JI et al: Pathologic and clinical findings to predict tumor extent of nonpalpable (stage T_{1c}) prostate cancer, *JAMA* 271:368, 1994.

41. Walsh PC: Why make an early diagnosis of prostate cancer? *J Urol* 147:853, 1992.

42. Simpson KN, Brown RE: Cost effectiveness of adding prostate specific antigen (PSA) test to digital rectal examination (DRE) for early detection of prostate cancer, *J Urol* 149:413A, 1993 (abstract).

43. Littrup PJ, Goodman AC, Mettlin CJ: The benefit and cost of prostate cancer early detection: the investigators of the American Cancer Society–National Prostate Cancer Detection Project, *CA Cancer J Clin* 43:134, 1993.

LUNG CANCER

Henry Wagner, Jr.
John C. Ruckdeschel

> *If discoursing on a difficult problem were like carrying weights, when many horses can carry more sacks of grain than a single horse, I would agree that many discourses would do more than a single one; but discoursing is like coursing, not like carrying, and one Barbary courser can go faster than a hundred Frieslands.*
>
> Galileo Galelei: The tester. Cited by Calvino I: *Six memos for the next millennium*, New York, 1993, Vintage.

Lung cancer kills one person in the United States every five minutes.[1] It is the most frequent cause of cancer death in both men and women. The grim toll exacted by this disease has increased during the past decade despite dramatic progress in our understanding of the molecular mechanisms that underlie its development and progression and modest but demonstrable progress in its treatment. Although the incidence of lung cancer appears to have decreased in white males, it continues to rise in nonwhite males and in females.

> *Although it has been plainly evident for several decades that the vast majority (about 90%) of cases of lung cancer are caused by cigarette smoking and that the most effective means of controlling lung cancer is prevention and reduction of tobacco use, such strategies have been of only modest success to date.[2-10]*

Furthermore, smokers who quit remain at an increased though gradually declining risk of lung cancer over at least the next decade.[11-15] For those individuals who have wisely become former smokers, early detection and treatment of the cancers that they may still develop remain the best hope of further reducing their risk of death from lung cancer.

The unsatisfactory results of treating clinically advanced disease have motivated clinicians and epidemiologists to explore several strategies for the diagnosis and treatment of lung cancer at an earlier time in its development. These may be divided into three themes:

- Early detection programs for the evaluation of patients presenting with ambiguous symptoms.
- True screening programs for the evaluation of asymptomatic individuals felt to be at high risk for lung cancer.
- Early intervention strategies aimed at stopping or reversing the processes involved in lung carcinogenesis before the development of invasive malignancy.

Because lung cancer usually develops in individuals with a history of current or past cigarette smoking, many of whom have respiratory symptoms such as shortness of breath or chronic cough, the distinction between screening and early detection is easily blurred. Individuals presenting for screening programs may in fact have been motivated by subtle changes in their baseline cough or sputum production (or by a family member's prodding that such a change has occurred), and may thus not truly represent the larger population of smokers and ex-smokers from whom they are drawn. The inclusion of such individuals tends to increase the apparent yield of screening programs while underestimating the difficulties of obtaining participation in such programs by individuals who are truly either asymptomatic or with stable chronic symptoms.

PRESENTATION, STAGING, AND TREATMENT OUTCOME

In the United States data from several large state tumor registries as well as the experience of large cancer centers give a good picture of current lung cancer occurrence and treatment.[16] Table 6-1 shows the distribution by stage of 170,000 cases of lung cancer diagnosed in 1993.[17] Although a small but growing proportion of patients with stage III disease (a favorable subset with minimal weight loss and good performance status) may be cured by aggressive multimodality therapy, including both local and systemic components, only those patients with stage I or II disease are classically considered to have resectable cancer with a high probability of cure (Table 6-2). T_3N_0 and N_1 disease, although grouped in stage IIIA, has a more favorable prognosis than $T_{1-3}N_2$ disease and should be considered separately from the rest of stage IIIA.

> *Considering as truly early presentations only those patients with T_1N_0 disease, about 75% of patients with lung cancer currently present with more advanced disease.*

The use of the word *early* to describe radiographically detectable lung cancer is somewhat of an oxymoron.

TABLE 6-1

STAGE DISTRIBUTION OF LUNG CANCER AT PRESENTATION

Stage and clinical operability group	Cases per year (United States)
T_1N_0	19,600
T_1N_1, T_2N_0, T_2N_1	25,900
IIIA resectable	10,500
IIIA partially resectable	7000
IIIB nonresectable	7000
IV	100,000
TOTAL	170,000

From Holmes EC: *Adv Oncol* 9:15, 1993.

TABLE 6-2

FIVE-YEAR SURVIVAL FOR CLINICAL AND SURGICAL TNM SUBSETS

TNM subset	Clinical			Surgical		
	Number	Percentage surviving	Median survival (months)	Number	Percentage surviving	Median survival (months)
$T_1\ N_0\ M_0$	591	61.9	60+	429	68.5	60+
$T_2\ N_0\ M_0$	1012	35.8	26	436	59.0	60+
$T_1\ N_1\ M_0$	19	33.6	20	67	54.1	60+
$T_2\ N_1\ M_0$	176	22.7	17	250	40.0	29
$T_3\ N_0\ M_0$	221	7.6	8	57	44.2	26
$T_3\ N_1\ M_0$	71	7.7	8	29	17.6	16
Any $N_2\ M_0$	497	4.9	11	168	28.8	22
Any M_1	1166	1.7	6	—	—	—
TOTAL	3753			1436		

From Mountain CF: *Chest* 89(suppl):225S-233S, 1986.

To be detectable on routine chest x-ray, in the favorable circumstance of a peripheral nodule that does not overlie shadows of rib or mediastinal structures, a lesion has to be about 1 cm in size. Such a mass typically contains 10^9 tumor cells, representing about 30 doublings under an ideal condition of no cell loss.

Such conditions never occur in human tumors, and a comparison of actual and potential doubling times would suggest that cell loss factors in the range of 80% to 90% are not uncommon.[18] At this point the "early" tumor has undergone most of its life span, both chronologically and in terms of number of doublings (although the number of cells undergoing division is now greater). This long preclinical history for even the smallest radiographically detectable tumors gives ample opportunity for the mutational appearance and clonal selection of phenotypes with diverse cell surface antigen expression; resistance to xenobiotics by mechanisms such as active transport out of the cell mediated by p170, MRP, and other transporter systems; amplification of DNA coding for target enzymes such as dihydrofolate reductase (DHFR)[19]; and other mechanisms that confer resistance to a variety of treatment modalities.[20-21]

The TNM staging system, although reasonably applicable to patients with non–small cell lung cancer (NSCLC), is not generally used for patients with small cell lung cancer (SCLC). At the time of the most recent revision of the staging system, the importance of local control in achieving long-term survival in SCLC was not so well recognized as it is now. With the exception of the patient presenting with an incidental peripheral nodule and negative surgical exploration of the hilar and mediastinal nodes, all patients with SCLC should be considered to have systemic disease at time of presentation. The distinction between limited and extensive disease then collapses to a comment on the sensitivity of the imaging and other technology used to search for it. For example, with computed tomography (CT) and magnetic resonance imaging (MRI) of the abdomen and brain there is far less limited disease now than in the era of radionuclide imaging of these sites, and with use of monoclonal antibody or polymerase chain reaction (PCR) evaluation of bone marrow biopsies there should be even less in the future. In this disease, as well as other malignancies, these changes in stage distribution based on increasing sensitivity of staging techniques must be factored in when we report apparent progress in treatment of subsets of patients based on stage grouping over time. At least a portion of the difference may simply be due to the "Will Rogers effect" brought about by this shift in stage classification.[22]

Shifts of stage distribution brought about by increased sensitivity for early diagnosis, although introducing other potential complications of survival analysis from lead

> *time bias and length biased sampling,[23-25] should not be confused with the shifts in staging classification.*

In the case of changes in diagnostic sensitivity, clinicians are intervening in the disease process at an earlier time, which may result in either a real therapeutic gain if effective therapies are available (such as treating disease before it has metastasized when tumor burden is small or before the tumor has developed drug resistance mechanisms) or an apparent one from the lead time gained in time from diagnosis to time of death. In contrast, by shifting patients from one stage to another by the use of more sensitive imaging techniques for staging but not changing the time of initial diagnosis, we are simply counting up the survival data of the same group of patients in a different manner.

Table 6-2 summarizes treatment outcome (in terms of 5-year survival) by stage for NSCLC. These figures are taken from the clinical database on which the new international staging system was based and are reasonably representative of what can be obtained with good standards of practice in staging and treatment.[26] They do not reflect the modest but real improvements in median and long-term survival now being reported for the use of adjuvant chemotherapy in combination with either surgical resection or definitive radiation therapy for locally advanced (predominantly stages IIIA and IIIB) disease.[21,27-29]

> *In selected series with meticulous surgical staging of the mediastinum, the survival for patients with $T_1N_0M_0$ disease is higher, up to 80% in the series of the Lung Cancer Study Group.[30] This rather encouraging figure is in contrast to the widespread perception of lung cancer as a dismal and untreatable disease.*

Survival for patients with $T_1N_0M_0$ lung cancer is comparable to that of those with $T_1M_0N_0$ breast cancer. The problem, and the reality behind the impression of untreatability, is that only a small percentage of patients with lung cancer are detected at this stage. Once regional nodal metastases have developed or have become detectable histologically the survival percentages decrease. It would thus seem a reasonable hypothesis that a procedure or set of procedures which could detect patients with lung cancer before the development of nodal metastases would significantly improve survival. It also appears that patients with lung cancer by and large will have a recurrence within the first 3 years after diagnosis if they are going to relapse. True late failures, defined as occurring after 5 or more years of disease-free survival after apparently successful treatment, as seen in adenocarcinomas of the breast and prostate, are quite uncommon in lung cancer. Second primary neoplasms of the lung, esophagus, and head and neck sites are a problem, however, and in aggregate have an incidence of about 2% to 3% per year.[31-34] Thus the impact of screening and early detection programs ought to be demonstrable with relatively modest durations of follow-up, unlike the situation in cancers of breast and prostate, whose more indolent disease course mandates longer follow-up to determine effects on survival.

CAUSATION AND EPIDEMIOLOGY

Less than a century ago lung cancer was a rare disease. The current worldwide epidemic of lung cancer, with over 2 million deaths estimated for the year 2000, is the direct result of aggressive marketing of addictive tobacco products, primarily cigarettes.[35,36] Although an effective strategy for lung cancer treatment and control includes a broad spectrum of activities, including research on palliative treatment of advanced disease, curative treatment of earlier but overt disease, early detection of preclinical disease, and secondary chemoprevention, it is inarguable that the greatest long-term reduction in lung cancer mortality will come from a decrease in the number of individuals who smoke.

In the United States lung cancer is most commonly diagnosed in the seventh decade.[37-39] Past studies have considered lung cancer predominantly a disease of males; the three large prospective trials of radiographic and cytologic screening conducted in the United States were limited to male smokers. However, with the increase in cigarette smoking by women starting in the 1940s, this situation has changed dramatically. Deaths from lung cancer overtook those of breast cancer for U.S. women in the 1980s.[16]

> *Although present smoking behavior in the United States has shown a decline in smoking prevalence among white males, smoking has continued to increase among women, and recent data have suggested a disturbing leveling off or even reversal in the tendency to decreased smoking in young women.[10,40-43]*

The advertising of cigarettes by youth-oriented cartoon animals, associating them with sporting events or teams (such as the Virginia Slims women's tennis tournament), circumventing bans on advertising by sponsoring such events and plastering product logos on the stadium or racing cars, as well as intentionally manipulating nicotine levels in cigarettes to optimize addictive potential should be held directly responsible (and liable) for most of this increase.[9,36]

At present about 25% of the adult population of the United States smokes, and an additional 40 to 50 million are former smokers.[15] It has been recognized for some time that the relative risk of developing lung cancer in former smokers declines with time after cessation.[13,14,44] The absolute risk may plateau or even rise as previously undetected lung cancers become clinically manifest. Recent analysis of data from the American Cancer Society Cancer Prevention Study II has quantified the extent of this change and demonstrated clearly that, though the risk of subsequent development of lung cancer declines regardless of the age of smoking cessation, the greatest gains are seen for those quitting at an earlier age, and that this difference is significant even when correcting for the number of years smoked.[15] This time-dependent reduction in risk was seen for both men and women.

BIOLOGY

Although it is common to refer to lung cancer as a single diagnostic entity, the lung is anatomically and physiologically at least three separate organs. The trachea and main bronchi are normally lined by squamous epithelium and also contain neuroendocrine cells. The predominant types of tumor seen in the large central airways are squamous cell carcinoma and small cell carcinoma. As one proceeds distally, there is a transition to adenomatous lining cells in intermediate bronchi and bronchioles with papillary cells characteristically present in the terminal alveoli. The predominant histology seen in peripherally arising lung cancers is adenocarcinoma, which morphologically can be divided into solid and bronchoalveolar types. At the cellular level these tumors arise from Type II pneumocytes, which normally produce surfactant. The bronchoalveolar carcinomas are believed to arise from Clara cells, which are involved in xenobiotic metabolism. Each of these cell types has associated characteristic differentiation markers that may form the basis for both detection and therapeutic strategies (Table 6-3).

In addition to these three classic histologic types of squamous cell, adenocarcinoma, and small cell carcinoma, about one fifth of lung carcinomas are large cell undifferentiated tumors that cannot be assigned to one of the above lineages. All of these histologic types can be found admixed within a single tumor, consistent with a model of their development from a common stem cell of variable differentiation potential. The usual anatomic distribution of the different tumor histologies may derive from the normal distribution of partially committed cell lineages, from variable penetration of different components of cigarette smoke to different regions of the lung, and from possible differences in local metabolic transformation of procarcinogens and effects of the extracellular matrix and paracrine growth factors on carcinogenesis.[45]

These distributions of normal cell and tumor types are typical rather than absolute. Lung cancers of all cell types may be found in any location in the tra-

---

TABLE 6-3

MARKERS OF LUNG CANCER DIFFERENTIATION

Neuroendocrine	Squamous	Adenomatous
Chromogranin A	Cytokeratin	Clara 10-kd protein
Leu 7	Involucrin	Surfactant-associated protein
Neuron-specific enolase	Epidermal growth factor receptor	Carcinoembryonic antigen
Dopa-decarboxylase		*ras* Oncogene
	Transglutaminase	

From Mulshine JR et al: *J Cell Biochem Suppl* 16G:183, 1992.

cheobronchial tree and lung. This classification implies that, though there may be some very early events common to the development of all types of lung cancer, further preneoplastic and neoplastic development can follow along several divergent lines, and screening strategies should be able to detect each of these. The observation that there has been a shift in the proportion of lung cancers of the various histologic types over the past several decades, with the predominant cell type changing from squamous cell to adenocarcinoma, should be accounted for in a proper theory of lung cancer initiation and promotion.[46]

In considering the various genetic and phenotypic differences between normal and malignant lung tissue, it is helpful to keep several questions in mind[47]:

- Which genetic events are causative and which bystander?
- Is there an obligate sequence of genetic events (i.e. early vs. late events), or is the cumulative mutational burden the relevant causative factor?
- If there is a required or usual sequence, can early events be used as early detection markers?
- Are some later events (such as *mdr* amplification, *ras* activation) prognostic markers independent of stage and histology?
- Can an understanding of early events lead to chemoprevention strategies?

GENETIC CHANGES

Early cytogenetic analysis of lung cancer cell lines as well as fresh tumor specimens showed that chromosome abnormalities are frequent and that certain nonrandom losses of genetic material are recurring themes.[48,49] Over ensuing decades these lesions have come closer to molecular delineation, as tumor suppressor genes that map to the characteristic chromosome deletions as well as point mutations not readily detectable by cytogenetic analysis and activating mutations of oncogenes are described. Although a number of specific lesions have come to be well characterized in both SCLC and NSCLC, the sequence of their mutation in the carcinogenic process, as well as the need for any specific mutation, is somewhat less well defined at present for lung cancer than for cancer of the colon.[50-52]

Tumor Suppressor Genes

Rb Gene

Abnormalities in the retinoblastoma tumor suppressor gene (Rb), which is located at 13q14, are common in lung cancer. Analysis of mRNA transcripts has shown loss of expression in about 60% of SCLC and 10% of NSCLC. About 75% of the SCLC lines expressing gene product produce an abnormal protein. The normal Rb gene product undergoes cycles of phosphorylation and dephosphorylation during the cell cycle, and in the dephosphorylated state binds to and inactivates the E2F transcription factor. Recent studies have shown that Rb also can interact with some mammalian D-type cyclins (D2 and D3 but not D1) and may normally function to restrain cells from premature progression through G1.[53-56] Cyclin D2 could phosphorylate Rb and thus abrogate its inactivation of E2F.

> *Although Rb inactivation is one of the most common genetic changes seen in human lung cancer, the time at which it occurs in carcinogenesis is unknown at present.*

Recent studies in SCLC lines with multiple genetic alterations have shown that reversal of Rb inactivation markedly reduces their growth in agar and tumorigenicity in mice.[57] Rb mutations specific for lung cancer are not well characterized, and the large size of the Rb gene and its product also complicate its genetic analysis and use in screening.

p53

The role of the p53 gene product has been a matter of considerable uncertainty and confusion over the past decade.[58-60] For some time p53 was thought to be an activating oncogene because transfection of cells with p53 in cooperation with another mutated protooncogene such as *ras* could lead to transformation.

> *Recent analysis has shown that wild type p53 functions as a cell cycle regulator and will normally delay replication in the face of unrepaired DNA damage.*

Loss of normal p53 function is common in human tumors, one of the most commonly described genetic changes, and this loss may arise through inactivation of both alleles or by the production of a dominant negative mutant in one.

Like the Rb protein, p53 can complex with and inactivate the SV40 large T protein and transforming proteins of other DNA viruses. Recent data suggest that p53 can also complex with endogenous transcription factors and alter their binding to promoter sites.[56,61]

The normal cellular function of p53 remains tantalizingly obscure. Somewhat unexpectedly, p53 "knockout" mice are viable, grow to maturity, and are fertile. They do, however, have a high incidence of tumors later in life. Thus p53 clearly is not required for normal development (although its functions may be, and may be provided redundantly by other genes in these mice). The high incidence of tumors in these animals parallels the observation that individuals with the Li-Fraumeni syndrome, who have a high incidence of tumors (usually involving breast, brain, and soft tissue sarcoma, leukemia, and adrenocortical carcinoma) can often be shown to have germ-line p53 mutations.

> *One key role of the p53 gene product is in apoptosis. The elimination of normal p53 function in mice prevents their thymocytes from undergoing their usual apoptotic response to ionizing radiation.*

They can, however, undergo apparently normal apoptosis in response to glucocorticoids.[62,63] Because a number of commonly used chemotherapeutic agents, as well as ionizing radiation, produce apoptosis-mediated cell death, mutational loss of p53 function may represent both a marker of carcinogenesis and a prognostic factor–predicting response to therapy. Current clinical data on this point are controversial.

Mutations in p53 are common in both NSCLC and SCLC. The percentages reported have varied considerably in different series, in large part because of methodologic differences. The tissue half-life of many mutant p53s is considerably longer than that of the normal protein, so many studies have used tissue detection of p53 gene product by immunohistochemical staining as an indication of p53 mutation. However, such an assumption will miss some p53 mutations that lead to complete lack of gene product, a functionally abnormal gene product with a normal half-life, or production of a functional gene product that is sufficiently changed in structure to be no longer recognized by the antibodies used for detection. False positive results could be obtained in situations in which normal p53 is produced in high amounts in proper response to DNA damage that has been produced, and allowed to persist, through other mechanisms.

Both p53 and Rb are involved in regulation of the cell cycles through their effects on the activity of E2F transcription factors. Rb blocks the activity of the E2F transcription factors when it is hypophosphorylated. The phosphorylation state of Rb normally is under the control of the cyclin-dependent kinase (CDK) system. In response to damage to the genome (through sensing and effector mechanisms not fully elucidated), p53 accumulates in an active form and acts as a transcription factor to induce expression of p21, an inhibitor of CDK. This inhibition results in the failure of Rb to become hyperphosphorylated, and thus remaining in its hypophosphorylated state, it remains bound to the E2F factors, inhibiting them and preventing the cell from crossing the G1/S transition.[56]

9p Deletions

The p16 gene located on 9p21 is associated with familial melanoma.[64] Deletions in this region are also seen in about one third of cell lines derived from both SCLC and NSCLC, with the deletions involving the regions coding for the interferon gene complex.[65] The prevalence of such deletions in intact tumor, as opposed to cell lines, is not known.

3p Deletions

Visible loss of chromatin bands from chromosome 3 was identified as a common genetic abnormality in lung cancer, and subsequent investigations using more sensitive techniques such as restriction fragment polymorphism analysis have identified changes in this region, with resultant loss of heterozygosity

(LOH), in almost all cases of SCLC and about 50% of NSCLC.[48,66,67] Although a number of genes of known biologic activity, including the retinoic acid receptor β, are present in the regions commonly deleted, none has to date been identified as a tumor suppressor.

Several other tumor suppressor genes and oncogenes are under investigation in lung cancer. The *MCC* and *APC* genes located on the long arm of chromosome 5 have had their roles in colorectal carcinogenesis lucidly delineated by Vogelstein and his colleagues.[68,69] The roles of these genes in lung cancer are less clear, with two groups recently reporting LOH in 23 of 76 cases (30%) or 3 of 26 cases (11.5%).[68,69]

In the majority of cases studied, inactivation of the tumor suppressor gene system occurs through the loss of one allele by deletion at a germ line level and functional inactivation of the other via a point mutation, which leads to loss of function. In some cases, however, a single mutation can lead to a dominant negative phenotype. One mechanism by which this may occur involves the production of an abnormal subunit for an enzyme that is polymeric in its active form. Through formation of inactive polymers, the inactive subunit can produce a substantial loss of enzymatic activity. In situations where polymers containing the mutant monomer are inactive but very stable, other monomers are either trapped in inactive complexes or rapidly degraded and may result in near total loss of function.

Dominant Oncogene Mutations

ras *Gene Family*

The *ras* oncogene was first identified as a transforming gene in virally induced rat sarcomas. The Harvey and Kirsten sarcoma viruses were identified as containing highly homologous genes (v-H- *ras* and v-K-*ras*) and soon afterward their counterparts were identified in normal cells (H-*ras*-1, K-*ras*-2, N-*ras*).[70,71] The *ras* gene product has been identified as a 21-kd polypeptide with marked structural homology to the G proteins involved in transmembrane signal coupling between membrane receptors and intracellular protein kinases.

In their normal function these proteins bind and hydrolyze guanosine triphosphate (GTP). When activated by binding of ligand to an associated receptor, a conformational change in the G protein activates both downstream signaling through *raf* kinase, phosphatidylinosotol-3-OH kinase, neurofibromin, and other not yet characterized pathways. This signaling appears to be mediated via direct interaction with a stretch of amino acids in the *ras* protein (residues 32 to 40) known as the effector region and does not appear to involve either kinase or phosphatase action by *ras,* which appears instead to play a role in the membrane localization of these downstream effector proteins. Inactivation of the active conformation of *ras* is modulated by several GTPase-activating proteins (GAPs), which promote GTP hydrolysis by *ras.* With the cleavage of GTP to guanosine diphosphatase (GDP) the *ras* protein reverts to the inactive conformation, and the cycle is completed.[72-74] Transforming *ras* genes are mutated in one of several specific positions (codons 12 and 59 in the viral genes, codons 12, 13, or 61 in spontaneous human tumors), which leads to a change in the *ras* protein conformation such that it can bind but no longer hydrolyze bound GTP and is thus always in the activated signaling state.[75] There are differences in the patterns of nucleotide substitution at these sites for tumors arising in different anatomic sites, suggesting differences in the mutagens involved in the lung and the GI tract.[50]

> *Mutations of ras occur commonly in several types of human tumors, including adenocarcinomas of the colon, pancreas, and lung. In lung adenocarcinomas they are found in about one third of cases and are highly associated with present or past cigarette smoking.[76,77]*

Although most commonly seen in adenocarcinomas, *ras* mutations have been reported in large cell and squamous cell carcinomas of the lung (both of native tumor specimens and cell lines) but are rare in small cell carcinoma.[78-81] By themselves, *ras* mutations appear insufficient to transform cell lines to a fully malignant state and require cooperation with other oncogenes such as *myc*.[82,83] The presence of mutationally activated *ras*, however, appears to be a poor prognostic factor in patients with either metastatic or resectable NSCLC.[84,85]

myc

The *myc* gene product is a nuclear phosphoprotein. It has been tentatively identified as a transcription factor through sequence homology to known transcription factors, although details of its role remain unclear. Three related genes have been identified: c-*myc*, N-*myc*, and L-*myc*, which in humans map to different chromosomes.[86]

Structural variants of *myc* have not been described in human lung cancer, but *myc* amplification and overexpression are reported in a number of human malignancies with neuroendocrine features, including neuroblastoma, retinoblastoma, and SCLC. Amplification of *myc* is particularly common in the intermediate or variant type of SCLC, which clinically is characterized by greater radiation and drug resistance than classic SCLC.[87-95]

Review of several studies of the frequency of *myc* overexpression or amplification indicates that these changes appear more common in cell lines than in fresh tumor specimens and in material taken from patients in relapse than in at time of initial diagnosis. This would suggest that *myc* amplification generally occurs late in the development of malignancy and may not be a particularly useful early marker. In cell lines that have amplification of *myc* (which is usually extrachromosomal), treatment with hydroxyurea has been shown to eliminate these extra gene copies and restore a less virulent phenotype to the cell line.[19] Such strategies suggest that, even if the detection of *myc* amplification and overexpression is not useful as screening, its modulation may have therapeutic benefit.

HER2/neu Gene

The HER2/neu protooncogene codes for a protein with sequence homologies to other tyrosine kinase growth factor receptors. It has been found to be overexpressed in about 30% of NSCLC, primarily adenocarcinomas. Such overexpression correlates with a poorer prognosis.[96-98] In adenocarcinoma of the breast, such HER2/neu overexpression not only heralds a poor outcome, but also identifies a subgroup of patients who benefit from dose-intense adjuvant chemotherapy.

Genetic Changes in Preinvasive Lesions

The previous sections have discussed genetic changes characterized in clearly malignant invasive tumors. Since such lesions do not arise in a single step from normal epithelium, but rather by the accumulation of multiple mutations in the context of a process of field carcinogenesis, it is reasonable to suspect that some of these genetic changes are found in other respiratory epithelium that is either morphologically normal or shows atypia short of frank malignancy.[99] Several recent studies[100] have convincingly demonstrated that such is indeed the case. Hyperplastic and dysplastic changes as well as aneuploidy are seen widely in the respiratory tract in patients with lung cancer of all histologies.

> *Sunderasan et al.[101] have shown that p53 mutations and deletions in 3p can be detected in preinvasive lesions of the bronchus adjacent to invasive cancer, and Rusch et al.[102] have made similar observations for the epidermoid growth factor receptor.*

A similar pattern is emerging for patients with squamous carcinoma and adenocarcinoma of the esophagus. The frankly malignant lesion arises from the midst of an epithelium with a diversity of molecular lesions, including mutations in *ras* and p53.[103,104]

Use of Molecular Markers in Screening

The polymerase chain reaction (PCR) allows detection of very small amounts of specific DNA sequences in the presence of a large excess of DNA lacking such sequences. It can be both highly sensitive, detecting one abnormal cell in a background of 10^6 normal cells, and highly specific, with some control over such stringency by the conditions used for hybridization. PCR forms a part of a core technology that may be able to revolutionize screening at a molecular level.

For such an approach an ideal marker genetic change should appear early in the carcinogenic process yet be specific for malignancy, or at least a high likelihood of subsequent malignant development. (See discussion concerning screening for cancer versus screening for carcinogenesis.) It should be detectable in body tissues that are easily and repeatedly obtainable by relatively noninvasive and inexpensive procedures, such as exfoliated cells or peripheral blood versus tissue obtained by bronchoscopic biopsies. The genetic change should be one readily detectable by automated or semiautomated methods, and structural changes in coding regions of the sequence may well be better targets than changes that alter gene regulation. Finally, situations in which a limited number of genetic changes account for the majority of tumors (the Pareto principle at a molecular level) are appealing because they limit the number of mutant sequences that have to be screened for.

For the above reasons genetic changes in *ras* have been an appealing target. As noted above, mutational activation of *ras,* which occurs in about 30% of lung adenocarcinomas as well as in high frequencies in adenocarcinomas of the bowel and pancreas, almost always involves point mutation at codons 12, 13, or 61.

Sidranski et al.[105] first demonstrated that *ras* mutations could be identified in exfoliated cells present in the stool of patients with resectable and potentially curable colon cancer. Subsequently Tobi et al.[106] were able to detect *ras* mutations at codon 12 in exfoliated colonic mucosa in 40% of clinically normal individuals at high risk for developing colorectal cancer because of strong family history or a personal history of adenomas. Others have reported detection of mutant *ras* in gastric aspirates and stool specimens of patients with pancreatic cancer.[107,108]

Several recent reports extend these data to lung cancer.

Kelly et al.[109] have demonstrated the feasibility of detecting ras mutations in cells obtained by sputum cytology in patients with known lung cancer, and Mills et al.[110] have made similar observations using cells from bronchoalveolar lavage fluid.

In an extension of this methodology to patients without diagnosed malignancy but at risk, Mao et al.[111] examined sputa that had been obtained during the Johns Hopkins Lung Project with a percentage of patients having gone on to develop adenocarcinoma. Of 15 patients so identified, analysis of the resected tumor specimen showed mutated *ras* or p53 in 10. In eight of these 10 the same mutation could be demonstrated in sputum samples that had been obtained at least 1 year before clinical diagnosis.

Sorenson et al.[112] have taken advantage of the fact that healthy individuals as well as those with cancer have small amounts of soluble DNA fragments in their circulation by developing a PCR assay to look for *ras* mutations (codon 12) in patients with lung cancer. They have reported preliminary findings indicating the feasibility of such detection in patients with known lung cancer and are extending the methodology to look at high-risk individuals.

These are all preliminary studies of limited numbers of patients, and most have used detection of *ras* mutations that are present in only about 30% of lung cancers. Substantial technical issues remain to be resolved before they can be more widely implemented.[113-115] There is little reason to doubt, however, that these or similar tests will be available on the internist's lab order sheet in the near future. There will arise substantial questions as to their interpretation, and initial caution is in order.[116] As noted above, these genetic changes are seen in both invasive tumors and preneoplastic epithelium.

HISTORICAL SCREENING STUDIES—NONRANDOMIZED

In the 1950s several nonrandomized trials of screening for lung cancer were conducted in the United States and Europe. A number of these were founded on large population-based tuberculosis screening programs. The trials done in Philadelphia[117] and London[118,119] all used chest photofluorograms obtained at 6-month intervals. These studies found that about half the cancers detected in these populations were found by the screening examinations, the remainder being identified on interval chest radiographs obtained for evaluation of symptoms. Although the resectability rate of the cases detected on the screening examinations was about 30%, the overall resectability for all cases was only 20%, which did not appear different from historical results in unscreened patients.

In an attempt to clarify some of the questions raised by these nonrandomized studies, the National Cancer Institute sponsored lung cancer screening trials that were conducted in the 1970s in three institutions: Johns Hopkins University Lung Project (JHLP), Mayo Clinic Lung Project (MLP), and Memorial-Sloan Kettering Cancer Center Lung Project (MSKLP).[120-122] In addition to these three U.S. studies, a randomized trial has been conducted in Czechoslovakia.[123] There are also several recent carefully conducted case-control studies from Europe and Japan. The individual trials differed somewhat in their design (Table 6-4).

Both the JHLP and the MSKLP trials were designed to evaluate the incremental benefit of adding sputum examination to chest x-ray. Patients in the control group were offered annual chest x-ray, whereas those in the screening group were offered both sputum cytology and chest x-ray every 4 months. Thus the

---

TABLE 6-4

PROSPECTIVE TRIALS OF SCREENING FOR LUNG CANCER

Study	No.	Eligibility	Group	Cases detected	Mortality
MLP	10,933	Male smokers	Prevention	91	n/a
	4618	Over 45 years old	Screen	206	3.2
	4593		Control	160	3.0
JHLP	5226	Male smokers	Screen	194	3.4
	5161	Over 45 years old	Control	202	3.8
MSKLP	5072	Male smokers	Screen	144	2.7
	4968	Over 45 years old	Control	144	2.7
Czechoslovakia	6364	Male smokers	Prevention	19	n/a
	3172	Over 40 years old	Screen	108	3.6
	3174		Control	82	2.6

MLP, Mayo Clinic Lung Project; *JHLP,* Johns Hopkins University Lung Project; *MSKLP,* Memorial-Sloan Kettering Cancer Center Lung Project

comparison is between the different frequencies of screening chest x-ray with or without sputum examination.

Of the U.S. studies, only the MLP trial was designed to compare a policy of intensive dual screening with both chest x-ray and sputum cytology examinations every 4 months to unscreened management. The unscreened group, however, was advised to obtain annual chest x-ray and sputum cytology as part of routine medical care, but patients were not reminded to comply with this initial recommendation. Thus this study can be seen as comparing two different frequencies of recommended screening and compliance.

The outcomes of these studies have been presented in several formats, as results of the initial prevalence examinations in the cohorts to be screened, the follow-up of the patients detected during the screening period, and overall pooled results of the three trials. The general observations and conclusions of the three trials are clear, but their interpretation has been somewhat controversial. In summarizing a discussion by the presenters of the results of these three trials, the chairman noted that they were in broad agreement with the following:

> *"Within the trials there was no advantage in terms of mortality reduction to the group offered intensive screening in the Mayo study, with 4 monthly sputum cytology and chest radiology, while in the Johns Hopkins and Memorial Sloan-Kettering studies, there was no advantage to the group that received sputum cytology in addition to annual chest x-ray examinations."[124] The trials as designed did not, however, address or resolve the question of whether any pattern of surveillance chest x-ray was better for high-risk populations than a policy of obtaining such studies only when patients presented with symptoms.*

In the discussion accompanying the presentation of the results of these trials at the Fourth World Conference on Lung Cancer in 1986, it was clear that strong and divergent opinions remained on this point.

Taken together, the three studies that comprise the National Cancer Institute collaborative trial led to the following conclusion:

> *Although the screening approaches available at that time could lead to the detection of presymptomatic lung cancer, particularly squamous cell carcinoma, at an earlier stage than in the control group, with resultant higher*

> *rates of resectability and survival for the cases in the screened group as compared with the cases in the control group, the overall survival for the screened population was not superior to that of the controls.*

This led to adoption of policies discouraging routine chest x-ray and sputum screening, and these tests were dropped from the recommendations of the American Cancer Society. These interpretations and actions led, in many circles, to an unwarranted nihilism regarding all aspects of lung cancer detection and treatment from which clinical practice is only now starting to emerge.

It must be noted that none of the U.S. randomized trials actually compared a policy of screening versus no intervention in the absence of symptoms. The trial that most closely approached this design was the Czechoslovak one in which all enrolled men underwent an initial prevalence examination, following which the control group had no other planned intervention for 3 years. Screened individuals had chest x-ray and cytology every 6 months. In the initial 3 years of the study 36 lung cancers were detected in the study group versus 19 in the controls, and survival of these patients with lung cancer was superior in the intervention group than for the controls. But the overall death rate from lung cancer was greater, although not significantly (28 versus 18 cases), in the study group ($P = .18$). At 3 years, chest x-ray and sputum cytology were performed for both groups, with annual chest x-ray afterward. At 6 years, follow-up mortality was the same for the two groups.

To a large degree the issues and populations studied in these trials, which were designed in the late 1960s and conducted in the early 1970s, are not entirely pertinent for the mid-1990s. The screened populations were all male, most still smoking, and often with other tobacco-related illnesses that led to a high frequency of interval chest x-rays in addition to the screening examinations that were performed.

> *The present situation for screening is more likely to be a man or woman in the 40s or 50s, a former smoker with a history of 15 to 25 pack-years, and often without significant acute illnesses requiring close medical attention.*

In addition to this shift in demographics, there has also been a change in the dominant histology of newly diagnosed lung cancer. During the period of the U.S. collaborative trial the majority of cases in both the screened and unscreened groups were squamous cell carcinoma, and the predominance of this histology was noted in settings that varied from the baseline prevalence studies to the distribution of patients presenting with symptomatic unresectable disease.[122,125-127] In the past decade this pattern has clearly changed, for unclear reasons, to one in which adenocarcinoma is the predominant histology in trials of patients with both unresectable and resectable disease. Adenocarcinomas of the lung have, in the past, been more common in women, but they have now become the predominant histology for both sexes in the United States.[46,128,129] European series continue to report higher incidences of squamous cell carcinoma, and the reasons for these differences, possibly related to differences in the particulate size of inhaled carcinogens as well as genetic differences in susceptibility to carcinogenic processes in the different regions of the lung, remain poorly understood. This is the population in which screening is likely to be of benefit.

TUMOR MARKERS

Various substances elaborated by tumor cells or by the host reaction to them have been proposed over the years to be tumor markers that might be used either to screen for malignancy or follow its course under treatment. With the exception of α-fetoprotein or β-human chorionic gonadotropin (HCG) in nonseminomatous germ cell tumors or β-HCG in choriocarcinoma, most proposed tumor markers have either lacked specificity or have not become elevated early enough in the course of tumor development to be clinically useful. Controversy over the proper use of prostate-specific antigen screening in a disease with a very variable virulence and natural history, and in which many affected individuals will die with, rather than of, prostate cancer, also points out the need to link diagnostic and therapeutic strategies; early diagnosis without effective or appropriate treatment is not necessarily beneficial. For lung cancer, without evidence that nonintervention is clinically useful, early detection should clearly imply early treatment.

In lung cancer several tumor markers have been proposed either to follow disease status or for screening. Both carcinoembryonic antigen (CEA) and neuron-specific enolase (NSE) are commonly elevated in lung cancer (the former in all histologies, the latter primarily in SCLC) but have not been reliably elevated in patients with minimal disease to allow for early detection either de novo or of relapse in patients who have undergone surgical resection or had complete response to chemotherapy.[130]

Newer approaches to the development of serum techniques for early tumor detection have focused on detection of growth factors produced by tumors. Most small cell carcinomas and about 15% of non–small-cell carcinomas are under autocrine growth stimulation mediated by gastrin-releasing peptide (GRP). Early studies that attempted to use this as a marker were not particularly successful, in part due to its very short serum half-life. If assays are performed for its prohormone (Pro-GRP), which has a longer half-life, much better specificity and detectability have been reported.[131] The ratio of Pro-GRP/GRP in tumor tissue is 1.2:1 but it is 76:1 in blood. An enzyme-linked immunoassay has been developed for Pro-GRP that takes 2 hours, costs $5, and can detect basal Pro-GRP levels in normal subjects. Using a cutoff of 40 pg/ml, investigators reported elevations in 0.5% of normal controls, 0.8% of nonmalignant pulmonary disease, 67% of patients with SCLC, with similar results for pure and mixed histologies.

Whether this test will show sufficient specificity and sensitivity for screening remains to be determined. Initial mass screening studies in Japan have reported a detection rate of about 0.04%. Aguayo[132] reported that bronchial washing and urine Pro-GRP levels are elevated in smokers, but serum levels are not.

IDENTIFICATION OF HIGH-RISK GROUPS

If screening tests were developed that had no cost and absolute specificity, there would be little need to consider limiting them to high-risk populations. A high true negative rate would be both expected and acceptable and, with absolute specificity, there would be no problem with false positive results. These conditions are not met by any present tests nor are they likely to be met in the near future.

The identification of groups of individuals at a higher risk of developing lung cancer than the general population is important for developing screening techniques for at least three reasons:

1. Testing of proposed new screening methods, intermediate markers, or risk intervention strategies in high-risk groups will be more efficient than in the general population.

2. Use of high-risk populations will reduce the frequency of false positive tests, which under many circumstances will far exceed the frequency of true positives. False positive results are harmful in that they invoke what is often a costly evaluation to exclude the presence of malignancy, and they produce considerable anxiety in the individuals so labeled.

3. Individuals at high risk for the development of lung cancer may be more willing than the population at large to participate in screening and prevention strategies that are invasive or unpleasant. Even in evaluating less invasive techniques (such as induced sputum) correlation with more invasive and nonroutine information (for example, bronchoalveolar lavage fluid) may well be of value in developing and validating new methods.

Several approaches have been taken to identify individuals and groups at high risk. These have classically included demographic factors (male gender, age), smoking history, and occupational history (asbestos, uranium mining, chloromethyl ether exposure).

The observation that lung cancer develops in only about 10% to 15% of smokers has prompted the search for additional risk factors. In addition to exposure to other carcinogens (either additive or synergistic), a further potential source of variability in risk derives from differences in the metabolic conversion of procarcinogens to active carcinogens, or the degradation and excretion of active carcinogens. During the past decade much interest has focused on members of the cytochrome p450 group of enzymes. There is normally considerable phenotypic variability in the activity of this system, which may be assessed either functionally, by rates of metabolism of certain test substances such as debrisoquine, or by direct structural analysis of enzyme isotypes. Although initial reports[133-136] suggested that slow metabolizers were at significantly altered risk, more recent, larger studies[137] have failed to confirm these and fail to establish this specific metabolic phenotyping as a valid indicator of risk. Although the value of this particular predictive test has failed attempts at confirmation, the more general concept may be valid and simply require better ways of measuring carcinogen exposure at the molecular level. This may be done either at the level of assay of the appropriate enzymes involved in the metabolism of key carcinogens, or by looking more directly at such DNA damage as adduct formation or production of double minute chromosomes. Spitz et al.[138] have recently reported that patients with curatively treated upper aerodigestive cancers whose periph-eral lymphocytes were hypersensitive to in vitro mutation induction by bleomy-cin had a significantly higher incidence of synchronous or metachronous sec-ond primary malignancies than those with lower mutagen sensitivity. Mutagen sensitivity did not correlate with age, sex, smoking status, or tumor stage. It is important to verify this finding and extend such studies to prospective monitor-ing of populations at high risk of developing their first malignancy. The ability to use an easily obtained and renewable tissue such as peripheral lymphocytes fa-cilitates tests of this sort for both the individual patient and the longitudinal stud-ies, where there may be concern about changes in mutagen sensitivity over time.[139]

A further approach to defining an individual at high risk is to identify those genetic changes which may facilitate the occurrence, retention, or misre-pair of somatic mutations in a fashion independent from exposure to exogenous mutagens. The delineation of the mutator phenotype and its role in the develop-ment of human colorectal adenocarcinoma, as well as evidence that not only the frequency of occurrence but also the efficiency of repair of various types of p53 mutations is important in their transforming ability, suggests that this may be an extremely powerful approach. Such changes may antedate more specific changes in the activation of oncogenes or tumor suppressor gene inactivation and provide a simpler unitary point of intervention for prevention strategies.

PROSPECTS FOR NEW SCREENING APPROACHES

Although the large trials of screening by chest x-ray and morphologic examination of exfoliated cells may be criticized for their lack of statistical power to detect small differences in mortality, they were still hampered by technolo-gies that are at best capable of detecting nodules exceeding 2 cm or exfoliated cells that are frankly malignant. Although these findings may be early in com-parison to the typical presentation of lung cancer in unscreened patients, they are very late in the biologic history of the disease. Major improvements in out-come require that investigators detect earlier biologic markers.

Immunostaining of Sputum Specimens

One approach to improving the sensitivity of analysis of examination of exfoliated cells is immunostaining of sputum. Tockman et al.[140] reported a tan-talizing finding that immunostaining of cytologically atypical sputa obtained and archived in the JHLP was able to predict which patients would go on to develop invasive carcinoma, with a lead of about 20 months before clinical diagnosis. These investigators used a pair of monoclonal antibodies, one raised against a squamous cell line and the other raised against a small cell cancer line, to exam-ine preserved sputa from 26 patients who were known to have subsequently developed lung cancer and 43 specimens from participants who did not develop cancer. The results of this are shown in Table 6-5. This dual antibody panel was able to detect both small cell and non–small cell histologies. The likelihood that a premalignant specimen from a patient (from this population of patients with cytologic atypia) who subsequently developed invasive cancer would stain posi-tively with one or both of the antibodies was highly significant ($P = .0001$).

TABLE 6-5

MONOCLONAL ANTIBODY STAINING OF ATYPICAL SPUTUM

	Lung cancer	No lung cancer	Total
Satisfactory	20	5	25
	2	35	37
SUBTOTAL	22	40	62
Unsatisfactory	4	3	7
TOTAL	26	43	69

From Tockman MP et al: An approach to the clinical application of a lung cancer biomarker. In Srivastava S et al, editors: *Early detection of cancer: molecular markers,* Armonk, NY, 1994, Futura Publishing.

This finding requires both validation and evidence that if earlier detection is possible, it will be therapeutically beneficial. To facilitate these studies, the Lung Cancer Early Detection Working Group (LCEDWG) has begun a prospective trial of evaluation of patients with previously resected $T_{1-2}N_0M_0$ NSCLC. This group is at high risk, approximately 3% per year, of developing second lung cancers (as well as other aerodigestive tumors), which will reduce the number of cases required for validation of this concept.[141,142] Patients are being evaluated by annual induced sputum, which is investigated both by conventional cytologic analysis as well as immunostaining. As of the end of 1993 this trial had accrued 580 of a planned 1000 participants, with completion of accrual expected to take a further 2 years.[32] An important correlative study is collecting bronchoalveolar lavage fluid from these patients for analysis of tumor growth factors, analysis of oncogene mutations in exfoliated cells, and other possible early tumor markers.

Fluorescence Bronchoscopy

It has been recognized for some years that a variety of substances will preferentially accumulate in neoplastic and preneoplastic tissues. Several fluorescent porphyrin derivatives have been developed that show such selectivity. In an attempt to determine the minimum dose of these agents needed for detection of neoplastic bronchial mucosa, Lam et al.[143-145] observed that there were differences in the intensity and wavelength of the intrinsic fluorescence of normal and atypical bronchial mucosa.[142-144] Initial studies were done using nonimaging ratio fluorimetry, but subsequently they have developed a fluorescence bronchoscope that allows real time video display of false color images based on ratios of fluorescence at two different wavelengths. This allows for the localization and biopsy of areas of bronchial epithelium that appear normal under conventional white light bronchoscopy but display abnormal fluorescence characteristics. In preliminary studies of 53 patients and 41 volunteers, they reported that, although white light and fluorescence bronchoscopy had similar specificity of 94%, the sensitivity of the fluorescence bronchoscopy was 72% compared with 48% for white light bronchoscopy.[146,147]

Before fluorescence bronchoscopy can be adopted more widely, several questions remain to be answered. Although it appears that the technique can identify areas of epithelial abnormality not seen on conventional bronchoscopy, the true sensitivity (compared to biopsy) is unknown. Prospective correlation of fluorescence bronchoscopy and biopsy with examination of the entire bronchial tree removed in patients undergoing resection would be a valuable way of ascertaining such sensitivity information. Although the technique has appeared to be useful in the experience of its developers, its more general applicability with both pulmonologists and pathologists less committed to development of such new methods is uncertain. Multiinstitution confirmatory studies comparing white light and fluorescence bronchoscopy are currently under way in the United States and Canada, and the wider application of bronchoscopy should await the results of these studies.

Intervention Strategies in High-Risk Populations

> *There is emerging consensus that carcinogenesis, rather than cancer, is the appropriate target for the major focus of our clinical investigations.*

In the past, scientists have concentrated on the end result (tumor, lump, shadow on x-ray), rather than the molecular or cellular processes that underlie and antedate it. Such a developmental and preventive approach is particularly appealing in the setting of a carcinogenic process that involves a broad field of tissue, as does the respiratory epithelium, and where multifocal disease (either synchronous or metachronous) is common, since about 3% per year of patients who survive their first case of lung cancer go on to develop a second one.[12,31,33,34,148]

A large body of in vitro and animal data has shown key roles for retinoids in facilitating normal differentiation of squamous epithelia and in reversing premalignant changes. Pioneering studies in head and neck cancer by Hong et al.[149] have demonstrated both a reversal of leukoplakia and a reduction in the risk of second malignancies in patients given rather high doses of 13-*cis*-retinoic acid. Current confirmatory trials in head and neck cancer are being conducted with somewhat lower and better tolerated drug doses.

In lung cancer a similar strategy is rational, and preliminary data are encouraging. Pastorino et al.[150] randomized 307 patients who had undergone curative resection for stage I NSCLC to observation or treatment with daily oral retinoyl palmitate for 1 to 2 years. After a median follow-up of 46 months, 48% of the control patients and 37% of the treated group had developed recurrence or a second primary tumor. Looking only at second primary tumors in the "field of prevention" (lung, head and neck, bladder), there was a statistically significant reduction from 25 to 13 events in the treated group. Neither local recurrence nor distant metastasis was significantly reduced by treatment. These encouraging results were achieved with modest toxicity; about 10% of patients discontinued treatment because of objective or subjective toxicity.

These results should not, however, be interpreted as mandating the routine use of chemopreventive agents. Two recent reports suggest caution in our approach to implementing chemoprevention strategies based on our present understandings and agents.

Several retrospective studies of dietary habits of smokers who did or did not develop lung cancer suggested a protective effect for consumption of carotenoids, and to a smaller extent, α-tocopherol. In 1985 a joint United States–Finnish trial was begun to prospectively evaluate the effects of dietary supplementation with β-carotene, α-tocopherol, or both in male smokers age 50 to 69. Using a two-way randomization design, a total of 29,133 patients were entered. As reported in 1994, a total of 876 new cases of lung cancer have been observed.[151] No reduction in incidence was seen in the men receiving α-tocopherol (change in incidence 2%; 95% confidence interval (CI) = 14% to 12%). Surprisingly, an increased incidence of lung cancer was seen in the men randomized to receive β-carotene (change in incidence 18%; 95% CI = 3% to 36%). Overall mortality was significantly higher in the men receiving β-carotene (95% CI = 1% to 16%; P = .02). The increased incidence and mortality were surprising and contrasted to results from animal data, other human trials using β-carotene, and to results of retrospective studies correlating dietary intake with risk of lung cancer. It may well be that the apparent harmful effects seen in this study were due to chance; however, it is unlikely that a strong protective effect was missed. It may be that the effective agent(s) in a diet high in the fruits and vegetables identified in epidemiologic studies or that the results of a long period of dietary ingestion are poorly predictive for the effects of a shorter and later pharmacologic intervention.

Lee et al.[152] have recently reported a prospective trial of the use of isotretinoin in a population of heavy smokers. This was an attempt to replicate in a controlled trial observations from earlier uncontrolled European trials that the use of the retinoid etretinate led to reductions in squamous metaplasia. Patients were randomized to treatment with isotretinoin (1 mg/kg) or placebo for 6 months and were evaluated by regular bronchoscopy with biopsies taken from multiple sites. The major study endpoint was change in bronchial metaplasia. The overall metaplasia index decreased over time for both the treatment and control groups, although the change was significant only for the control group, and the difference in the change in metaplasia index for the two groups was not significant. Significant reductions in dysplasia were seen in 54.3% of the isotretinoin subjects and 58.8% of controls. A confounding factor was the cessation of smoking by a large number of members of both the treatment and control groups; significant reductions in metaplasia were seen only in those subjects who continued to smoke. It is not clear from this trial whether the use of the metaplasia index as an intermediate marker was an unfortunate choice or whether the pharmacologic intervention was ineffective. One valuable lesson is that changes in smoking (and possibly dietary) behaviors that may accompany participation in trials of chemopreventive agents may well alter the processes of carcinogenesis and need to be carefully analyzed in phase III trials.

The take-home message from these two "negative" trials is not that chemoprevention has failed, but rather that it remains an area warranting increased laboratory and clinical investigation. Aside from heeding parental advice to eat our vegetables, there is little specific guidance we can give at present regarding dietary or pharmacologic manipulations that should be taken to reduce the risk of lung cancer.

Cautions in Application of New Screening Methods for Preneoplasia

The rapid development of highly specific and sensitive tools for detection of genetic changes in respiratory epithelium must be applied with speed and caution in the clinic. There is little if anything in biology with absolute specificity. Cancer represents a maladaptive choreography (to the individual organism, although not necessarily to the species) of the usual repertoire of cellular responses and processes. Even structurally abnormal oncogene products (such as mutated *ras* gene product) work their harm by performing a normal function (signaling for cell growth) in improper circumstances (the absence of an activating ligand for a growth factor receptor). The line between malignancy and premalignancy is likely to be ill marked and may shift over time. There is likely to be benefit both in approaches that aim for early detection and intervention in what is clearly malignant as well as detection and interference with the process of carcinogenesis, but it is essential that we be clear as to which of these processes we are dealing with. Acceptable costs, both social and individual, are likely to be different for the two approaches.

The high incidence and lethality of lung cancer have prompted a variety of therapeutic and diagnostic approaches to reduce this appalling toll. We recognize that primary prevention through the reduction of cigarette smoking is likely to be the most successful strategy in achieving this goal.

> *However, were all current smokers to quit today, we would still face more than a million cases of lung cancer developing over the next decade from cigarettes already smoked.*

No screening strategy has yet been shown in a prospective trial to reduce lung cancer mortality.

> *The three prospective trials conducted in the United States as well as the Czechoslovak trial all showed that screening of a high-risk group of male smokers 45 years of age or older could alter the usual composition of newly diagnosed patients, with a shift to earlier stage at diagnosis and greater resectability for the screened cases.*

These gains, which are consistent with the shifts that would be seen from lead time bias and length biased sampling, did not translate to consistent benefit either in survival of the detected cases or in a reduction in mortality for the population as a whole.

CONCLUSIONS

What have I learned but the proper use for several tools?
Snyder G: *Axe handles,* San Francisco, 1983, North Point Press.

At the present time, no strategy of screening large populations of smokers or ex-smokers has been shown to be of benefit in reducing overall mortality from lung cancer. This should not be interpreted as a demonstration that the concept is without worth, but rather as an indication of the blunt diagnostic and therapeutic tools that we have used to date, and an impetus to improve these. While we await improvements in these technologies, what recommendations should be make for the concerned individual, smoker or former smoker, who asks about the value of screening at the present time?

On a general health policy level, present data do not support implementing screening policies based on regular chest x-ray and sputum cytology in older male smokers, the populations that have been addressed in the published trials. One can argue that any possible benefit of screening for these individuals would have been masked by other smoking-related mortalities and that benefit might have been seen even with the same crude tools had they been applied to a younger population of ex-smokers. Nor should these data lead primary physicians to think that an indolent approach to symptoms consistent with lung cancer can be neglected or indolently evaluated in the patient at risk.

> *Although past screening programs have failed to reduce the mortality of screened populations, there is reason to believe that these studies may not apply to the present situation. We have a somewhat different population to screen, with an increasing number of former rather than current smokers.*

There has been some small but real progress in the treatment of lung cancer even when diagnosed by conventional (nonscreening) methods. Most critically, our understanding of the early molecular and cellular events in lung cancer development are providing us with tools that can allow for the detection of preneoplastic or early neoplastic changes at a time when the tumor burden is several logs less than with present radiographic detection, and with the promise of a greater therapeutic efficacy. As methods are developed to arrest or reverse some of these molecular events, we will have made a key step from early detection to prevention. The potential for application of these new technologies to today's clinical trials and tomorrow's clinical practice, rather than the disappointing results of the past, should leave us with a mood of realistic optimism in the role of screening and early intervention in lung cancer. This does not negate the primacy of risk reduction by smoking avoidance, or the need for research in areas of economics, politics, and behavioral change in which our tools are to date less honed than those of molecular biology.

REFERENCES

1. Boring C, Squires T, Tong T: Cancer statistics, 1992, *CA Cancer Clin J* 42:19, 1992.
2. Baquet C et al: *Cancer among blacks and other minorities: statistical profiles,* Washington, DC, 1986, National Cancer Institute.
3. Brown C, Kessler L: Projections of lung cancer mortality in the United States, *J Natl Cancer Inst* 80:43, 1988.
4. Burns D: Positive evidence on effectiveness of selected smoking prevention programs in the United States, *J Natl Cancer Inst Monogr* 12:17, 1992.
5. Castonguay A: Methods and strategies in lung cancer control, *Cancer Res (suppl)* 52:2641s, 1992.
6. Cullen J, McKenna J, Massey M: International control of smoking and the US experience, *Chest* 89(suppl):206s, 1986.
7. Gritz E: Lung cancer: now, more than ever, a feminist issue, *CA Cancer Clin J* 43:197, 1993.
8. Horm J, Kessler L: Falling rates of lung cancer in men in the United States, *Lancet* 1:425, 1986.
9. Pierce J, Thurmond L, Rosbrook B: Projecting international lung cancer mortality rates: first approximations with tobacco-consumption data, *J Natl Cancer Inst Monogr* 12:45, 1992.
10. Resnicow K, Kabat G, Wynder E: Progress in decreasing cigarette smoking, *Important Adv Oncol* 1991:205, 1991.
11. Lubin J, Blot W: Lung cancer and smoking cessation: patterns of risk, J Natl Cancer Inst 85:422, 1993 (editorial).
12. Richardson G et al: Smoking cessation significantly reduces the risk of second primary cancer in long-term cancer-free survivors of small cell lung cancer (SCLC), *Proc Am Soc Clin Oncol* 12:326, 1993.
13. Higgins I, Wynder E: Reduction in risk of lung cancer among exsmokers with particular reference to histologic type, *Cancer* 62:2397, 1988.
14. The health benefits of smoking cessation: a report of the Surgeon General, 1990, US Department of Health and Human Services.
15. Halpern M, Gillespie M, Warner K: Patterns of absolute risk of lung cancer mortality in former smokers, *J Natl Cancer Inst* 85:457, 1993.
16. Boring C, Squires T, Tong T: Cancer statistics 1993, *CA Cancer J Clin* 43:7, 1993.
17. Holmes E: Postoperative chemotherapy for non-small cell lung cancer, *Chest* 103:30s, 1993.
18. Kerr K, Lamb D: A comparison of patient survival and tumour growth kinetics in human bronchogenic carcinoma, *Br J Cancer* 58:419, 1988.
19. von Hoff D et al: Elimination of extrachromosomally amplified MYC genes from human tumor cells reduced their tumorigenicity, *Proc Nat Acad Sci USA* 89:8165, 1992.
20. Cole SPC: The 1991 Mark Frost Award: multidrug resistance in small cell lung cancer, *Can J Physiol Pharmacol* 70:313, 1992.
21. Doyle LA: Mechanisms of drug resistance in human lung cancer cells, *Semin Oncol* 20:326, 1993.
22. Feinstein A, Sosin D, Wells C: Stage migration and new diagnostic techniques as a source of misleading statistics for survival in cancer, *N Engl J Med* 312:1604, 1985.
23. Helzlsouer K: The challenges of population screening. In Srivastava S et al, editors: *Early detection of cancer: molecular markers,* Armonk, NY, 1994, Futura Publishing.
24. Hulka B: Cancer screening: degrees of proof and practical application, *Cancer* 62:1776, 1988.
25. Shepherd F: Screening, diagnosis, and staging of lung cancer, *Curr Opinion Oncol* 5:310, 1993.
26. Mountain C: Prognostic implications of the international staging system for lung cancer, *Semin Oncol* 15(3):236, 1988.

27. Dillman R et al: A randomized trial of induction chemotherapy plus high-dose radiation versus radiation alone in stage III non-small cell lung cancer, *N Engl J Med* 323:940, 1990.

28. Dillman R et al: Randomized trial of induction chemotherapy plus radiation therapy vs RT alone in stage III non-small cell lung cancer (NSCLC): five-year follow-up of CALGB, *Proc Am Soc Clin Oncol* 12:329, 1993 (abstract 1092).

29. Roth JA et al: A randomized trial comparing perioperative chemotherapy and surgery with surgery alone in resectable stage IIIA non-small cell lung cancer, *J Natl Cancer Inst* 86:673, 1994.

30. Rossell R et al: A randomized trial comparing preoperative chemotherapy plus surgery with surgery alone in patients with non-small cell lung cancer, *N Engl J Med* 330:153, 1994.

31. Richardson G et al: Second tumors are the major cause of late mortality in long term survivors of small cell lung cancer, *Lung Cancer* 7:175A, 1991.

32. Tockman M et al: The early detection of second primary lung cancers by sputum immunostaining, *Chest* 106:385s, 1994.

33. vanBodegon P et al: Second primary lung cancer: importance of long-term follow-up, *Thorax* 44:788, 1989.

34. Johnson B et al: Risk of second cancers (SC) in long-term survivors of small cell lung cancer (SCLC), *Lung Cancer* 11(supplement 1):220, 1994 (abstract).

35. Stjernsward J, Stanley K: Lung cancer: a world wide health problem, *Lung Cancer* 4:P11, 1988.

36. Mackay J: US tobacco export to third world: third world war, *J Natl Cancer Inst Monogr* 12:25, 1992.

37. Chin HW: Bronchogenic carcinoma in geriatric population, *Proc Am Soc Clin Oncol* 12:342, 1993.

38. Peto R, Parish S, Gray R: There is no such thing as aging, and cancer is not related to it. In Likhachev A, Anisimov V, Montesano R, editors: *Age-related factors in carcinogenesis,* IARC Scientific Pub No 58, Lyon, France, 1985, International Agency for Research on Cancer.

39. Davis K: Get ready for the era of geriatric care, *Geriatrics* 38:34, 1983.

40. Garfinkel L, Silverberg E: Lung cancer and smoking trends in the United States over the past 25 years, *CA Cancer Clin J* 41:137, 1991.

41. Garfinkel L, Stellman S: Smoking and lung cancer in women: findings in a prospective study, *Cancer Res* 48:6951, 1988.

42. Pierce J, Fiore M, Novotny T: Trends in cigarette smoking in the United States: projections to the year 2000, *JAMA* 261(1):61, 1989.

43. Steinfeld J: Combating smoking in the United States: progress through science and social action, *J Natl Cancer Inst* 83:1126, 1991.

44. Huber G, Shafer D, Pandina R: Tobacco smoking, smoking cessation, nutrition, and metabolism: importance to smoking cessation strategies, *Semin Respir Med* 11:69, 1990.

45. Mulshine J et al: Candidate biomarkers for application as intermediate end points of lung carcinogenesis, *J Cell Biochem (suppl)* 16G:183, 1992.

46. Devesa S, Shaw G, Blot W: Changing patterns of lung cancer incidence by histological type, *Cancer Epidemiol Biomark Prev* 1:29, 1991.

47. Birrer M, Brown P: Application of molecular genetics to the early diagnosis and screening of lung cancer, *Cancer Res* (suppl) 52:2658s, 1992.

48. Whang-Peng J et al: Specific chromosome defect associated with human small cell lung cancer: deletion 3p(14-23), *Science* 215:181, 1982.

49. Whang-Peng J et al: Non-random structural and numerical chromosome changes in non-small cell lung cancer, *Genes Chrom Cancer* 3:168, 1991.

50. Carbone D, Minna J: The molecular genetics of lung cancer, *Adv Intern Med* 37:153, 1992.

51. Gazdar A: The molecular and cellular basis of human lung cancer, *Anticancer Res* 13:261, 1994.

52. Minna J: The molecular biology of lung cancer pathogenesis, *Chest* 103:449s, 1993.

53. Dowdy S et al: Physical interaction of the retinoblastoma protein with human D cyclins, *Cell* 73:499, 1993.

54. Ewen M et al: Functional interactions of the retinoblastoma protein with mammalian D-type cyclins, *Cell* 73:487, 1993.

55. Ewen M: The cell cycle and the retinoblastoma protein family, *Cancer Metastasis Rev* 13:45, 1994.

56. Picksley S, Lane D: p53 and Rb: their cellular roles, *Curr Opinion Cell Biol* 6:653, 1994.

57. Ookawa K et al: Reconstitution of the Rb gene suppresses the growth of small cell lung carcinoma cells carrying multiple genetic alterations, *Oncogene* 8:2175, 1993.

58. Montenarh M: Biochemical, immunological, and functional aspects of the growth suppressor/oncoprotein p53, *Crit Rev Oncogenesis* 3:233, 1992.

59. Hollstein M et al: p53 Mutations in human cancers, *Science* 253:49, 1991.

60. Tominaga O et al: p53: From basic research to clinical applications, *Crit Rev Oncogenesis* 3:257, 1992.

61. Pietenpol J, Vogelstein B: No room at the p53 inn, *Nature* 365:17, 1993.

62. Lowe S et al: p53 And apoptosis, *Nature* 362:842, 1993.

63. Clarke A et al: p53 And apoptosis, *Nature* 362:849, 1993.

64. Cannon-Albright L et al: Assignment of a locus for familial melanoma, *MLM*, to chromosome 9p13-22, *Science* 258:1148, 1992.

65. Olopade O et al: Homozygous loss of the interferon genes defines the critical region on 9p that is deleted in lung cancers, *Cancer Res* 53:2410s, 1993.

66. Kok K et al: A gene in the chromosomal region 3p21 with greatly reduced expression in lung cancer is similar to the gene for ubiquitin-activating enzyme, *Proc Natl Acad Sci USA* 90:6071, 1993.

67. Brauch H et al: Molecular analysis of the short arm of chromosome 3 in small-cell and non-small-cell carcinoma of the lung, *N Engl J Med* 317:1109, 1987.

68. Fong K, Zimmerman P, Smith P: Loss of heterozygosity at the *MCC/APC* loci and prognosis in restricted non-small cell lung cancer, *Lung Cancer* 11:9, 1994 (abstract 030).

69. D'Amico D et al: Polymorphic sites within *APC* and *MCC* loci reveal infrequent loss of heterozygosity in primary human non-small cell lung cancer, *Lung Cancer* 11:12, 1994 (abstract 42).

70. Downward J: The *ras* superfamily of small GTP-binding proteins, *Trends Biochem Sci* 15:469, 1990.

71. Bos J: *ras* Oncogenes in human cancer: a review, *Cancer Res* 49:4682, 1989.

72. Feig L: The many roads that lead to *ras*, *Science* 260:767, 1993.

73. Khosravi-Far R, Der C: The *ras* signal transduction pathway, *Cancer Metastasis Rev* 13:67, 1994.

74. Moodie S, Wolfman A: The 3 Rs of life: *ras, raf,* and growth regulation, *Trends Genetics* 10:44, 1994.

75. Krengel U et al: Three-dimensional structures of H-*ras*p21 mutants: molecular basis for their inability to function as signal switch molecules, *Cell* 62:539, 1990.

76. Slebos R et al: Relationship between K-*ras* oncogene activation and smoking in adenocarcinoma of the human lung, *J Natl Cancer Inst* 83:1024, 1991.

77. Westra W et al: K-*ras* oncogene activation in lung adenocarcinomas from former smokers, *Cancer* 72(2):432, 1993.

78. Rodenhuis S et al: Mutational activation of the K-*ras* oncogene: a possible pathogenetic factor in adenocarcinoma of the lung, *N Engl J Med* 317:929, 1987.

79. Rodenhuis S et al: Incidence and possible clinical significance of K-*ras* oncogene activation in adenocarcinoma of the lung, *Cancer Res* 48:5738, 1988.

80. Rodenhuis S, Slebos R: Clinical significance of *ras* oncogene activation in human lung cancer, *Cancer Res* (suppl) 52:2665s, 1992.

81. Mitsudomi T et al: Mutations of *ras* genes distinguish a subset of non-small-cell lung cancer cell lines from small-cell lung cancer cell lines, *Oncogene* 6:1353, 1991.

82. McKenna W et al: Synergistic effect of the v-*myc* oncogene with H-*ras* on radioresistance, *Cancer Res* 50:97, 1990.

83. Mabry M et al: v-Ha-*ras* oncogene insertion: a model for tumor progression of human small cell lung cancer, *Proc Natl Acad Sci USA* 85:6523, 1988.

84. Mitsudomi T et al: *ras* Gene mutations in non-small-cell lung cancers are associated with shortened survival irrespective of treatment intent, *Cancer Res* 51:4999, 1991.

85. Slebos R et al: K-*ras* oncogene activation as a prognostic marker in adenocarcinoma of the lung, *N Engl J Med* 323:561, 1990.

86. Alt F et al: The human *myc* gene family, *Cold Spring Harbor Symp Quant Biol* 51:931, 1986.

87. Bergh J: Gene amplification in human lung cancer: the *myc* family genes and other proto-oncogenes and growth factor genes, *Am Rev Respir Dis* 42:20, 1990.

88. Brennan J et al: *myc* Family DNA amplification in 107 tumors and tumor cell lines from patients with small cell lung cancer treated with different combination chemotherapy regimens, *Cancer Res* 51:1708, 1991.

89. Johnson B et al: *myc* Family oncogene amplification in tumor cell lines established from small cell lung cancer patients and its relationship to clinical status and course, *J Clin Invest* 79:1629, 1987.

90. Johnson B et al: *myc* Family DNA amplification in small cell lung cancer patients' tumors and corresponding cell lines, *Cancer Res* 48:5163, 1988.

91. Little C et al: Amplification and expression of the c-*myc* oncogene in human lung cancer cell lines, *Nature* 306:194, 1983.

92. Wong AJ et al: Gene amplification of c-*myc* and N-*myc* in small cell carcinoma of the lung, *Science* 233:461, 1986.

93. Takahashi T et al: Expression and amplification of *myc* gene family in small cell lung cancer and its relation to biological characteristics, *Cancer Res* 49:2683, 1989.

94. Reference deleted in proofs.

95. Yoshimoto K, Hirohashi S, Sekiya T: Increased expression of the c-*myc* gene without gene amplification in human lung carcinoma and colon cancer cell lines, *Jpn J Cancer Res* 77:540, 1986.

96. Kern J et al: Mechanisms of pl 85HER2 expression in human non-small cell lung cancer lines, *Am J Respir Cell Mol Biol* 6:359, 1992.

97. Kern J et al: pl 85neu expression in human lung adenocarcinoma predicts shortened survival, *Cancer Res* 50:5184, 1990.

98. Tateishi M et al: Prognostic value of c-*erb*B-2 protein expression in human lung adenocarcinoma and squamous cell carcinoma, *Eur J Cancer* 27:1372, 1991.

99. Slaughter D, Southwick H, Smejkal W: "Field cancerization" in oral stratified squamous epithelium: clinical implications of multicentric origin, *Cancer* 6:963, 1953.

100. Gazdar A et al: Extensive areas of dysplasia and aneuploidy of the entire bronchial mucosal tract accompanies non-small cell lung cancers and provides evidence for the field cancerization theory, *Proc Am Soc Clin Oncol* 12:334, 1993.

101. Sundaresan V et al: p53 And chromosome 3 abnormalities, characteristic of malignant lung tumours, are detectable in preinvasive lesions of the bronchus, *Oncogene* 7:1989, 1992.

102. Rusch V et al: Differential expression of the epidermal growth factor receptor and its ligands in primary non-small cell lung cancers and adjacent benign lung, *Cancer Res* 53:2379, 1993.

103. Jaskiewicz K, DeGroot K: p53 Gene mutants expression, cellular proliferation and differentiation in oesophageal carcinoma and non-cancerous epithelium, *Anticancer Res* 14:137, 1994.

104. Sorsdahl K et al: p53 And *ras* gene expression in human esophageal cancer and Barrett's epithelium: a prospective study, *Cancer Detect Prev* 18:179, 1994.

105. Sidranski D et al: Identification of *ras* oncogene mutations in the stool of patients with curable colorectal tumor, *Science* 256:102, 1992.

106. Tobi M, Luo F-C, Ronai Z: Detection of k-*ras* mutation in colonic effluent samples from patients without evidence of colorectal carcinoma, *J Natl Cancer Inst* 86:1007, 1994.

107. Tada M et al: Detection of *ras* gene mutations in pancreatic juice and peripheral blood of patients with pancreatic adenocarcinoma, *Cancer Res* 53:2472, 1993.

108. Caldas C et al: Detection of K-*ras* mutations in the stool of patients with pancreatic adenocarcinoma and pancreatic ductal hyperplasia, *Cancer Res* 54:3568, 1994.

109. Kelly K: Evaluation of k-*ras* mutations in sputum samples by single-stranded conformation polymorphism, *Lung Cancer* 11(suppl 1):225, 1994 (abstract).

110. Mills N et al: *ras* Oncogene detection in bronchoalveolar lavage fluid from patients with lung cancer, *Lung Cancer* 11(suppl 1):41, 1994 (abstract).

111. Mao L et al: Detection of oncogene mutations in sputum precedes diagnosis of lung cancer, *Cancer Res* 54:1634, 1994.

112. Sorenson G et al: Detection of mutated k-*ras* sequences in blood from patients with pulmonary carcinoma, *Lung Cancer* 11(suppl 1):57, 1994 (abstract).

113. Mao L, Sidranski D: Cancer screening based on genetic alterations in human tumors, *Cancer Res* 54:1939s, 1994.

114. Sidranski D: Molecular screening: how long can we afford to wait, *J Natl Cancer Inst* 86:955, 1994.

115. Mulshine J et al: Global strategies for the early detection of epithelial cancers. In Srivastava S et al, editors: *Early detection of cancer: molecular markers,* Armonk, NY, 1994, Futura Publishing.

116. Ruckdeschel J: Cellular characterization of lung cancer: a caveat, *Chest* 104:331, 1993.

117. Boucot K, Horie U, Sokoloff M: Lung cancer detected by survey methods, *Am J Public Health* 49:793, 1959.

118. Brett G: Bronchial carcinoma in men detected by selective and unselective miniature radiography: a review of 228 cases, *Tubercle* 40:192, 1959.

119. Nash F et al: South London lung cancer study, *Br Med J* 2:715, 1968.

120. Sanderson D: Lung cancer screening: the Mayo study, *Chest* (suppl) 89:324s, 1986.

121. Tockman M: Survival and mortality from lung cancer in a screened population, *Chest* 89:324s, 1986.

122. Martini N: Results of the Memorial Sloan-Kettering study in screening for early lung cancer, *Chest* (suppl) 89:325s, 1986.

123. Kubik A et al: Lack of benefit from semiannual screening for cancer of the lung: follow-up report of a randomized controlled trial on a population of high-risk males in Czechoslovakia, *Int J Cancer* 45:26, 1990.

124. Miller A: Lung cancer screening: summary, *Chest* 89:325s, 1986.

125. Eddy D: Screening for lung cancer, *Ann Intern Med* 111:232, 1989.

126. Flehinger B et al: Early lung cancer detection: results of the initial (prevalence) radiologic and cytologic screening in the Memorial Sloan-Kettering study, *Am Rev Respir Dis* 130:555, 1984.

127. Flehinger B et al: Screening for lung cancer: the Mayo lung project revisited, *Cancer* 72:1573, 1993.

128. Wu A et al: Secular trends in histologic types of lung cancer, *J Natl Cancer Inst* 77:53, 1986.

129. El-Torky M, El-Zeky F, Hall J: Significant changes in the distribution of histologic types of lung cancer, *Cancer* 65:2361, 1990.

130. Hansen M, Pedersen A: Tumor markers in patients with lung cancer, *Chest* (suppl) 89:219s, 1986.

131. Miyake Y, Kodama T, Yamaguchi K: Pro-gastrin-releasing peptide (31-98) is a specific tumor marker in patients with small cell lung carcinoma, *Cancer Res* 54(8):2136, 1994.

132. Aguayo S et al: Urinary levels of bombesin-like peptides in asymptomatic cigarette smokers: a potential risk marker for smoking related diseases, *Cancer Res* 52(suppl):2727s, 1992.

133. Law M, Hetzel M, Idel J: Debrisoquine metabolism and genetic predisposition to lung cancer, *Br J Cancer* 59:686, 1987.

134. Caporaso NE, Tucker MA, Hoover RN: Lung cancer and the debrisoquine metabolic phenotype, *J Natl Cancer Inst* 82:1264, 1990.

135. Speirs C et al: Debrisoquine oxidation phenotype and susceptibility to lung cancer, *Br J Clin Pharmacol* 29:101, 1990.

136. Benitez J et al: Polymorphic oxidation of debrisoquine in lung cancer patients, *Eur J Cancer* 27:158, 1991.

137. Shaw G et al: Debrisoquine metabolism and lung cancer risk, *Proc Am Assoc Cancer Res* 35:1753a, 1994.

138. Spitz M et al: Mutagen sensitivity as a risk factor for second malignant tumors following malignancies of the upper aerodigestive tract, *J Natl Cancer Inst* 86:1681, 1994.

139. Olden K: Mutagen hypersensitivity as a biomarker of genetic predisposition to carcinogenesis, *J Natl Cancer Inst* 86:1660, 1994.

140. Tockman M et al: Sensitive and specific monoclonal antibody recognition of human lung cancer antigen on preserved sputum cells: a new approach to early lung cancer detection, *J Clin Oncol* 11:1685, 1988.

141. Tockman M et al: Considerations in bringing a cancer biomarker to clinical application, *Cancer Res* (suppl) 52:2711s, 1992.

142. Tockman M et al: An approach to the clinical application of a lung cancer biomarker. In Srivastava S et al, editors: *Early detection of cancer: molecular markers,* Armonk, NY, 1994, Futura Publishing.

143. Hung J et al: Autofluorescence of normal and malignant bronchial tissue, *Lasers Surg Med* 11:99, 1991.

144. Lam S et al: Detection of early lung cancer using low dose Photofrin II, *Chest* 97:333, 1990.

145. Lam S, Hung J, Palcic B: Mechanism of detection of early lung cancer by ratio fluorometry, *Laser Life Sci* 4:67, 1991.

146. Lam S et al: Detection of dysplasia and carcinoma in situ by a lung imaging fluorescence endoscope (LIFE) device, *Lasers Surg Med* 12(4):40, 1992.

147. Lam S et al: Detection of dysplasia and carcinoma in situ using a lung imaging fluorescence endoscope device, *J Thorac Cardiovasc Surg* 105(6):1035, 1993.

148. Heyne K et al: The incidence of second primary tumors in long-term survivors of small cell lung cancer, *J Clin Oncol* 10:1519, 1992.

149. Hong W et al: Prevention of second primary tumors with isotretinoin in squamous-cell carcinoma of the head and neck, *N Engl J Med* 323:795, 1990.

150. Pastorino U et al: Adjuvant treatment of stage I lung cancer with high-dose vitamin A, *J Clin Oncol* 11:1216, 1993.

151. The Alpha-Tocopheral Beta Carotene Cancer Prevention Study Group: The effect of vitamin E and beta-carotene on the incidence of lung cancer and other cancers in male smokers, *N Engl J Med* 330:1029, 1994.

152. Lee J et al: Randomized placebo-controlled trial of isotretinoin in chemoprevention of bronchial squamous metaplasia, *J Clin Oncol* 12:937, 1994.

153. Feld RA, Rubenstein L, Thomas PA: Adjuvant chemotherapy with cyclophosphamide, doxorubicin, and cisplatin in patients with completely resected stage I non-small cell lung cancer, *J Natl Cancer Inst* 85:299, 1994.

OVARIAN CANCER

James V. Fiorica
William S. Roberts

EPIDEMIOLOGY

Ovarian cancer is the most common cause of death among gynecologic malignancies and the fourth most common cause of cancer death in American women. In 1994 an estimated 24,000 new cases of ovarian cancer were diagnosed, and approximately 13,600 women died of the disease. In the United States the lifetime risk from birth to age 85 is approximately 1.5%. Ovarian cancer incidence appears to be highest in North America and Northern Europe and lowest in Japan, and it occurs more commonly in white women. The mean age at diagnosis is 59 years, and the incidence increases with age and peaks in the eighth decade. The incidence rate of ovarian cancer increases from 15.7 per 100,000 per year in the 40 to 44 age group to a peak rate of 54 per 100,000 per year in the 75 to 79 age group. The surveillance, epidemiology and end results program (SEER) of the National Cancer Institute (NCI) reports the average annual age-adjusted incidence was 13.7 per 100,000 during 1987. The prevalence is 30 to 50 per 100,000 women in the United States.[1]

Multivariate analysis shows that International Federation of Gynecology and Obstetrics (FIGO) stage, age, lymph node status, grade, histology, presence of ascites, and race are all predictors of survival. The 5-year survival varies from 87.8% for stage Ia to 18% for stage IV disease, with an overall 5-year survival rate of 37%. The age-adjusted mortality is 28.4 per 100,000 per year for women over age 50 years.[2]

THEORIES OF CAUSE AND NATURAL HISTORY

Epithelial ovarian cancers are believed to arise from embryologic derivatives of the ovarian surface epithelium. Epidemiologic factors associated with a reduced risk of ovarian cancer are also generally associated with a decrease in ovulation.

Because of this ovarian cancer, etiologic theories are often grouped into three categories: (1) incessant ovulation, (2) increased exposure to circulating pituitary gonadotropins, and (3) the presence of ovarian inclusion cysts, possibly secondary to minor trauma or increased proliferation of epithelium. An increased galactose consumption and a decreased galactose-1-phosphate uridyl transferase activity have also been implicated as possible etiologic factors.

The natural history of ovarian cancer appears to begin with malignant transformation of the epithelial lining of inclusion cysts within the ovarian stroma. The cells replicate, the tumor penetrates through the ovarian capsule, and malignant cells generally spread throughout the peritoneal lining of the pelvis and abdomen. At this point the cells may attach directly to the adjacent organs of the pelvis or the small or large intestines, or they may circulate in a clockwise fashion with the peritoneal fluid to the pericolic gutters and diaphragmatic surfaces or omentum, where implants may grow.

In addition, the malignant cells may follow the ovarian blood supply and lymphatic channels to spread retroperitoneally superiorly along the aorta and vena cava or inferiorly down the infundibulopelvic ligament to the pelvic lymph nodes.

> *Only 25% of women with newly diagnosed ovarian cancer present with stage I disease; 75% present with malignant cells outside the ovaries at the time of diagnosis.*

Therefore strategies must be developed for prevention or early diagnosis to control this disease process.

T A B L E   7 - 1

CRITERIA FOR AN EFFECTIVE SCREENING TEST

- Large burden of disease
- Recognizable preclinical stages
- Curative potential much greater in early stages
- Acceptable to the screener and the person being screened
- Improvement in cause-specific mortality

From Hulka BS: *Cancer* 62:(suppl 8):1776, 1988.

EFFICACY OF SCREENING
Requirements

Frequently the medical and lay communities assume that early diagnosis of cancer of any type automatically benefits the patient and that any diagnostic test which can identify early stages of disease must therefore be useful for screening. However, this is not necessarily the case; certain requirements must be met (Table 7-1).[3]

An optimal screening test is distinguished by high specificity, sensitivity, patient acceptance, and ease of performance.

Based on the prevalence of ovarian cancer among American women, it is estimated that the positive predictive value of a screening test for ovarian cancer at 99% specificity in women ages 45 to 74 is approximately 4% (24 false positives for each case of ovarian cancer). No single test achieves this level of specificity; therefore, unless there is a careful selection of screening tools and patient population, the result would be several unnecessary laparoscopies or laparotomies and their associated patient morbidity and financial costs. It is possible that an algorithm combining two or more screening tests could be identified that would improve the test characteristics. This, however, would necessitate a prospective randomized trial.

Screening Test: Pelvic Examination

The pelvic examination is currently the standard for screening women with ovarian cancer. It has a sensitivity of 67% for detecting a 4×6 cm mass. Over a 15-year period, MacFarlane et al[4] found only six ovarian cancers among 1319 women who had undergone a total of 18,753 pelvic examinations.

Therefore the pelvic examination alone is of limited value as a screening tool for the detection of early ovarian cancer.

T A B L E   7 - 2

CAUSES OF CA-125 ELEVATION

Benign	Malignant
Endometriosis	Epithelial ovarian carcinoma
Pelvic inflammatory disease	Germ cell tumors
Leiomyoma	Gonadal stromal tumors
Adenomyosis	Endometrial adenocarcinoma
Ectopic pregnancy	Cervical adenocarcinoma
Cystadenoma	Fallopian tube carcinoma
Liver disease	Mixed müllerian tumor
Pancreatitis	Biliary tract tumors
Peritonitis	Hepatic tumors
Renal failure	Pancreatic carcinoma
Cirrhosis of the liver	Breast carcinoma
First-trimester pregnancy	Colon carcinoma
	Lung carcinoma

From Squatrito RC, Buller RE: *Female Patient* 19:14, 1994.

Biochemical Test: CA-125

The ideal tumor marker would specifically detect a malignancy and would not be present in nonmalignant tissues. Unfortunately, no current test exists that fulfills this description. Most tumor markers are nonspecific in that they are found in multiple types of malignancies as well as normal and benign tissues (Table 7-2). A number of tumor markers have been studied for ovarian carcinoma, including CA-125, TAG72, NBK70, CA15-3, CA19-9, urinary gonadotropin fragment (UGP), and placental alkaline phosphatase (PLAP).[5] Table 7-3 summarizes their characteristics.

The most extensively studied ovarian cancer–associated antigen is CA-125, a high molecular weight glycoprotein that is recognized by the murine OC125 monoclonal antibody as an immunogen. A normal cutoff value of 35 U/ml is generally accepted.

> *CA-125 levels are elevated (>35 U/ml) in more than 85% of women with ovarian cancer. CA-125 correlates with the stage of disease in that it is elevated in 90% of stage II, III, IV disease but in only 50% of stage I disease.*

The three largest studies in the world literature pertaining to serum CA-125 measurements are the Janus study,[6] The Royal London Hospital study,[7] and the Stockholm study.[8] The Janus study used a serum blood bank of 39,300 stored samples; 105 of the represented women developed ovarian cancer. Age-matched controls were assayed for CA-125. The Royal London Hospital study is a prospective evaluation of 22,000 postmenopausal women using CA-125 and ultrasound in the screening for ovarian cancer. This is an ongoing study, with CA-125 the primary screen and ultrasonography the secondary test in the screening project.

TABLE 7-3

SUMMARY OF TUMOR MARKERS IN OVARIAN EPITHELIAL CARCINOMAS

Tumor marker	Description
CA15-3	Tumor-associated antigen in milk fat globule membrane found in adenocarcinoma of breast, lung, ovary, pancreas; most useful for breast cancer
CA19-9	Antigen recognized by monoclonal antibody; useful for colon, gastric, lung, pancreatic, ovarian, and endometrial cancer; best for pancreatic; most likely positive in well-differentiated carcinoma; may be useful for mucinous ovarian cancer for which CA-125 is not elevated
NB/70K	Glycoprotein from human ovarian carcinoma; elevated in advanced disease and in some cervical and endometrial carcinomas
PLAP (placental alkaline phosphatase) plus PLAP-like alkaline phosphatase	Most useful for endometrial carcinoma of ovary; not elevated as often as CA-125 for ovarian carcinomas
TAG 72	A glycoprotein surface antigen (monoclonal antibody B72.3), found to react to ovarian and colon cancer; linked to radionuclides (^{111}In, ^{131}I) for radioimmunodetection of ovarian cancer
UGF (urinary gonadotropin fragment)	Derived from β-human chorionic gonadotropin (free β-subunit plus asialo free β-subunit; elevated in urine of patients with gynecologic malignancies (ovarian, endometrial, cervical, and vulvar carcinoma)

From Herbst AL: *Am J Obstet Gynecol* 170:1103, 1994.

In the Stockholm study Einhorn et al. evaluated 5550 healthy asymptomatic women with a serum CA-125 test. Elevations were followed clinically with ultrasound and serial CA-125 measurements.

The Janus study detected eleven cases of ovarian cancer at the prevalence screen. Another three presented as interval cases within 12 months of the screen. Five presented as interval cases 12 to 24 months after screening, yielding a sensitivity of 79% at 1 year and 58% at 2 years of follow-up. Einhorn found 175 elevated CA-125 levels in the 5500 women age 40 and older who were screened. Of these, six of the nine cases of ovarian cancer occurred where there was an elevated CA-125, yielding a similar sensitivity.

The specificity of serum CA-125 estimation among postmenopausal women was 98% in the Royal London Hospital study. The CA-125 has a lower specificity in premenopausal than postmenopausal women, presumably because of a rise in levels associated with menstruation and benign disorders. The specificity is similar to the specificity of ultrasound alone and would not be acceptable in general population screening. With a prevalence of 40 per 100,000 per year in women older than 45, and a specificity of 98%, 50 false positive results would occur for each case of ovarian cancer (Table 7-4).[9]

Di-Xia[10] evaluated patients with elevated CA-125 levels and pelvic masses. He found a false positive rate of 40% at a level over 35 U/ml. When the

TABLE 7-4

PREOPERATIVE CA-125 FOR PELVIC MASSES

	Sensitivity	Specificity	Positive predictive value	Negative predictive value
Premenopausal				
Malkasian et al.	.60	.89	.49	.93
Finkler et al.	.50	.69	.36	.77
Patsner et al.	.65	.78	.67	.83
Consensus	.58	.79	.51	.84
Postmenopausal				
Malkasian et al.	.78	.97	.98	.72
Finkler et al.	.84	.92	.94	.80
Patsner et al.	.77	.81	.87	.68
Consensus	.80	.90	.93	.73
Overall				
Vasilev et al.	.78	.78	.28	.97
Ovarian Neoplasms Only	.73	.81		
Over 50 Years of Age	1.00	.98		

From Squatrito RC, Buller RE: *Female Patient* 19:26, 1994.

cutoff was raised to higher levels, the sensitivity was reduced, as was the false positive rate. Some investigators have used multiple tumor markers to enhance the specificity of screening. In the Royal London Hospital study the best combination was CA-125 and OVX1. The combination of either a CA-125 level over 25 U/ml or an OVX1 level over 12 U/ml achieved a sensitivity of 80% and a specificity of 91%. Soper et al.[11] added TAG72 and CA15-3 to CA-125 and found the sensitivity for detection of malignancy was 81%, with a specificity of 100% for those over 50 years of age.

On the horizon is the development of a new antigen, CA-130, located in the same glycoprotein as CA-125 but at a distinct ectopic site. The CA-130 site is recognized by two different monoclonal antibodies. Hosono[12] evaluated 8000 samples and found that, when the CA-130 was used together with a CA-125 level, the specificity and positive predictive value of CA-125 were enhanced.

The ideal screening program should be safe, noninvasive, and inexpensive.

The sole use of tumor markers such as CA-125 would be inexpensive, but on the basis of current data it would not provide adequate specificity for mass screening.

Diagnostic Test: Transvaginal Ultrasonography

Transabdominal ultrasonography (TAS) and transvaginal ultrasonography (TVS) have been studied as noninvasive screening tools. TVS is currently the preferred modality. The potential success of ultrasound imaging is based on its ability to detect early morphologic changes accompanying ovarian oncogenesis.

Campbell[13] published a prospective study of ultrasound ovarian cancer screening. He screened 5479 women (age 18 to 78) using TAS and found 326 (5.9%) with persistently abnormal ovarian morphology. At laparotomy five stage I ovarian cancers, of which there were three borderline tumors, four metastatic ovarian cancers, and 255 benign ovarian lesions were found. The odds of detecting ovarian cancer were one in 67.

Van Nagell[14] evaluated 3220 asymptomatic postmenopausal women with TVS. In 44 women (1.4%) morphologic ovarian abnormalities were detected, only 16 of which were clinically appreciated. These patients were taken to surgery, where 41 benign ovarian pathologies, two stage I ovarian cancers (one granulosa, one epithelial), and one stage IIIb ovarian cancer were found. Twenty-one serous cystadenomas were found, thereby possibly preventing a premalignant condition from proceeding to cancer.

Morphologic scoring systems are being developed to improve the accuracy of TVS. The three criteria being evaluated are size/volume, papillary projections from the cyst wall, and cyst complexity. Papillary projections correlated highly with malignancy, being the most ominous and reliable finding.[15] Karlan et al.[18] have all proposed morphologic scoring systems to predict malignancies in the ovary. Of the 11,283 women scanned, the overall specificity was approximately 96% with a positive predictive value of 3.1% (Table 7-5). Morphology indices are difficult to standardize and are associated with an increased risk of false negative studies.

The use of color Doppler imaging (CDI) has been coupled with TVS to detect specific flow patterns associated with malignancy. Dividing cancer cells are believed to produce an angiogenesis factor that stimulates new blood vessels. The resultant vascular tumor bed is morphologically abnormal because it lacks intimal smooth muscle, which is necessary for increasing peripheral vascular resistance. Arteriovenous communications are also common within the tumor bed, resulting in a large diastolic flow component that can be expressed as resistance index or pulsatility index.[16]

The use of CDI has reduced the false positive rate of ovarian cancer detection but at an additional expense to the patient. Because of the low prevalence of disease in the general population, some studies have focused on high-risk populations such as older women or women with a family history of the disease. Bourne and Campbell[16] screened 1601 women ages 17 to 29 with a family history of ovarian cancer by TVS and CDI. All patients with abnormal TVS received CDI and a morphology index as the secondary screen. Of these, 909 women (57%) required follow-up scans, but only 61 patients (3.8%) ultimately went to surgery for exploration. Six ovarian cancers were found, three of which were of low malignant potential (five stage I and one stage III).

Karlan[18] screened 597 women (age 35 to 80) with a family history of ovarian cancer, endometrial cancer, or colon cancer using TVS and CDI. Of these, 115 individuals (19%) of the scans were initially abnormal. Nineteen patients

TABLE 7-5

PROSPECTIVE ULTRASOUND SCREENING TRIALS

Authors	Number of women (age)	Ultrasound technique	Number of surgeries	Number of cases	Number Stage I OV CA (grade)	Specificity OV CA (%)	PPV OV CA (%)
Campbell (1989)	5749 (18-78)	TAS	326	9 (5 OV CA, 4 metastatic)	5 (3 gr 0)	97.7	1.5
DePriest, van Nagell (1993)	3220 (33-90)	TVS, MI	44	3	2 (1 granulosa)	98.7	6.8
Bourne, Campbell (1993)*	1601 (17-79)	TVS, CDI, MI	61	9† (6 OV CA, 3 metastatic)	5 (3 gr 0)	96.5	9.8
Karlan (1993)	597 (35-80)	TVS, CDI	19	1	1 (gr 0)	97	5.3
Muto (1993)*	386 (20->60)	TVS, CDI	36‡	0	0	90.7	—
TOTALS	11,283§		486	22	13 (5 invasive epithelial CA)	95.8	3.1

From Karlan BY, Platt LD: *Gynecol Oncol* 55:529, 1994.
*Repeat ultrasound required in 19% to 57% of participants.
†Three interval stage III ovarian cancers found in 22 to 44-month follow-up.
‡Operative small bowel injury requiring reexploration.
§Number needed to treat (NNT) (all) 32 (range: 20 to 58); NNT (family history) 17 (range: 8 to 41).
PPV, Positive predictive value; *TAS,* transabdominal sonography; *TVS,* transvaginal sonography; *MI,* morphology index; *CDI,* color Doppler imaging.

went to surgery, and one stage I borderline ovarian cancer, one stage I, grade 3 endometrial cancer, and 18 benign adnexal pathologies were found.

Muto[19] used TVS and CDI on 386 patients (age 20 to over 60) with a family history of ovarian cancer. Fifteen patients had persistent ovarian masses and went to surgery. All of these masses were benign. Twenty-one additional patients underwent surgery because of other study parameters, but to date no ovarian cancers have been reported.

Table 7-5 summarizes all of the above reports. At 1 year of follow-up all of the studies showed sensitivities of approximately 100%. The sensitivities and positive predictive values are shown in the table. Only 13 stage I ovarian cancers were found, and of these only five were epithelial histology, among the 11,283 women screened, including 486 surgical procedures. Thirty-two surgeries (95% CI = 8 to 41) were required to diagnose one stage I ovarian cancer. If screening is done only on women with a family history of ovarian cancer, 17 surgeries (95% CI = 8 to 41) would be required to find one stage I cancer.

The above studies have taught us the following:

> *TVS screening is optimal in postmenopausal women, in whom ovarian volume does not vary on a physiologic basis. When applied to the premenopausal age group, 60% of ovarian abnormalities disappear spontaneously and no cancers are detected.*

Screening women over age 50 increases the positive predictive value. However, familial ovarian cancer occurs at a lower median age (47 years versus 59 years), making it difficult to design a screening program.[20] A standardized morphology index may help to identify a true high-risk patient requiring surgery. The screening interval is unknown because the lag time for ovarian cancer to develop and metastasize remains unknown. New technologies, including three-dimensional ultrasonography coupled with CDI, may decrease the false positive rates of ovarian cancer screening.

Other Diagnostic Tests: Computed Tomography, Magnetic Resonance Imaging, and Positron Emission Tomography

Other radiologic techniques, including computed tomography (CT), magnetic resonance imaging (MRI), and positron emission tomography (PET), are sometimes helpful in the identification and follow-up of bulky ovarian cancer with metastatic disease or ascites. Their role in screening is of limited value.

Because of the subtle differences of x-ray attenuation in soft tissues and the gastrointestinal tract, CT scanning is associated with a high false negative rate in early ovarian cancer. CT scanning appears more sensitive than ultrasound but is associated with a lower specificity.[21] In addition, the necessity of using intravenous contrast to optimize its use in gynecology, combined with the cost of CT scanning, makes this modality unacceptable as a screening tool.

MRI offers a multiplanar noninvasive evaluation of soft tissue masses in the pelvis by measuring differences in hydrogen content, magnetic relaxation times, and the blood flow through the tissue.[22] MRI is most notable for delineation of endometriosis and mature cystic teratomas. Both MRI and CT have a low sensitivity for identifying peritoneal implants. Because of the low sensitivity and high cost, MRI is also unacceptable as a screening modality.

PET images tissue based on its biochemistry. Using 2-^{18}F-fluoro-2-deoxy-D-glucose (FDG), PET has successfully visualized primary and metastatic ovarian carcinomas. As new radiopharmaceuticals are developed to improve resolution and sensitivity, PET scans may prove valuable in the evaluation of the adnexa.[23]

Monoclonal Antibodies

Monoclonal antibodies directed against cancer-associated antigens have been combined with γ-emitting radionuclides to visualize some solid tumors, including breast cancer, colorectal cancer, and prostate cancer.[24] At least 17 different monoclonal antibodies have been characterized that are reactive with epithelial ovarian cancer, and at least eight of these have been administered to ovarian cancer patients. In patients with known ovarian cancer, the true positive rate has been 80% to 95%. A false negative rate of 10% to 20% and a false positive rate of 50% are noted in the scans performed. The false negative scans include tumor metastasis under 1 cm, tumor necrosis, and undifferentiated tumors for the B72.3 antibody studies.[25] Immunoscintigraphy using ^{111}In CYT-103 (with radiolabeled TAG72 monoclonal antibody) and the B43.13 antibody combined with whole body imaging using single positron emission computed tomography (SPECT) have been performed in known ovarian cancer patients. However, these tests are costly and the studies are in their preliminary stages of development.[26]

IDENTIFICATION OF A HIGH-RISK POPULATION

> *Probably the most significant risk factor for ovarian cancer is advancing age.*

The risk of developing ovarian cancer increases from 15.7 per 100,000 women to 54 per 100,000 with increasing age from 40 to 79 years. Other risk factors include nulliparity, North American or Northern European descent, a personal history of endometrial, colon, or breast cancer, and a family history of ovarian cancer. There is inconsistent evidence regarding the use of fertility drugs as an isolated risk factor. Age of menarche, age at menopause, age at first birth, estrogen replacement therapy, and smoking appear to have little or no effect on risk. Increasing the number of pregnancies (whether full term or not), increasing the length of oral contraceptive use, and increasing the duration of lactation are protective factors, supporting the theory of incessant ovulation in the development of ovarian cancer. It is unclear whether there is an association of talc exposure with ovarian cancer. Four case-control studies reported an excess risk of ovarian cancer associated with perineal talc exposure, although it was not statistically significant.[27]

> *In summary, risk factors for ovarian cancer development are related to ovarian activity, and factors associated with reduced ovulation are associated with a reduced risk.*

GENETICS

With available tools screening for ovarian cancer in the general population, regardless of age, is not recommended. Nonetheless, certain small high-risk segments of the population that may benefit from screening can be identified.

> *One of the clear risk factors for the development of epithelial ovarian cancer is a family history of the disease. About 7% of ovarian cancer patients report a family history.*

Of these patients, 90% report only one relative. The lifetime risk for the development of ovarian cancer is related to the number of first-degree relatives (mother, sister, daughter) with ovarian cancer as well as the identification of a specific inheritable syndrome. The magnitude of this risk is illustrated in Table 7-6.[28] The age of onset of ovarian cancer in the family history is also of major import in determining a lifetime risk. Houlston[29] estimated a lifetime risk of 20% in first-degree relatives of women who develop ovarian cancer before the age of 45. This was based on an analysis of 391 pedigrees from women who were self-referred to an ovarian cancer screening clinic. Because of self-referral bias the estimate of 20% may be inflated, but the importance of early age of onset in the family history remains.

TABLE 7-6

SIGNIFICANCE OF FAMILY HISTORY OF OVARIAN CANCER IN DEGREE OF RISK

Number of first-degree relatives with ovarian cancer	Lifetime risk %
0	1.6
1	5
2	7
Definite hereditary syndrome	40

Estimates of the contribution of specific hereditary ovarian cancer syndromes to the total ovarian cancer burden vary from less than 1% to 10%.

Three syndromes have been identified to date. These include the site-specific ovarian cancer syndrome, the breast-ovarian cancer syndrome, and the Lynch type II syndrome, which is characterized by early onset colon cancer and an excess of ovarian and endometrial cancers.

As is typical of hereditary cancer syndromes in general, all of these syndromes are characterized by early age of onset.

The mean age of onset of ovarian cancer in the general population is 59, compared with 50.6 in the breast-ovarian cancer syndrome, 49 in the site-specific ovarian cancer syndrome, and 45 in the Lynch type II syndrome. Statistical analysis of these age differences reveals a highly significant difference between the age of onset in the general population and the age of onset in the hereditary syndromes as a whole.[30,31] In addition, the differences between the syndromes were significant, although the *P* value was only .05. These syndromes are characterized as well by an autosomal dominant inheritance pattern with regard to the major cancer in the group. In other words, this is true for ovarian cancer in the site-specific syndrome, breast cancer for the breast-ovarian cancer syndrome, and colon cancer for the Lynch type II syndrome. The exact risk of ovarian cancer development in the latter two syndromes is not known, although it is clearly in excess of the general female population without heredity cancers. With an autosomal dominant inheritance pattern, 50% of patients with the site-specific ovarian cancer syndrome will inherit the trait. The penetrance of the trait is thought to be about 80% so the risk of developing the disease is about 40%.

The diagnosis of a hereditary ovarian cancer syndrome requires the construction of an informative pedigree from the family history. Many obstacles make this process difficult, if not impossible (Table 7-7). Unfortunately, genetic markers have not been discovered that can identify patients with a hereditary syndrome, with the possible exception of the breast-ovarian cancer syndrome. King et al.,[32] using genetic linkage analysis, identified chromosome 17q12-21 as the location of the BRCA1 gene. BRCA1 appears to encode a tumor suppressor gene. The functional BRCA1 protein is present in normal breast and ovarian epithelial tissue and is altered, reduced, or absent in some breast and ovarian tumors. It is estimated that BRCA1 mutation female carriers experience an 85% risk of developing breast and/or ovarian cancer. At the moment, carriers of this gene can be identified only in special research settings. Screening for BRCA1 mutations is likely to be the first widespread presymptomatic genetic test that finds its way into general medical practice. Extensive counseling will be necessary by the ge-

TABLE 7-7

FACTORS ASSOCIATED WITH DIFFICULTY IN DETERMINATION OF FAMILIAL ORIGIN OF OVARIAN CANCER

Small family size
Families that have predominately male offspring
Unknown paternity of offspring
Difficulty of obtaining medical records
Premature death preventing genetic expression of ovarian cancer
Patient refusal to give information
Physician noncooperation
Misclassification of ovarian cancers as nonovarian cancers
Ignorance of patients as to the cause of death of family members

neticists and treating physician, since disclosure of such information would have substantial psychologic and economic ramifications.[33-35]

In women whose family history clearly reveals a specific hereditary syndrome, screening is warranted. This policy is best summarized in the following statement from the National Institutes of Health (NIH) consensus conference on ovarian cancer held in April of 1994.

> *"There are no data demonstrating that screening these high-risk women reduces their mortality from ovarian cancer. Nonetheless, annual rectovaginal examination, CA-125 determination, and transvaginal ultrasonography are recommended in these women until childbearing is completed or at age 35, at which time prophylactic bilateral oophorectomy is recommended to reduce this risk."*

Prophylactic oophorectomy unfortunately is no guarantee that these patients will not develop a peritoneal carcinomatosis. Primary peritoneal neoplasms may occasionally arise from coelomic epithelium. It is possible that residual embryonic tissue may have given rise to neoplasia that resembles ovarian carcinoma. The exact risk of this occurrence is largely unknown.[36] Piver[37] reported six cases in 324 women from the Gilda Radner Familial Ovarian Cancer Registry who underwent prophylactic oophorectomy, with follow-up ranging from 1 to 27 years.

Neither screening nor prophylactic oophorectomy is recommended for women with one first-degree relative with ovarian cancer. The possible exception to this would be the woman whose relative developed ovarian cancer before the age of 45. Piver[38] has recommended screening and prophylactic oophorectomy in women with two or more first-degree relatives with ovarian cancer. This seems reasonable, although the great majority of these women do not have a family pedigree documenting a specific hereditary syndrome. Lynch et al.[39] recommended prophylactic oophorectomy only in patients who approach a 50%

TABLE 7-8

ACOG RECOMMENDATIONS FOR PROPHYLACTIC OOPHORECTOMY

Confirmation of Indication

A physician may recommend prophylactic bilateral oophorectomy based on documentation of any one of the following:
- Two or more first-degree relatives with epithelial ovarian cancer suggesting either maternal or paternal transmission
- Pedigree of multiple occurrences of nonpolyposis colorectal cancer, endometrial carcinoma, and ovarian cancer (Lynch syndrome II)
- Pedigree of multiple cases of breast or ovarian cancer

Action Before Procedure
- Obtain pedigree of the patient's family history of cancers, especially those of the ovary, breast, bowel, or endometrium
- Seek documentation that the affected relatives' malignancies were actually of ovarian epithelial origin
- Document counseling with patient regarding her relative risk for cancer and risk by age of occurrence, including the potential benefits of oral contraceptive use
- Document patient's childbearing history and her understanding that the procedure results in sterility
- Counsel patient that oophorectomy does not eliminate her risk of peritoneal papillary serous adenocarcinoma

Unless otherwise stated, each numbered item must be present.

From American College of Obstetricians and Gynecologists: *Prophylactic oophorectomy,* ACOG Technical Bulletin 111, Washington, DC, 1987, The College.

risk for development of ovarian cancer and who have completed their families. This is particularly important in women in direct cancer-prone lineage of breast-ovarian cancer families who have already manifested breast cancer. These women are obligate gene carriers, and prophylactic oophorectomy is of the highest importance. The current recommendations by the American College of Obstetricians and Gynecologists regarding a prophylactic oophorectomy to prevent epithelial ovarian cancer are shown in Table 7-8.[40]

MOLECULAR BIOLOGY AND OVARIAN CANCER SCREENING

Tumor development has been associated with aberrant, dysfunctional expression and/or mutation of various genes. This can include oncogene overexpression, amplification, or mutation; aberrant tumor suppression (antioncogene) expression, or mutation; and the inappropriate expression of cytokines and growth factors, or cellular receptors for cytokines and growth factors.

Because ovarian epithelium must proliferate to heal cyst rupture (from processes such as ovulation), ovulation must be associated with the growth and/or differentiation of ovarian epithelial cells. Cytokines and growth factors, including transforming growth factors (TGF-α) and IL-6 have been found in ovarian follicular fluid. With repeated ovulation and healing there exists a greater chance of a genetic accident in DNA replication that could activate an oncogene or inactivate a tumor suppressor gene.

Aberrant expression of various oncogenes in ovarian cancer includes HER2/neu, c-*fms, ras, myc, myb,* macrophage colony-stimulating factor (M-CSF). In addition to HER2/neu being overexpressed in breast cancer, normal ovarian epithelium expresses low to moderate levels. HER2/neu is overexpressed in 30% of ovarian malignancies and appears to be highly indicative of a poor prognosis and survival. When HER2/neu overexpression was seen, these ovarian cancer cells were more resistant to tumor necrosis factor (TNF) or lymphokine-activated killer cell mediated lysis.[41] Both M-CSF and *fms* are expressed in many ovarian cancer cells. The levels of *fms* transcripts correlate strongly with high-grade and advanced clinical stage ovarian cancers.

The p53 tumor suppressor gene, on chromosome 17p, is overexpressed in 30% to 50% of ovarian cancers. The p53 gene product appears to regulate cellular growth and development. Mutations result in a dominant transformed phenotype, preventing the formation of a functional DNA-binding, regulatory complex.

The retinoblastoma (Rb) locus is another antioncogene that is seen in ovarian cancer.

Growth factors and cytokines play an important role in the development and growth of cancer. Epithelial ovarian cancer may in fact be a cytokine-propelled disease.

Transforming growth factor-β (TGF-β), epidermal growth factor (EGF), and TGF-α are among the growth factors that have been evaluated. Tumor necrosis factor (TNF-α, interleukin-1 (IL-1), M-CSF, and IL-6 are cytokines that may also play important roles in ovarian cancer. M-CSF is elevated in 70% to 80% of ovarian cancers and produces other cytokines, including IL-1 and IL-6, whose exact roles are unclear. M-CSF may modify the tumor cell environment, resulting in enhanced tumor cell growth.

The cytokine IL-10 has been found, along with other cytokines, in the peritoneal cavity. IL-10 is believed to be a cytokine synthesis inhibitory factor, suppressing the release of IL-1, IL-6, IL-8, and TNF-α. Studies are under way to determine whether a specific cytokine/tumor marker/acute phase reactant pattern could be useful in monitoring the progress of patients with ovarian cancer. The levels of various cytokines in ascites are also being evaluated to determine if certain cytokines could result in a peritoneal environment that is immunodeficient and unresponsive and promotes tumor growth.[42]

PRIMARY CARE GUIDELINES

Ovarian cancer is the fourth leading cause of cancer death in American women. It is a particularly difficult disease to manage, since 70% of women have metastatic disease at the time of diagnosis and the overall 5-year survival is only 37%. If appropriate tools can be identified, screening in ovarian cancer would be useful, since 85% to 90% of patients diagnosed with early-stage disease survive.

Pelvic examination is clearly an inadequate screening tool. Tumor markers have been tested, most notably serum CA-125. The sensitivity and specificity are inadequate for screening, particularly in premenopausal women. The specificity improves markedly in postmenopausal women; however, with the prevalence of the disease the false positive to true positive ratio is 50 to 1. Another problem with serum CA-125 is that 50% of patients diagnosed with early stage ovarian cancer do not have an elevated value.

Various imaging tests have been suggested. Ultrasound, particularly TVS, is the most accurate modality. Screening of over 11,000 women with pelvic ultrasonography has been reported in the medical literature. As with serum CA-125, specificity was inadequate for screening, and there was an unacceptably high false positive rate. This remained true even if morphology indices and CDI were added.

Routine screening for ovarian cancer in the general population is not recommended by the American College of Obstetrics and Gynecology (ACOG).[43] The Society of Gynecologic Oncologists (SGO) concur that there are insufficient data to recommend any routine screening for ovarian cancer. There has been interest in looking at high-risk groups for screening. Advancing age and a family history of ovarian cancer are clear risk factors for developing the disease. Nonetheless, screening women over the age of 50 and those with a family history of the disease presents the same problems with specificity and false positive rate as general screening. For this reason the Early Detection Branch of the NCI has launched a large randomized clinical trial to screen for prostate, lung, colon, and ovarian cancers. This trial will include 74,000 postmenopausal (over age 60 years) women randomized to screening or to routine care. The endpoint will be patient mortality, the testing will include CA-125 and TVS, and the patients will be followed for at least 10 years.

> *Screening is recommended for some very high-risk patients. Those patients with a specific inheritable ovarian cancer syndrome and women with two first-degree relatives with epithelial ovarian cancer clearly should be screened. The current recommendation for those patients is annual rectovaginal examination, serum CA-125, and TVS until childbearing is complete or the woman reaches 35 years of age. At that point prophylactic oophorectomy is recommended.*

Further research in ovarian cancer screening includes new tumor markers and imaging tools. It also includes a multiyear randomized study sponsored by the NCI comparing annual pelvic examination only with a combination of pelvic examination, serum CA-125, and TVS. Prevention of ovarian cancer is an important adjunct to screening. Oral contraceptives have been shown to have a protective effect. As of yet, there is no recommendation regarding the use of oral contraceptives as a preventive measure. This concept, however, clearly deserves further study.

REFERENCES

1. Boring CC et al: Cancer statistics, 1994, *CA Cancer J Clin* 44:7, 1994.
2. Thigpen T et al: Age as a prognostic factor in ovarian carcinoma: the Gynecologic Oncology Group experience, *Cancer* 71:606, 1993.
3. Hulka BS: Cancer screening: degrees of proof and practical application, *Cancer* 62(suppl 8):1776, 1988.
4. MacFarlane C, Sturgis MC, Fetterman FC: Results of an experience in the control of cancer of the female pelvic organs: in report of a 15-year research, *Am J Obstet Gynecol* 69:294, 1956.
5. Herbst AL: The epidemiology of ovarian carcinoma and the current status of tumor markers to detect disease, *Am J Obstet Gynecol* 170:1099, 1994.
6. Zurawski VR et al: Elevated CA-125 levels prior to diagnosis of ovarian neoplasia: relevance for early detection of ovarian cancer, *Int J Cancer* 42:677, 1988.
7. Jacobs I et al: Prevalence screening for ovarian cancer in postmenopausal women by CA-125 measurement and ultrasonography, *Br Med J* 306:1030, 1993.
8. Einborn N et al: Prospective evaluation of serum CA-125 levels for early detection of ovarian cancer, *Obstet Gynecol* 80:14, 1992.
9. Patsner B, Mann WJ: The value of preoperative serum CA-125 levels in patients with a pelvic mass, *Am J Obstet Gynecol* 159:873, 1988.
10. Di-Xia C et al: Evaluation of CA-125 levels in differentiating malignant from benign tumors in patients with pelvic masses, *Obstet Gynecol* 72:23, 1988.
11. Soper JT et al: Preoperative serum tumor–associated antigen levels in women with pelvic masses, *Obstet Gynecol* 75:249, 1990.
12. Hosono MN et al: Different antigenic nature in healthy women with high serum CA-125 levels, compared with typical patients with ovarian cancer, *Cancer* 70:2851, 1992.
13. Campbell S et al: Transabdominal ultrasound screening for early ovarian cancer, *Br Med J* 299:1363, 1989.
14. DePriest PD et al: Ovarian cancer screening in symptomatic postmenopausal women, *Gynecol Oncol* 51:205, 1993.
15. Granberg S, Wikland M, Jansson I: Macroscopic characterization of ovarian tumors and the relation to the histologic diagnosis: criteria to be used for ultrasound evaluation, *Gynecol Oncol* 35:139, 1989.
16. Carter J et al: Flow characteristics in benign and malignant gynecologic tumors using transvaginal color flow Doppler, *Obstet Gynecol* 83:125, 1994.
17. Bourne TH et al: Screening for early familial ovarian cancer with transvaginal ultrasonography and colour flow imaging, *Br Med J* 306:1025, 1993.
18. Karlan BY et al: A multidisciplinary approach to the early detection of ovarian carcinoma: rationale, protocol design and early results, *Am J Obstet Gynecol* 169:494, 1993.
19. Muto MG et al: Screening for ovarian cancer: the preliminary experience of a familial ovarian cancer center, *Gynecol Oncol* 51:12, 1993.
20. van Nagell JR Jr: Ovarian cancer screening, *Cancer* 68:679, 1991 (editorial).
21. Buy JN et al: Epithelial tumors of the ovary: CT findings and correlation with US, *Radiology* 178:811, 1991.
22. Brown HK et al: PC-based multiparameter full-color display for tissue segmentation in MRI of adnexal masses, *J Comput Assist Tomogr* 17:993, 1993.
23. Hubner KF et al: Assessment of primary and metastatic ovarian cancer by positive emission tomography (PET) using 2-[18F] deoxyglucose (2-[18f] FDG), *Gynecol Oncol* 51:197, 1993.
24. Cohen CJ, Jennings TS: Screening for ovarian cancer: the role of noninvasive imaging techniques, *Am J Obstet Gynecol* 170:1088, 1994.
25. Thor AD, Edgerton SM: Monoclonal antibodies reactive with human breast or ovarian carcinoma: in vivo applications, *Semin Nucl Med* 14:295, 1989.

26. Surwit EA et al: Clinical assessment of III-In-CYT-103 immunoscintigraphy in ovarian cancer, *Gynecol Oncol* 48:285, 1993.

27. Leung Y, DePetrillo AD: Etiology, epidemiology, risk and prognostic factors, screening and imaging of gynecologic cancers, *Curr Opin Oncol* 5:869, 1993.

28. Kerlikowske K, Brown JS, Grody DG: Should women with familial ovarian cancer undergo prophylactic oophorectomy, *Obstet Gynecol* 80:700, 1992.

29. Houlston RS et al: Risk of ovarian cancer and genetic relationship to other cancers in families, *Hum Hered* 43:111, 1993.

30. Lynch HT et al: Hereditary ovarian cancer: heterogeneity in age at diagnosis, *Cancer* 67:1460, 1991.

31. Lynch HT et al: Hereditary ovarian cancer: natural history, surveillance, management and genetic counseling, *Hematol Oncol Ann* 2:107, 1994.

32. Hall JM et al: Linkage of early onset breast cancer to chromosome 17q21, *Science* 250:1684, 1990.

33. Futreal PA et al: BRCA1 mutations in primary breast and ovarian carcinomas, *Science* 266:120, 1994.

34. Miki Y et al: A strong candidate for the breast and ovarian cancer susceptibility gene BRCA1, *Science* 266:66, 1994.

35. Biesecker BB et al: Genetic counseling for families with inherited susceptibility to breast and ovarian cancer, *JAMA* 269:1970, 1993.

36. Tobacman JK et al: Intraabdominal carcinomatosis after prophylactic oophorectomy in ovarian cancer-prone families, *Lancet* 2(8302):795, 1982.

37. Piver MS et al: Primary peritoneal carcinoma after oophorectomy in women with a family history of ovarian cancer: report of the Gilda Radner familial ovarian cancer registry, *Cancer* 71:2751, 1993.

38. Piver MS et al: Familial ovarian cancer: report of 653 families from the Gilda Radner familial ovarian cancer registry (1981-1991), *Cancer* 71:582, 1993.

39. Lynch HT et al: Genetics and gynecologic cancer. In Hoskins WJ, Perez CA, Young RC, editors: *Principles and practice of gynecologic oncology*, Philadelphia, 1992, JB Lippincott.

40. American College of Obstetricians and Gynecologists: Prophylactic bilateral oophorectomy to prevent epithelial ovarian cancer, *ACOG criteria set* no. 2, Washington, DC, 1994, The College.

41. Godwin AK, Hamilton TC, Knudson AJ Jr: Oncogenes and antioncogenes. In Hoskins WJ, Perez CA, Young RC, editors: *Principles and practice of gynecologic oncology*, Philadelphia, 1992, JB Lippincott.

42. Barton DPJ et al: Expression of interleukin-2 receptor alpha (IL-2Rα) mRNA and protein in advanced epithelial ovarian cancer, *Anticancer Res* 14:761, 1994.

43. American College of Obstetricians and Gynecologists: Routine cancer screening, *ACOG Technical Bulletin* no. 128, Washington, DC, 1993, The College.

SKIN CANCER AND MELANOMA

Rona M. MacKie
Howard K. Koh
Alan Geller
Douglas S. Reintgen

EPIDEMIOLOGY

The 5-year survival of all patients diagnosed with malignant melanoma has increased from 40% in 1940 to greater than 80% in 1990.

> *However, the death rate for melanoma has doubled in the last 35 years with increases of approximately 5% per year in the older white population.*

Melanoma may be one of the most extensively researched solid tumors because of the ease of diagnosis with a noninvasive skin examination and the ability to completely excise most tumors with a simple skin biopsy. Prevention, education, and early detection should decrease melanoma morbidity and mortality, since the cancer is visible and external, risk factors are well accepted, and early detection of melanoma is associated with a high 5-year survival rate.

The United States has spent $22 billion in the 20 years since President Nixon signed the National Cancer Act on December 23, 1971. Major advances in the basic science of cancer have followed, including the discovery of oncogenes and other genetic abnormalities, detection of growth factors with early clinical application, and the various immunotherapy approaches for treating cancer. Molecular biology techniques have resulted in a better understanding of malignant transformation. Despite these advances, the incidence of cancer has increased 15% over the past 20 years, and the death rate of some tumors, including melanoma, continues to rise. Today's discoveries in molecular biology may take at least 10 years to be realized in the clinical arena. Progress in the next decade will most likely be realized by the prevention and early detection of disease. Malignant melanoma is a tumor that lends itself to this approach.

Decreasing melanoma mortality can be achieved by either primary or secondary prevention. Primary prevention of melanoma centers on efforts to avoid excessive sun exposure and practice safe sun strategies. Secondary prevention concentrates on early detection, such as public and professional education on the features of early melanoma, the importance of self-examination, and seeking prompt treatment at an early, curable stage.

DEFINITIONS

The terms *case finding, screening,* and *surveillance* require definition. The formal definition of case finding is the incidental detection of cancer within the routine physical examination or physician visit for an unrelated medical complaint. *Screening* for melanoma involves the systematic cutaneous examination of a population. Population screening involves the systematic screening of a selected group from one geographic area, with individuals selected on the basis of age, sex, or other features. Screening may also be confined to those known to be at increased risk of melanoma, for example, those with a family history of melanoma, those who are known to have multiple nevi, or those who have other risk factors. *Surveillance* is the ongoing examination at regular intervals of individuals for the development of new pigmented lesions that may be early malignant melanoma. The interval at which surveillance examinations take place varies, ranging between 3 and 6 months. Surveillance is a labor-intensive exercise confined to a small number of centers examining individuals at an increased risk of developing primary malignant melanoma, including persons with one primary melanoma and individuals with a family history of melanoma and large numbers of benign nevi. Because these early detection methods involve the same screening method, that is, the visual skin examination, some may find the distinctions between these activities to be somewhat arbitrary.

Although earlier activities have attempted to show reductions in mortality from melanoma control programs, well-designed randomized controlled studies are necessary to prove this benefit.

EFFICACY OF SCREENING

The biologic and clinical behavior of melanoma supports a theoretical potential for screening, in that thin melanoma is often associated with cure, whereas thicker, more advanced disease is not. The need for screening is based on the increasing melanoma incidence and mortality rates (Figure 8-1). Melanoma now has an incidence and mortality that are increasing faster than any other cancer in the United States, except for lung cancer in women.

Unlike other cancer sites, the skin can be directly viewed, and thus almost all patients with the diagnosis have their primary lesion visible, with the remainder having unknown primary or mucous membrane melanomas.[1]

> *The screening skin examination is a simple visual inspection that is brief, noninvasive, inexpensive, and regarded as reliable in diagnostic settings.*

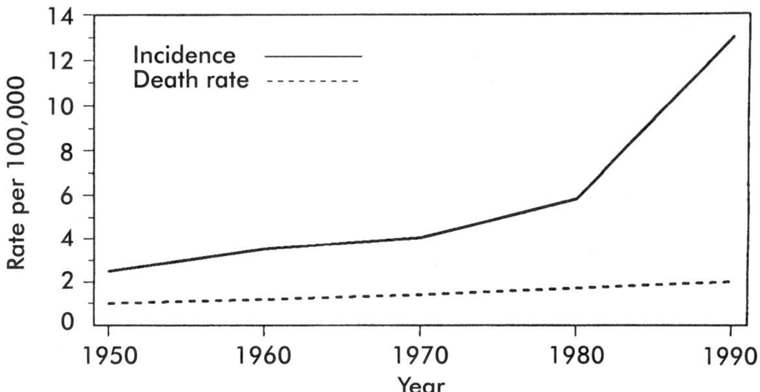

Figure 8-1   Increasing malignant melanoma incidence and mortality rates in the United States.

However, the quality of the screening test for melanoma varies widely and requires careful evaluation. Both Kelly[2] and Rigel[3] have documented the need for a total skin examination to find most cutaneous melanomas, and this recommendation seems to be accepted by most registrants at screening clinics.[4] Preliminary estimates from the American Academy of Dermatology/American Cancer Society (AAD/ACS) national skin cancer/melanoma screening project show that a thorough examination by trained dermatologists can be accomplished in an average of 7 minutes,[5] which also includes a discussion of the results of screening with the person undergoing the examination. Other examiners with different training may take longer.

> *The diagnostic step consists of a simple punch biopsy, and some centers have found it easy to incorporate the diagnostic biopsy in the screening clinic setting.*

Costs are also minimal, and an estimated $50 to $75 charge for a skin biopsy compares favorably to the diagnostic step for breast cancer, a needle-directed breast biopsy for a nonpalpable mammographic lesion, which may cost 30 to 70 times as much.

Melanoma is also theoretically conducive to screening because a detectable preinvasive phase corresponds to the noninvasive radial growth phase that may last months or even years.[6] This clinically apparent radial phase consists of horizontal growth of the melanoma without the potential for metastases.[7] Since the radial growth phase may last for years, the changes may be found during interval screening examinations.

Detection of Thin Melanomas

Further investigations also indirectly support the efficacy of screening for melanoma. Investigators have noted that thinner melanomas are found in screened populations,[8] in those diagnosed coincidentally on physical examination,[9] and when there is no delay between detection of a suspicious lesion and the physician visit.[10] The most intensely screened populations perhaps should be persons with a history of melanoma and those kindreds with the dysplastic nevus syndrome (DNS). Masri[11] describes a population of 555 individuals among 264 familial melanoma kindreds who were followed closely every 3 months. The average tumor thickness of the 48 index cases of melanoma in this population was 1.44 mm compared with 0.52 mm for 28 surveillance incident melanomas and 0.55 mm for 64 nonsurveillance incident melanomas ($P < .001$). The author concluded that surveillance on populations at high risk could have a beneficial effect.

Secondary Lesions

Patients with a history of one melanoma are also at an increased risk of developing another primary lesion. Rogers[12] estimates the lifetime cumulative incidence of second primaries to be 1.3% to 6.5%, whereas others have seen second and third primaries develop in 7% of their melanoma populations.[13] Patients with thin melanomas are more likely to be diagnosed with a second primary than to have the original thin lesion recur, if one estimates the chance of recurrence with a melanoma less than 0.76 mm to be less than 1% and the chance of a second primary to be 7%. In addition, the likelihood of second primaries in DNS has been reported to be 30%. These individuals have a 9 to 12.5 times higher risk of developing a second primary tumor when compared with individuals in the general population. Other high-risk groups for the development of second melanomas are populations who develop the disease at an early age or those who have a compromised immune system. Clinicians involved with these patients note that the second primary is always thinner than the first and potentially curable when tumor thickness is under 0.76 mm.

Prophylactic Lesion Removal

Another line of evidence to suggest the efficacy of screening and early removal of atypical pigmented lesions is the finding that if patients are kept free from atypical moles, they are also kept free from melanoma. Cohen[14] has recently reviewed his 14-year experience with prophylactic skin nevus removal. Seventy-five of 250 individuals with a history of melanoma underwent prophylatic removal of multiple skin nevi, and 28% of the lesions showed some atypia. Twelve melanomas were discovered, and it was estimated from previous reports of prevention of melanoma with dysplastic nevus removal[15] that four to six additional melanomas were prevented by excising precursor lesions. During the same period another 112 individuals without a history of melanoma underwent prophylactic lesion removal. Three cases of melanoma were found, and it was estimated that another three to five cases were prevented with the removal of the precursor lesion. An average of 2.7 lesions were removed among all screened patients. No melanoma-related deaths were reported during this 14-year period.

Tumor Thickness at Diagnosis

Another factor supporting melanoma screening is the intermediate end point for efficacy—the tumor thickness at diagnosis. Multiple regression analy-

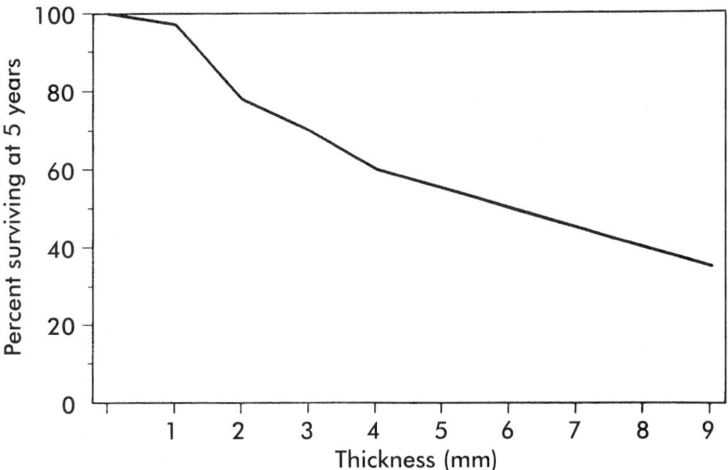

Figure 8-2   Breslow thickness versus survival. There is an almost linear relationship between increasing melanoma thickness and decreasing survival.

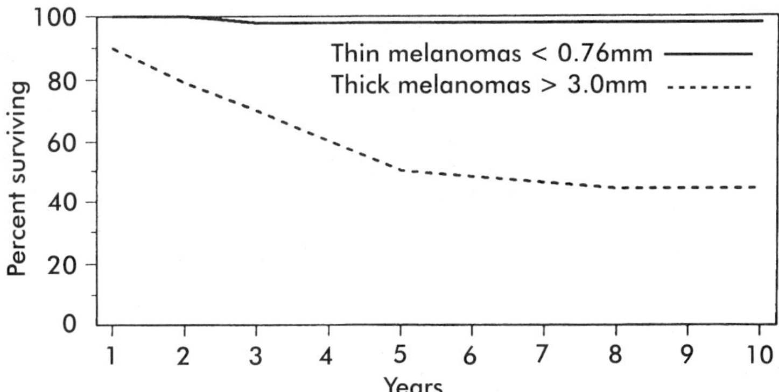

Figure 8-3   Survival versus tumor thickness in malignant melanoma. There exists a large separation between the thin curable lesions and intermediate or thick melanoma.

ses have repeatedly confirmed tumor thickness to be the most powerful prognostic factor for stages 1 and 2 melanoma.[16,17] Tumor thickness helps the clinician estimate the chance of occult nodal and systemic metastases, the need for elective node dissection, and, indeed, the eventual prognosis for the patient. There is a high correlation between tumor thickness and survival (Figure 8-2). Five-year survival for persons diagnosed with melanoma less than 0.76 mm is an estimated 96% compared with 30% for persons diagnosed with lesions greater than 4 mm (Figure 8-3).[18] Although the true power of a screening examination can be eventually judged only by survival data, investigators do not have to wait 5 or 10 years to measure the effectiveness of a program. A steady drop in mean tumor thickness at diagnosis and a drop in absolute numbers of thick lesions should lead to increasing survival of the screened population.

Australian Data

This phenomenon is illustrated by data from the Sydney, Australia, Melanoma Project. Australia has the highest incidence of melanoma of any location in the world because of its equatorial climate and an immigrant Celtic popula-

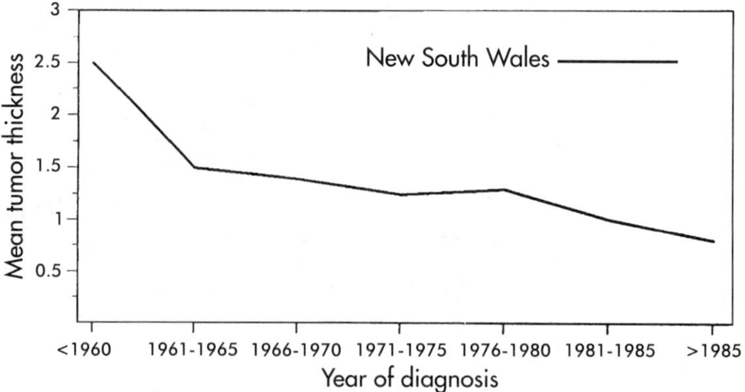

Figure 8-4   Data from the Sydney Melanoma Unit, NSW, Australia, showing a decreasing trend for melanoma tumor thickness at diagnosis that has resulted in an increase in survival of the group of melanoma patients diagnosed in the latter years.

tion. The mean tumor thickness at diagnosis in 1960 for this area was greater than 2.5 mm. In 1960 an intensive education campaign was instituted for the lay public and community physicians on the early signs of malignant melanoma. Almost immediately more patients were referred to skin cancer specialists, more melanomas were diagnosed, and the mean tumor thickness began to fall (Figure 8-4).[19] By 1986 the mean tumor thickness at diagnosis had decreased to 0.8 mm.[20] This was associated with an increased diagnosis of superficial spreading melanoma in the radial growth phase, a decrease in the diagnosis of ulcerated lesions, which have a worse prognosis, and an increase in survival. The 5-year survival before 1960 for stages 1 and 2 melanomas was 82%, improving to 94% in the last decade.

> *Thus the earlier decrease in tumor thickness at diagnosis seen in data from Australia eventually influenced the survival data.*

To date, however, the incidence of melanoma continues to rise in Australia, and the mortality rate remains stable.

Data from Scotland

Studies from other parts of the world confirm the increase in survival noted with the diagnosis of thinner melanomas. Early work in Scotland[21] showed that a high percentage of patients were presenting with thick melanomas, defined as tumor thickness greater than 1.5 mm. Eighty-four percent of individuals delayed seeking medical advice for more than 3 months after noticing a new or changing pigmented lesion. Patient delay was caused by a lack of knowledge of the consequences of a new or changing pigmented lesion. Armed with this data, a public and professional education campaign began in Glasgow.[22] The response and the resulting publicity led to a 380% increase in the number of patients referred to pigmented lesions clinics. This was associated with a doubling in the number of melanomas diagnosed per month compared with the period before the interventions. There was an overrepresentation of younger females and an underrepresentation of older males in the population attending the clinic.

> *An analysis of thickness of melanomas at diagnosis in the whole of Scotland from 1985 has shown a sustained and significant shift in favor of the diagnosis of thinner lesions.*

The percentage of detected tumors less than 1.5 mm in thickness rose from 38% in the 1979 to 1984 period to 54% in 1985 to 1989.[23]

> *Melanoma mortality trends show a downward slope for females in the west of Scotland, but the trend for males is still upward.[23,24]*

AMERICAN ACADEMY OF DERMATOLOGY SKIN CANCER EDUCATION AND SCREENING

The ideal study for skin cancer screening would be a randomized prospective trial. No such randomized trial currently exists in the United States or worldwide. In addition, case-control studies are not possible until the screening exposure becomes more prevalent. Short of this the AAD has promoted free melanoma and skin cancer education and screening programs as a demonstration project throughout the United States since 1985. In this effort local and national media disseminate public information about melanoma and skin cancer. In addition, volunteer dermatologists provide educational materials and free screenings (visual examinations) in special sessions open to the public. Education and screening for early detection are offered together because of the unique external and visible nature of the disease and to take advantage of the "captive" audience registered for the screening.

From 1985 to 1993 this volunteer effort has grown rapidly, providing more than 650,000 free screenings to at least 600,000 Americans. Screenings have averaged nearly 100,000 persons per year since 1990.

Education

AAD-sponsored skin cancer education primarily occurs during the spring of each year, when national and local media publicize the availability of free skin cancer screening programs and at the same time disseminate educational messages (through newspaper, radio, and television) alerting the public to the warning signs of skin cancer risk factors and the importance of early detection and sun protection. For example, in May 1992, 238 television stations in more than 150 U.S. cities (with populations greater than 50,000) carried skin cancer broadcasts during prime-time news coverage. These messages penetrated all 30 of the top television markets in the United States, reaching an estimated 50 million Americans. Further data are needed to determine how these messages affect knowledge, attitude, and behavior.

Screening Organization

Free screening programs are generally conducted in community hospitals, physician offices, area workplaces, and local shopping malls. Volunteer screening dermatologists provide educational materials and visually examine the skin for cancer (melanoma, basal cell carcinoma, squamous cell carcinoma) and precancerous lesions (atypical mole/dysplastic nevus). No biopsies or diagnostic studies are performed. Screening participants found to have lesions suspected of being cancerous or precancerous are asked to consult a dermatologist or their own family physician after the screen to obtain definitive diagnosis and appropriate treatment. AAD staff encourage persons to seek follow-up medical care and provide names of physicians in the area. All persons across the country with suspected melanoma receive telephone calls and letters to ensure rapid follow-up.

Screening Results

Local Programs

The national screening program in the United States, co-sponsored by the AAD and the ACS, has registered an increasing number of people each year in the program (Figure 8-5), suggesting the demand for this public service. The AAD program was not designed as a formal screening study, and the evaluation has been limited to preliminary analyses. Nevertheless, important questions can be answered with information from areas in which local follow-up was possible. Koh et al.[25] achieved 85% follow-up of 2560 patients screened in Massachusetts; 30% of the screened population had an abnormal examination and 0.3% had melanoma. An appropriate self-selection took place in that 86% of the registrants had one of the risk factors for melanoma and 78% had two.

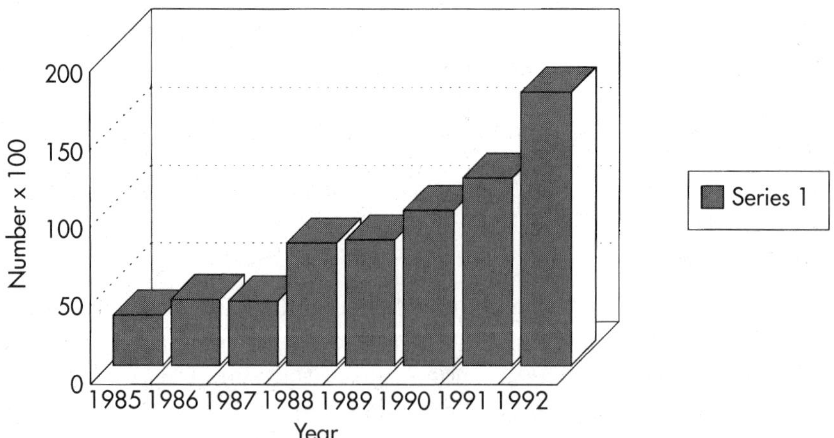

Figure 8-5   Number of registrants per year in the American Academy of Dermatology/American Cancer Society Screening/Education Project.

The screened population had a predominance of white, college educated women, and these investigators have questioned how to attract white men of low socioeconomic status.

Rigel[3] reported on a follow-up study from the 1986 Manhattan program, concentrating exclusively on the yield of biopsy-proven melanomas. Of the 2239 persons screened by dermatologists, 14 cases of melanoma were verified by biopsy. Other issues such as sensitivity, specificity, and compliance with follow-up were not addressed. Further evaluations must address questions such as the compliance with the referral recommendation, the rate of pathologically confirmed results, the sensitivity and specificity of the skin examination performed by various health care providers, and the cost-effectiveness of the program.[25]

Since 1985 dermatologists in the Tampa Bay, Florida, area have taken part in national AAD/ACS skin cancer/melanoma screening project. In 1991 the Moffitt Cancer Center (MCC) screened 234 patients during a 2-hour period. Five possible melanomas were discovered (2.1%), and 28 patients (12%) had a presumptive diagnosis of nonmelanoma skin cancer made.[5] The features of the screened population show that 92% were white and 37% had at least a high school education; 24% were blonde, and 36% had blue eyes. Of the screened population 71% had at least one blistering sunburn and 48% reported a mole change. There was a personal history of skin cancer in 12.9%, a personal history of melanoma in 3%, and a family history of melanoma in 11.5%. About 60% of the population used sunscreens. The high percentage of risk factors in this population (compared with the MCC general patient population) would suggest that there is some self-selection taking place in the screening program and that the Florida population is at high risk for the development of melanoma.

In 1991, over a 2-week period, dermatologists in the Tampa Bay area screened over 3387 individuals and identified 1.2% possible melanomas and 10.1% possible nonmelanoma skin cancers. The characteristics of this expanded population were similar to those screened at MCC, but because of the lack of follow-up, useful clinical information is minimal. There are 1.5 million people in the Tampa Bay area, so the annual screen reaches only 0.2% of the at-risk population.

Education and screening are difficult to separate. In 1987 MCC and the University of South Florida (USF) began a Cutaneous Oncology Program. This is a multidisciplinary clinic with representation from general surgery, plastic surgery, dermatology, pathology, radiology, and medical oncology. In 1995, 500 new melanoma patients were registered at the clinic, accounting for 20% of all the new cases of melanoma that were diagnosed in Florida and 1.5% of the new cases diagnosed nationally.[26] Each year MCC and USF cosponsor a melanoma conference that updates health care providers in Florida and the Southeast on the latest developments in the diagnosis and treatment of the disease. Talks on the differential diagnosis of pigmented lesions, the skin examination, and screening are included. In one sense the Tampa Bay area has a loosely screened population that is served by community physicians with a heightened appreciation for the importance of the skin examination as part of the routine physical. They are perhaps more knowledgeable in the early diagnosis of melanoma. In a retrospective computer-aided review, 607 patients over 4 years have been registered at the Melanoma Treatment Center at MCC and USF. The number of patients with localized disease (stages 1 and 2, negative regional nodes) was 516 (85%). For all stages of disease the 3-year actuarial survival for this loosely screened population was 85%. From the 1990 NCI SEER database, the percentage of melanoma patients diagnosed with localized disease is 77% and the 3-year survival for all stages of melanoma is 81%.[26] From the NCI database of 9879 patients registered with melanoma over a similar period, 75% have localized disease at diagnosis, and the 3-year survival for all stages of melanoma was 76%.[27] There were significant differences noted between the screened Florida population and the nationwide databases using an odds ratio statistic. This involved a higher percentage of patients diagnosed with localized disease ($P < .0001$) and a better survival ($P = .0001$) in the loosely screened, community physician–educated population.[28]

> *Although the comparisons are not ideal, it was concluded that screening and community-based education programs result in earlier diagnosis and improved survival rates.*

Melanoma screening may be worthwhile in a high-risk Florida population with a high incidence of melanoma.

National Programs

As the first step to achieve comprehensive ascertainment of those screened nationwide, the AAD used several follow-up systems for individuals with a screening diagnosis of melanoma in the 1989 to 1993 programs. A centralized follow-up program has now successfully contacted 97% of people in the 1992 to 1993 screened population with a suspected diagnosis of melanoma at the time of screening.[29] Preliminary results find that AAD skin cancer screenings appear to detect early melanoma (almost 99% of all screen-detected melanomas are stages 1 and 2), with fewer advanced melanomas identified compared to the 1990 U.S. SEER registry.

> *Specifically, of those persons with a screening diagnosis of melanoma attending the 1992 to 1993 AAD national programs, 257 melanomas have been confirmed, with all but four cases being diagnosed at a localized stage of disease (AJCC stages 1 and 2).*

Only 18 of the 257 melanomas (7%) discovered during this time have had melanoma thickness greater than 1.5 mm. Lesions that were either in situ or had tumor thickness less than 0.76 mm accounted for 77% of the screened detected melanomas. All but four persons had localized disease.

> *In comparison with 1990 SEER population-based data, screen-detected persons (1992 to 1993) had fewer advanced melanomas (P = .003).*

The investigators caution that the results are preliminary and, lacking a formal control group and without longer follow-up, they cannot make any projections about improved mortality. There is also the strong likelihood that self-selection bias and other screening biases exist.

Access to Screening

AAD screening programs for melanoma/skin cancer in the United States may serve as the sole opportunity for skin cancer examinations for some participants. In an analysis of insurance status and prior dermatologic care among participants (1992 and 1993), 80% of registrants reported not having a regular dermatologist, 52% would not have seen their physician without the screen, and 9% had no health insurance. About 80% were attending their first program, suggesting that screenings also offer an opportunity for many persons to receive their first professional, complete skin examination.

Future Studies

During the next few years further studies should examine issues including the following:

1. The benefit of educational campaigns, for example, can we measure an increase in high-risk persons seeking skin cancer examinations from nondermatologist physicians?
2. Melanoma mortality in intensely screened states versus states without intensive screening
3. Proportions of high-risk persons (for example, men at least 50 years of age) attending screening programs

Rigorous analysis of these and other issues should help determine the ultimate role of education and screening in reducing melanoma mortality.

MELANOMA PREVENTION AND EARLY DETECTION ACTIVITIES IN EUROPE

Melanoma control activities, including primary prevention and early detection programs, are ongoing in several European countries. Public health departments, dermatologists, and others have led campaigns to encourage sensible sun exposure.

One of the first early detection exercises in Europe was conducted by Cristofolini et al.[30] in the provence of Trentino in northern Italy. From 1977 to 1985 this group trained dermatologists in the earlier recognition of malignant melanoma, informed general practitioners of these activities, and led public education self-examination for melanoma using leaflets, conferences, television, and radio. The comparison population for this study comprised the adjacent neighboring areas of Veneto, Alto Adige, and Lombardia. Potential contamination from these adjacent areas was not addressed.

Expected and observed deaths in Trentino were compared for the period 1977 to 1985. For men the expected deaths numbered 40 and the observed 26; for women the expected deaths numbered 34 and the observed 26. Cristofolini et al.[31] estimated that 22 lives have been saved as a result of melanoma education. The cost of the campaign was $70,800, and the cost per year of life saved was calculated at $400.

In Scotland a similar campaign has taken place. In 1985 it was observed that a relatively high proportion of patients had melanoma diagnosed when it was thicker than 1.5 mm.[21,23] A campaign was therefore launched, first to improve early detection of malignant melanoma by those working in the primary care sector, and thereafter to offer public information on the features of early malignant melanoma and encourage rapid self-referral.

Five audit measures were built into the public education campaign: (1) a measure of increasing interest in malignant melanoma, (2) increasing referrals of true malignant melanoma, (3) an increase in the number of thin melanomas excised, (4) an absolute fall in the number of thick melanomas excised, and (5) a fall in melanoma mortality trends. From the early days of the campaign it was apparent that there was an increasing interest in melanoma with a sharp increase in the number of patients referred with histologically proven melanoma.

Comparison of the Breslow thickness of melanomas excised in the whole of Scotland from 1985 to 1987 with melanomas excised in the years 1980 to 1985 showed a significant increase in the proportion of thin tumors (less than 1.5 mm).

> *Thereafter this was followed by a fall in the absolute number of thick tumors in women but not in men, and subsequently by a downward mortality trend in women but not in men.*

In 1985 the rate per 100,000 female population of melanomas greater than 3.5 mm in tumor thickness was 2, and this rate fell to 1.5 by 1990. In addition, the mortality rate per 100,000 population due to melanoma for women in Scotland in 1985 was 1.7, decreasing to 1.5 in 1990.[31]

This campaign is one of the few that has been carefully audited from the outset and has shown clear evidence that public education using television, radio, newspapers, leaflets, posters, and other measures is an effective method of educating women with early malignant melanoma, but appears to have virtually no effect on men. The reasons for this sex difference are not immediately apparent. One feature, however, may be the extremely useful and informative wave of secondary education published in women's magazines. These may well be an underestimated avenue of health education.

Rampen et al.[32,33] offered screening in the town of Oss and Arahem, Netherlands, in 1989 and 1990, and 2564 individuals took advantage of the offer. One hundred three skin cancers were suspected in this population, and the cost of the campaign, including follow-up, was modest, being estimated at only $6000. Nine melanomas were pathologically confirmed.

Hoffman et al.[34] have reported on 1467 individuals in Bochum, Germany, who attended a screening clinic after publicity was generated. Fourteen pathologically confirmed melanomas were diagnosed in this population, with a ratio of 1 melanoma per 100 individuals examined.

In Austria campaigns conducted in 1988 and 1989 showed a sharp rise in the number of melanomas diagnosed, from 169 in 1988 to 213 in 1989.[35] The mean thickness of these melanomas fell from 1.4 to 1.1 mm. Since these campaigns a return to the earlier year pattern was seen, suggesting that regular reminder campaigns are necessary to maintain early detection activities.

Buillard et al.[36] reported screening activities in Basel, Switzerland. Programs began in 1986 with an augmentation campaign in 1989. A doubling in the number of newly diagnosed cases immediately after the 1986 campaign with a statistically significant drop in the age of diagnoses, and a nonsignificant drop in tumor thickness was reported. However, the recall campaign in 1989 did not appear to produce any significant changes.

In summary, many European countries are currently conducting early detection programs. These activities must be carefully audited and important issues for public education should be identified. Incidence and prevalence of melanoma should be enumerated, and tumor thickness in the population must be monitored for 3 to 4 years preceding any educational activity. Population-based thickness and mortality data must also be monitored upon completion of the intervention. Obtaining these data may be difficult in areas where office-based surgeons, dermatologists, and plastic surgeons may not report pathology findings to centralized cancer registries. Nevertheless, the overall impression is that early detection and melanoma publicity campaigns may lead to presentation of thinner melanomas. If all thin melanomas are lesions that would have in time become thicker tumors, then these activities should lead to a fall in melanoma-associated mortality.

PRIMARY PREVENTION OF MALIGNANT MELANOMA

Primary prevention of malignant melanoma is a long-term exercise. From what is known about the growth kinetics of malignant melanoma, it is likely that trends in falling melanoma mortality and falling tumor thickness might be seen within 3 to 5 years of mounting a public education campaign aimed at secondary melanoma, but the latent interval between receipt of an insult on the skin and development of melanoma may be longer than 20 years. Currently, programs in many European countries educate the public on safe sun exposure,[37] on the assumption that excessive exposure to natural ultraviolet radiation is the most important etiologic agent in developing malignant melanoma. Epidemiologic studies strongly support this hypothesis, with increasing evidence that sunlight exposure in early childhood is a significant risk factor for subsequent development of malignant melanoma. The exact wavelength and action spectrum for the development of malignant melanoma is not yet established.

> *Because of the recently recognized importance of avoiding excessive sun exposure in early life, emphasis also includes the education of young mothers and school-age children.*

A wealth of educational material is now available for primary school children in a variety of European languages. Educational materials stress safe sun approaches, including avoidance of noonday sun, the use of shade (such as trees or sun umbrellas), protective clothing, and frequent application of a high SPF sunscreen.

The field of assessment of primary prevention of melanoma is a new one, pioneered by Robin Marks and David Hill in Australia.[38]

> *Marks and Hill stress that knowledge and attitude changes precede behavioral change and emphasize the importance of age-appropriate material that does not arouse fear or alarm.*

Recently Boldeman et al.[39] illustrated the feasibility of delivering skin cancer education to schools, colleges of nursing science, preschool teachers, and pharmacies in Sweden. In 1993 the United Kingdom cancer research campaign mounted a "Play Safe in the Sun" activity similar to those promoted in Australia. These programs emphasize enjoyment of outdoor activities with appropriate precautions to prevent excessive sun exposure.

These activities are inherently more difficult to monitor and audit than early detection activities, but preliminary surveys in Australia indicate a greater awareness of the hazards of sun exposure. However, there is still considerable room for improvement in the public's knowledge of dangerous sun exposure. For example, a large survey of 22,000 individuals in the United Kingdom in 1993 found SPF 4 to be the most popular sunscreen.

Assessment of the efficacy of primary prevention campaigns is a long-term activity, involving rigorous monitoring of incidence and mortality trends. With increasing availability of leisure time and the possible effects of a fall in ozone levels in the northern hemisphere, it is possible that incidence rates will continue their upward trend of the last 20 years. In the short term, primary prevention campaigns may lead to a flattening of the incidence rate, although there has been no evidence of this to date.

Primary prevention activities also refer to the avoidance of excessive exposure to artificial ultraviolet (UV) radiation. In northern European countries sunbeds and sunlamps have been popular both during the winter months and more recently at all times of year to promote a year-round tan. Three case control studies from Canada, United Kingdom, and Sweden show that excessive use of UV sunbeds to be an additional risk factor for malignant melanoma. Primary prevention activities also should advise against excessive exposure to artificial UV radiation.

Targeting primary prevention messages to the high-risk population has been recommended. In Europe this appears an appropriate strategy because the incidence of melanoma, although rising rapidly, is still relatively low. In contrast, policy decisions in high-incidence countries (such as Australia) target all white persons. MacKie et al.[40] have identified four important independent risk factors, including total number of banal nevi, presence of freckling, presence of three or more clinically atypical or dysplastic nevi, and a history of three or more episodes of severe sunburn. A melanoma risk factor chart, in regular use in a number of clinics, categorizes the population into four main groups. The group with the most significantly increased risk of developing melanoma receives additional advice against excessive sun exposure and possibly surveillance. The chart has recently been extended and confirmed in a German population.[41,42]

Sun avoidance and sensible sun exposure are the mainstays of advice on primary prevention. Currently monitors to measure UV penetration of the skin are being evaluated.[43] Since no safe level of sun exposure has been determined, such monitors must be treated cautiously.

In conclusion, melanoma early detection and prevention in Europe is currently at a relatively early stage compared with that in Australia, but appropriate educational activities to decrease the incidence of melanoma and increase the knowledge of the public are being identified. It is essential that ongoing audit of the efficacy of these systems is conducted so that the most effective approaches can be widely disseminated to public and professional organizations.

PITFALLS OF SCREENING PROGRAMS

Screening for melanoma may not work. Certainly, the finding of amelanotic melanoma in 1% to 2% of the cases may decrease the sensitivity of the skin examination. A fraction of the melanomas, perhaps as many as two thirds of the lesions, arise de novo with no antecedent lesion. The radial growth phase may be too short to detect in a screening interval, although the weight of evidence is to the contrary. And finally, the early changes may be too subtle to be clinically apparent. Nevertheless, the increasing incidence of the disease, the growing understanding of the natural history of melanoma, the well-established effectiveness of treating early melanoma, and the availability of an acceptable, safe screening test are factors that simply do not exist for other cancers and favor the investigation of screening as an early detection for melanoma.

IDENTIFYING A HIGH-RISK POPULATION
DNS Population

> *Screening programs make the most sense if they can be directed at a high-risk population.*

This could include those kindreds with DNS, in whom 30% to 50% are expected to develop melanoma sometime in their life. Programs have been established in this population, and screening has resulted in the diagnosis of thin melanomas that are curable.[11]

History of Melanoma

Individuals with a history of melanoma are at a 9 to 12.5 times greater risk of developing a second primary when compared with the normal population.[12] The second primary lesion in programs that have the intensive follow-up program is always thinner than the first and curable[44] with simple excision with conservative margins. In fact, persons with a thin melanoma on initial diagnosis may have more of a chance of developing a second primary than dying of metastatic melanoma.[12]

This experience is reflected in data from the Cutaneous Oncology Clinic at MCC. Patients with melanoma who present to the MCC clinic are placed in an intensive follow-up/screening program that consists of physical examinations and liver function tests every 3 months for the first 2 years, since this is the interval in which up to 80% of the recurrences in malignant melanoma occur.[45] They are then followed every 6 months thereafter with blood work and chest x-rays. A retrospective computer-aided review showed that 43 patients (7%) developed a second primary lesion, whereas a smaller percentage were diagnosed with more than two primary melanomas. The second primaries were always thinner than the initial melanoma, with a mean tumor thickness of 1.79 mm for the first primary, 0.79 mm for the second primary, and 0.56 mm for the third melanoma. Likewise, the number of Clark level 1 lesions increased and the number of Clark level 4 and 5 lesions decreased when comparing the initial primary to the second and third melanoma. About 30% of the initial lesions were ulcerated, but none of the second and third primaries had this unfavorable prognostic factor. Since beginning the intensive follow-up of the melanoma patients, all the lesions diagnosed subsequently had tumor thicknesses under 1 mm and are considered curable. None of the multiple primary melanoma patients have developed metastatic disease in the local-regional distribution of the second and third primaries, and no patients have died in this series of metastatic disease.[44] It makes sense to screen this high-risk population.

Risk Factor Models

Other investigators[19,25,40,41,46] have identified risk factors for the development of malignant melanoma and have proposed mathematical models to identify the high-risk population suitable for screening. This identification improves the predictive value of a skin examination in the screening setting. The following variables have been identified as important risk factors for melanoma:

1. Total number of common nevi greater than 2 mm[41]
   a. Number of nevi on buttocks[46]
   b. Number of raised nevi on arms[46]
   c. More than 120 nevi between 1 and 5 mm (relative risk = 19.6)[46]
   d. More than five nevi between 5 and 10 mm (relative risk = 10)[40]
   e. One atypical nevus (relative risk = 2.77)[40]
2. Freckling tendency[40]
3. Number of clinically atypical nevi greater than 5 mm[40]

    4. a. History of severe sunburn[40]

       b. Propensity to sunburn[41]

    5. History of nonmelanocytic skin cancer[46]

    6. Time spent outdoors from the age of 10 to 24[46]

    7. Family history of melanoma[25,46]

    8. History of dysplastic nevus[25]

    9. Fair complexion[25]

    10. A changing mole[25]

Counting the number of raised nevi on the arms[46] has been suggested as a simple self-screening test to identify persons requiring physician examination. Prospective randomized controlled trials should assess the feasibility of this procedure so that models can be produced for the population screened. These models can then be applied to statewide and national programs. For example, MacKie et al.[40] followed 116 patients with three or more clinically atypical nevi for at least 5 years. Patients were examined and photographed every 3 to 6 months, and nevi undergoing change were excised for histologic diagnosis. Among 85 patients with no personal or family history of melanoma, five invasive melanomas developed during 583 person-years of follow-up. The expected number in this population was 0.05 and the relative risk was 92 ($P < .001$). There was a similarly increased risk among 24 patients with atypical nevi and a family or personal history of melanoma, with a relative risk reported to be 91. By comparison, no second melanoma developed among 25 patients with previous melanoma but a normal nevus pattern during 213 person-years of similarly intensive follow-up. The risk of melanoma was highest among seven patients with atypical nevi and a family history of melanoma (relative risk = 444). The median thickness of surveillance-detected melanomas was 0.75 mm. This study illustrates the ability to identify a high-risk population that can be followed to detect early, thin, curable melanomas.[40]

Environmental Factors

Screening programs may also consider targeting geographic areas with highest incidence or mortality rates. For example, in the Tampa Bay program the incidence of positive melanoma findings that were later pathologically confirmed for the same year was 1.2%, suggesting a greater incidence of disease in a higher risk population.[28] In fact, Florida has the highest rate of cancer per capita of any state; this has influenced the Florida Senator, Connie Mack, to sponsor The Cancer Screening Incentive Act.[47] This bill will provide a tax credit of up to $250 to reimburse the cost for those individuals who avail themselves of a cancer screening test. Indigent patients are also provided for in the bill: for those individuals who cannot afford a screening test or examination up front, the provider of the service will receive a tax benefit. Recent health care reform rhetoric has included funding for prevention and early detection programs.

Thick Melanoma Populations

High-risk populations may be identified by finding characteristics of patients with thick primary melanomas. In the MCC database 334 patients (220 men and 114 women) have presented with melanomas greater than 3 mm. Of the 220 men, 159 (72%) were over the age of 50 years with an average age of 59. Data from the National Center for Health Statistics indicated that men older than 50 comprise half of all melanoma deaths.[48]

> *It is apparent that males over the age of 50 would be a suitable high-risk population to screen in the Tampa Bay area.*

In 1993 MCC instituted the 5-day-a-week Lifetime Cancer Screening Center to screen persons with a family history of melanoma and men 50 years or older.

SCREENING EXAMINATION

A possible strategy for reducing the morbidity and mortality for melanoma is to incorporate the skin examination as part of the routine physical, since fewer than 20% of people have a regular dermatologist. Fletcher[49] has found that 85% of the population in the United States see a physician every 2 years for a routine physical examination, and routine physicals are among the 10 most common reasons for seeing a physician.[50] Primary care physicians already manage skin problems, and dermatologic complaints constitute 7% of all ambulatory patient visits.[25]

> *It is reasonable to teach community physicians the technique of a good skin examination and biopsy so that they will incorporate a thorough skin examination in routine physicals.*

The accuracy of the skin screening examination between dermatologists and nondermatologist physicians has been tested in two studies. Cassileth[51] compared the accuracy of identifying common skin lesions among a group of 105 nondermatologists, ranging from first-year residents to community physicians with 48 board certified dermatologists. Only 12% of the nondermatologists were able to correctly identify five of six melanomas, whereas 69% of the dermatologists did so. Ramsey[52] and Wagner[53] also found similar results. These results are not surprising, since a 1987 survey[54] of dermatology in the medical school curriculum showed that medical students spend a total of 0.24% of the overall medical school curriculum on dermatology. Future programs should train community physicians, physician assistants, and nurses to perform an accurate, high-quality examination.

The gold standard for the skin examination is the accuracy of the dermatologist's examination in a hospital or screening setting. Kopf[55] reports a sensitivity of 77%, specificity of 99%, and a positive predictive value of 80% in this setting. Others have reported much lower results. Epstein[56] states that he makes an accurate diagnosis of melanoma only 40% of the time. Bosch,[57] from the "freckle bus campaign" in the Netherlands, argued that general practitioners can be taught to detect melanoma and perform the diagnostic biopsy. Future studies should compare dermatologic examinations with those by newly trained non-dermatologist providers. Although intermediate and thick melanomas may be more obvious, provider education programs should teach the skills necessary to detect thin melanomas (< 0.76 mm) (Plates 1 to 3).

MOLECULAR BIOLOGY AND SCREENING

Genetic alterations are known to be intimately associated with the genesis and progression of human cancers, including malignant melanoma. With the advent of new molecular biology techniques and the discovery and cloning of genes that can identify persons with high susceptibility to certain cancers, it may soon become possible to screen large populations for susceptibility to disease with a simple blood test. These screening tests may be performed before patients develop the disease, even in utero. The ethical implications of this approach to screening will have to be established.

Identification of Melanoma/Dysplastic Nevus Gene

Initial reports[58] suggested that there was a linkage between cutaneous melanoma and the dysplastic nevus syndrome (CM/DNS gene) to markers located on the distal portion of the short arm of chromosome 1, a region frequently involved in karyotypic abnormalities in melanoma cells. Dracopoli et al.[59] examined loci on chromosome 1p for loss of constitutional heterozygosity (LOH) in 35 primary melanomas and 21 melanoma cell lines to analyze the role of these abnormalities in the malignant transformation. LOH was identified in 15 of 35 (43%) primary melanomas and 11 of 21 (52%) melanoma cell lines. Analysis of multiple metastases derived from the same patient and of melanoma and lymphoblastoid samples from a family with hereditary melanoma showed that the LOH at loci on the distal arm of 1p was a late event in tumor progression, rather than the second mutation that would occur if melanoma were due to a cellular recessive mechanism.

Investigative Efforts

The reported linkage of the CM/DNS gene to the short arm of chromosome 1 was questioned after the examination of three Utah kindreds with multiple cases of melanoma markers around this chromosomal region.[60] Family members in these kindreds were genotyped for the two chromosomal 1 markers previously reported to be closely linked to the melanoma foci, PND and D1S47. Both melanoma alone and a combined CM/DNS phenotype were analyzed; no evidence of linkage was found. By multipoint linkage analysis the CM/DNS locus was excluded from an area of 55 cM containing the PND-D1S47 region. Diagnostic or genetic heterogeneity was considered the explanation for the discrepancy between the observations. Subsequently, this same group[61] provided evidence that the locus for familial melanoma susceptibility was on chromosomal region 9p13-p22. Linkage analysis of 10 Utah and one Texas kindred with multiple cases

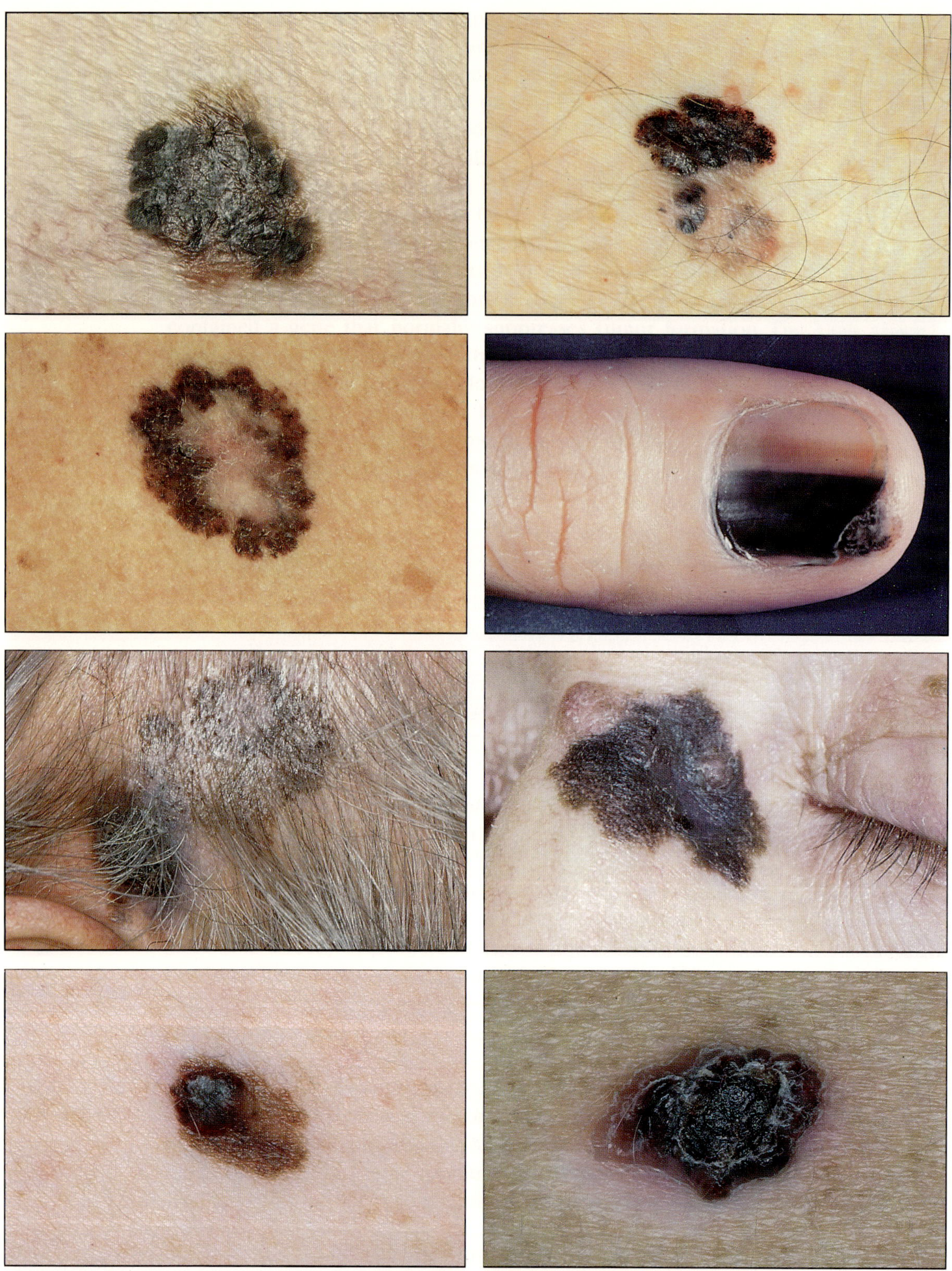

Plate 2 Some subtlety exists for the diagnosis of intermediate thickness melanoma (τ 0.76 mm but $\leq$ 4 mm in thickness). (From Kopf W, Friedman RJ, Rigel DS: *The many faces of malignant melanoma*, New York, 1985, The Skin Cancer Foundation.)

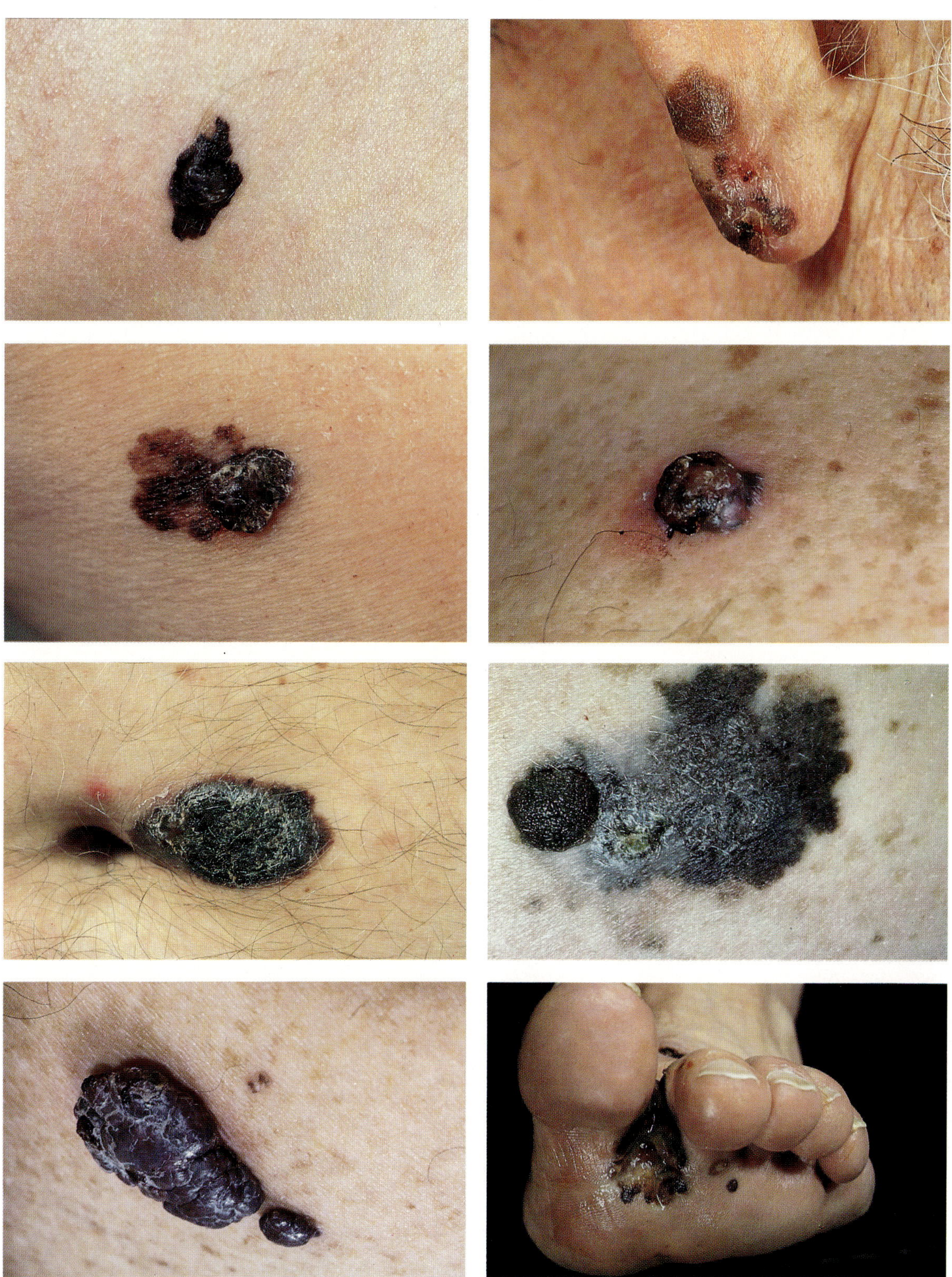

Plate 3   Thick (greater than 4 mm) melanomas have recognizable characteristics that are easy to diagnose. The *ABCD*s of melanoma diagnosis include a change in *A*symmetry of the lesion, irregular *B*order of the lesion, variegated *C*olor pattern, and a *D*iameter above 6 mm. (From Kopf W, Friedman RJ, Rigel DS: *The many faces of malignant melanoma*, New York, 1985, The Skin Cancer Foundation.)

chromosome 4 is lost (corresponds to the human 6q chromosome), the suppression of tumorigenicity is lost. Using a technique of microcell-mediated chromosome transfer of normal human chromosomes directly into murine melanoma cell lines, the effect was quite dramatic. In terms of cell morphology, parental cells grew quickly to confluence, forming foci even at low plating densities; in contrast, the introduction of chromosome 6 resulted in hybrids displaying a flattened stellate appearance and failing to produce foci even at high plating densities. The transformed cells do not express melanoma antigens because they become nonreactive with melanoma-associated monoclonal antibodies. In vivo assays are negative, since transformed cells do not form tumors when implanted into immunodeficient nude mice. This approach suggests that tumor suppressor genes play a critical role in melanoma tumorigenesis.

A novel approach using chromosome microdissection has identified previously cryptic chromosome alterations of potential significance in malignant melanoma. With this technique small amounts (40 fg) of DNA are captured to cause an artificial deletion in chromosome 6. These cells have similar properties to the melanoma cells. A candidate gene on chromosome 6 has been identified that confers the suppressor phenotype. This manganese superoxide dismutase gene is a mitochondrial matrix gene that maps to the distal arm of chromosome 6. A single copy of cDNA placed into melanoma cells suppresses the growth if the cDNA is expressed at high levels. It is also possible to reverse the phenotype.[67]

> *Ideally, a genetic predisposition to disease could be identified so that effective interventions could take place before the development of melanoma.*

Similar to the work that has occurred with colon cancer,[68] breast cancer,[69] and the MENII syndrome,[70] patients identified with the genetic predisposition for melanoma can be counseled for lifestyle changes (avoid UV light exposure) or placed on chemoprevention trials (retinoids).

Ethical Considerations

Molecular genetic screening, however, opens new areas of concerns. Recent advances in cancer genetics have raised the possibility of widespread DNA testing for the detection of the predisposition to cancer. Although alleviation of much human suffering may eventually result from these advances, a number of important questions must be addressed before widespread testing can be recommended[71]:

1. How many different mutations in the genes can be found, and what is the risk of cancer associated with each?
2. What are the technical and laboratory issues associated with the detection of mutations in the genes such as false positive and false negative results and quality control procedures?
3. How effective are interventions to prevent cancer morbidity and mor-

tality in high-risk families and in the general population? For a woman with breast cancer predisposition, tamoxifen or prophylactic mastectomies may be offered, but in conditions without effective intervention, such as muscular dystrophies, genetic screenings may have deleterious consequences.

4. How can education and genetic counseling about the complexities of DNA testing be provided to potentially large numbers of at-risk individuals, and how can informed consent be ensured?

5. How will the possibility of genetic discrimination against those found to be at high risk be avoided? For instance, will a predisposition to cancer be considered by insurance companies a preexisting condition and the identified people uninsurable? Will insurance companies cover interventions such as total thyroidectomies in children who have inherited the mutation for the MENII syndrome and medullary carcinoma, when the pathology specimen will identify only normal thyroid or C cell hyperplasia?

6. Will interruption of pregnancy be warranted for genetic defects found in utero?

Molecular genetic testing for a predisposition for certain cancers is an exciting area of research. The gathering of information and establishing the protocols that will be needed to safely integrate genetic testing and counseling for cancer risk into clinical practice can best be accomplished through a coordinated set of clinical research studies to be cosponsored by the NIH and the National Center for Human Genome Research.

GUIDELINES FOR PRIMARY CARE

> *If screening programs are to have an impact on the early detection of melanoma, primary care providers may need to incorporate the screening physical examination into their routine practice.*

Certainly, with the emphasis on primary care physicians as "gatekeepers" and the goal to increase primary care physicians to 55% of all medical school graduates by the year 2000, it is likely that future community physicians will be more likely to integrate the skin examination into routine practice. The diagnostic procedure, either a punch biopsy or small excisional biopsy, could be incorporated into the generalist's practice, provided that the lesion is not in an area of cosmetic or functional concern, such as the face or palms. Figure 8-6 outlines the management of the patient in a primary care setting. It depends on a number of areas, including (1) the ability of the primary care physician to accurately examine the skin and perform the diagnostic procedure, the skin biopsy, (2) the continued need for referral centers, staffed by skin cancer specialists, such as dermatologists, plastic surgeons, general surgeons (patients to be referred include those with suspicious moles on the face, palms, or soles or those with abnormal biop-

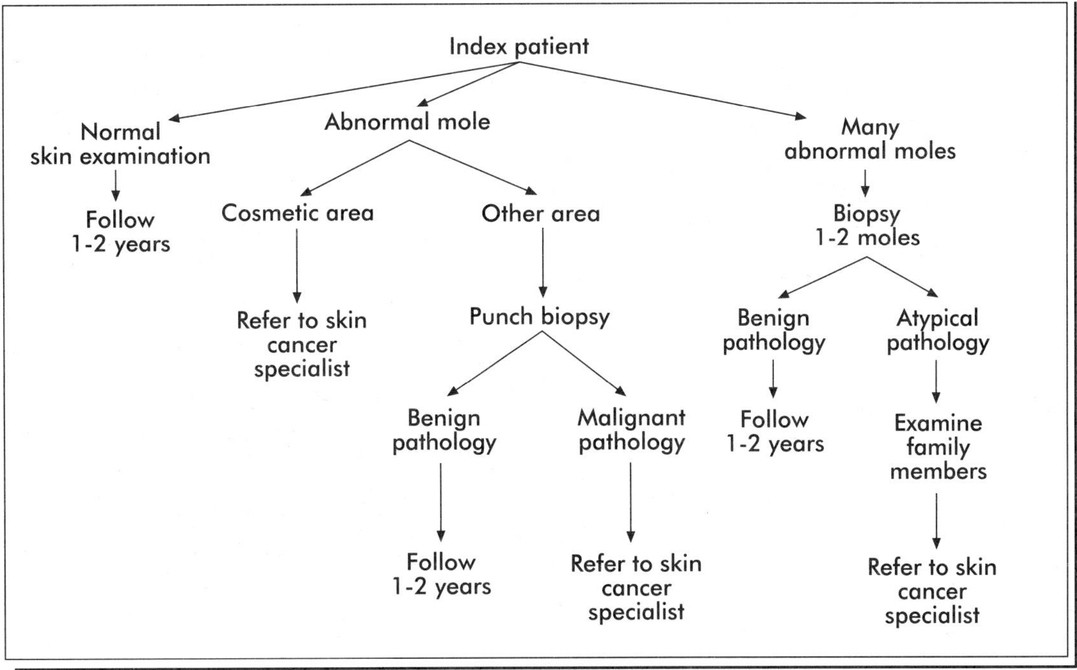

Figure 8-6   Flow diagram for skin screening in the primary care setting.

sies), and (3) a mechanism to screen family members and a forum for genetic screening and counseling.

FINANCIAL/HEALTH POLICY

The average age for melanoma patients presenting for the first time to a local clinic is 59 years for men and 50 years for women. Melanoma is a disease that affects people at the most productive periods of their life. In addition, the total cost for an initial office visit, diagnostic biopsy, and a 1-cm wide local excision under local anesthesia for a thin melanoma ranges from $500 to $1000. In contrast, the medical bill for an intermediate thickness melanoma that requires general anesthesia and a lymph node dissection is $10,000, and a 6-month course of chemotherapy for a stage 4 patient costs as much as $50,000. These figures do not include time lost from work, rehabilitation, and long-term follow-up. It becomes obvious that it would be cost-effective to diagnosis melanoma at the thin stage. If all patients had thin melanomas at diagnosis, a minimalistic approach to follow-up could be considered.

OUTLOOK FOR THE FUTURE

A number of studies would seem to be indicated before public health policy fully embraces the idea of screening for melanoma. The first question to be evaluated is the accuracy and integration of the nondermatologic skin examination. Eventually an efficacy study needs to be performed, otherwise skin cancer screening may not receive the attention that it deserves. A prospective, randomized controlled trial may be impossible to perform in the United States because of practice patterns and the saturation of the population with at least some information on the causes and concerns associated with skin cancer. In lieu of such a trial, enough indirect evidence may be accumulated from other experiences, such as in Scotland and Australia, where public and professional education have attempted to prove the efficacy of melanoma control programs. One possible future project is to compare the stage at diagnosis and the mortality of melanoma diagnosed on the west coast and east coast of Florida. The west coast has a fledgling education/screening project established for the last 6 years, whereas no such organized program exists on the east coast. Results of this study may give indirect evidence of screening efficacy in a high-risk area.

Cost-effectiveness studies and outcome measures of screening for melanoma should also be pursued, particularly with cost-cutting measures sought by health care reform. It is increasingly important for physicians to be able to generate this data, compare outcomes, and provide financial information to third-party companies to document low-cost quality care.

With the advent of molecular genetic screening, patient populations may be screened with a simple blood test for a predisposition to cancer. Tests similar to a chemistry panel may be ordered in the not too distant future that measure an individual's predisposition to a number of cancers. This cancer profile can then be used to counsel the patient and perhaps intercede in the disease process before the development of occult cancer. Lifestyle counseling, such as avoiding sun exposure and self-screening, can be recommended to persons with a predisposing genetic defect for melanoma. Likewise, chemoprevention trials may be performed for high-risk individuals. As in the recently funded chemopreventive trial for breast cancer using the antiestrogen tamoxifen, agents such as the retinoids may be useful in preventing skin cancers and melanoma.

The minimum intervention for individuals predisposed to melanoma would be an intensive follow-up program, such as programs for patients with a history of melanoma and those families affected with DNS. Primary prevention programs with behavioral interventions as well as chemopreventive trials and early detection programs will all play an invaluable role in stemming the epidemic of this cancer.

REFERENCES

1. Reintgen DS et al: Malignant melanoma with an unknown primary, *Surg Gynecol Obstet* 156:335, 1983.
2. Kelly JW: The management of early skin cancer in the 90's, *Aust Fam Physician* 19:1714, 1990.
3. Rigel DS et al: Importance of complete skin exam for the detection of malignant melanoma, *J Am Acad Dermatol* 14:857, 1986.
4. Boyce JA, Bernhard J: Total skin exam: patient reactions, *J Am Acad Dermatol* 14:280, 1986.
5. *Greater Tampa Bay Skin Cancer/Melanoma Screening Project,* American Cancer Society-Florida Chapter, January 1992.
6. Mihm MC Jr, Fitzpatrick T: Early detection of malignant melanoma, *Cancer* 37:597, 1976.
7. Clark WH et al: The histogenesis and biologic behavior of primary malignant melanoma of the skin, *Can Res* 29:705, 1969.
8. Cristofolini M et al: Community detection of early melanoma, *Lancet* 1:18, 1986.
9. Rampen FH, Rumke P, Hart AA: Patient's and doctor's delay in the diagnosis and treatment of cutaneous melanoma, *Eur J Surg Oncol* 15:143, 1989.

10. Temoshek L et al: Factors related to patient delay in seeking medical attention for cutaneous malignant melanoma, *Cancer* 54:3048, 1984.

11. Masri GD et al: Screening and surveillance of patients at high risk for melanoma result in detection of earlier disease, *J Am Acad Dermatol* 22:1042, 1990.

12. Rogers GS: *Follow-up studies: second primary melanoma,* Paper presented at NIH Consensus Development Conference on Early Melanoma, Bethesda, Md, 1992.

13. Hieken T, Ridgeway C, DasGupta T: Multiple primary malignant melanoma. Forty-sixth annual symposium, Society of Surgical Oncology, Los Angeles, 1993 (abstract).

14. Cohen MH et al: Surgical prophylaxis of malignant melanoma, *Ann Surg* 213:308, 1991.

15. Kraemer KK et al: Dysplastic nevi and cutaneous melanoma risk, *Lancet* 2:1076, 1983.

16. Day CL et al: Prognostic factors for patients with clinical stage 1 melanoma of intermediate thickness (1.51-3.99 mm): a conceptual model for tumor growth and metastasis, *Ann Surg* 195:35, 1982.

17. Balch CM et al: An analysis of prognostic factors in 8500 patients with cutaneous melanoma. In Balch C et al, editors: *Cutaneous melanoma,* Philadelphia, 1992, JB Lippincott.

18. Breslow A: Thickness, cross sectional areas and depth of invasion in the prognosis of cutaneous melanoma, *Ann Surg* 172:902, 1970.

19. Balch CM et al: A multifactorial analysis of melanoma. II. Prognostic factors in patients with stage 1 (localized) melanoma, *Surgery* 86:343, 1979.

20. Balch CM et al: Changing trends in cutaneous melanoma over a quarter of a century in Alabama, USA, and New South Wales, Australia, *Cancer* 52:1748, 1983.

21. Roush GC et al: Screening for melanoma. In Balch C et al, editors: *Cutaneous melanoma,* Philadelphia, 1992, JB Lippincott.

22. Doherty VR, MacKie RM: Reasons for poor prognosis in British patients with cutaneous malignant melanoma, *Br Med J* 292:987, 1986.

23. MacKie RM, Hole D: Audit of public education campaign to encourage earlier detection of malignant melanoma, *Br Med J* 304:1012, 1992.

24. Doherty VR, MacKie RM: Experience of a public education program on early detection of cutaneous melanoma, *Br Med J* 297:388, 1988.

25. Koh HK et al: Evaluation of melanoma/skin cancer screening in Massachusetts: preliminary results, *Cancer* 65:375, 1990.

26. Boring CC et al: Cancer statistics 1994, *CA Cancer J Clin* 44:7, 1994.

27. Steele GD et al: Clinical highlights from the National Cancer Data Base: 1994, *CA Cancer J Clin* 44:71, 1994.

28. Reintgen DS et al: Prevention and early detection of melanoma: a surgeon's perspective, *Semin Surg Oncol* 9:174, 1993.

29. Koh HK: Melanoma education and screening in the US: third international conference on melanoma, *Melanoma Res* 3:7, 1993 (abstract).

30. Cristofolini M et al: Analysis of the cost effectiveness ratio of the health campaign for the early diagnosis of cutaneous melanoma in Trentino, Italy, *Cancer* 71:370, 1993.

31. MacKie R, McHenry P, Hole D: Accelerated detection with prospective surveillance for cutaneous malignant melanoma in high risk groups, *Lancet* 341:1618, 1993.

32. Rampen FHJ, van Huystee BEWL, Kiemeney LALM: Melanoma/skin cancer screening clinics: experiences in the Netherlands, *J Am Acad Dermatol* 25:776, 1991.

33. Rampen FJH et al: Lack of selective attendance of participants at skin cancer/melanoma screening clinics, *J Am Acad Dermatol* 29:423, 1993.

34. Hoffmann K et al: A local education campaign on early diagnosis of malignant melanoma, *Eur J Epidemiol* 9:591, 1993.

35. Pehamberger H et al: Immediate effects of a public education campaign on prognostic feature of melanoma, *J Am Acad Dermatol* 29:106, 1993.

36. Bulliard J-L et al: Prevention of cutaneous melanoma: an epidemiological evaluation of the Swiss campaign, *Rev Epidemiol Sante Publique* 40:431, 1992.

37. MacKie RM et al: Report on consensus meeting of the EORTC melanoma group on edu-

cational needs for primary and secondary prevention of melanoma in Europe, *Eur J Cancer* 27:1317, 1991.

38. Marks R, Hill D: The outcomes of melanoma education programs in Australia: third international conference on melanoma, *Melanoma Res* 3:7, 1993.

39. Boldeman C et al: Primary prevention of malignant melanoma in the Stockholm Cancer Prevention Programme, *Eur J Cancer Prev* 2:441, 1993.

40. MacKie RM, Freudenberger T, Aitchison TC: Personal risk factor chart for melanoma, *Lancet* 2:487, 1989.

41. Garbe C et al: Risk factors for developing cutaneous melanoma and criteria for identifying persons at risk: multicenter case-control study of the central malignant melanoma registry of the German Dermatological Society, *J Invest Dermatol* 102:695, 1994.

42. Garbe C et al: Associated factors in the prevalence of more than 50 common melanocytic nevi, atypical melanocytic nevi, and actinic lentigines: multicenter case-control study of the central malignant melanoma registry of the German Dermatological Society, *J Invest Dermatol* 102:700, 1994.

43. Moseley H, MacKie RM, Ferguson J: The suitability of SunCheck patches and Tanscan cards for monitoring the sunburning effectiveness of sunlight, *Br J Dermatol* 128:75, 1993.

44. Reintgen DS et al: Multiple primary melanomas: Evidence for the efficacy of screening and evidence against the minimalistic approach to cancer follow-up care. Forty-sixth annual symposium, Society of Surgical Oncology, Los Angeles, 1993 (abstract).

45. Reintgen DS et al: Recurrent malignant melanoma: the identification of prognostic factors to predict survival, *Ann Plast Surg* 28:45, 1992.

46. Groh JJ et al: Count of benign melanocytic nevi as a major indication of risk of nonfamilial melanoma, *Cancer* 69:387, 1990.

47. Reintgen DS: Innovative cancer screening legislation, *Ann Plast Surg* 28:2, 1992.

48. National Center for Health Statistics: Vital statistics mortality data, multiple causes of death detail, Hyattsville, Md, 1987, US Dept of Health and Human Services.

49. Fletcher S: The periodic health examination and retrieval medium, *Ann Intern Med* 101:866, 1984.

50. Hingson R et al: In sickness and in health, St Louis, 1981, Mosby.

51. Cassileth BR et al: How well do physicians recognize melanoma and other problem lesions? *J Am Acad Dermatol* 14:555, 1986.

52. Ramsay DL, Fox AB: The ability of primary care physicians to recognize the common dermatoses, *Arch Dermatol* 117:620, 1981.

53. Wagner RF et al: Resident's corner: diagnosis of skin diseases—dermatologists versus nondermatologists, *J Dermatol Surg Oncol* 11:476, 1985.

54. Ramsay DL, Mayer F: Material survey of undergraduate dermatologic medical education, *Arch Dermatol* 121:1529, 1985.

55. Kopf A, Mintzis M, Bart R: Diagnostic accuracy in malignant melanoma, *Arch Dermatol* 111:1291, 1975.

56. Epstein E: Thoughts on melanoma, *Dermatol Clin* 2:171, 1984.

57. Bosch MM, Bom ME: Malignant melanoma in a primary care pathologic-anatomical laboratory in 1988 and the freckle bus year. *Med Tijdschv Geneskel* 134:2051, 1990.

58. Green MH et al: Familial cutaneous melanoma: autosomal dominant trait possibly linked to the RH locus, *Proc Natl Acad Sci USA* 80:6071, 1983.

59. Dracoploi NC et al: Loss of alleles from the distal short arm of chromosome 1 occurs late in melanoma tumor progression, *Proc Natl Acad Sci USA* 86:4614, 1989.

60. Cannon-Albright LA et al: Evidence against the reported linkage between cutaneous melanoma-dysplastic nevus syndrome locus to chromosome 1p36, *Am J Hum Genet* 46:912, 1990.

61. Cannon-Albright LA et al: Assignment of a locus for familial melanoma MLM to chromosome 9p13-p22, *Science* 258:1148, 1992.

62. Kamb A et al: Analysis of the p16 gene (CDKN2) as a candidate for the chromosome 9p melanoma susceptibility locus, *Nature Genet* 8:22, 1994.

63. Serrano M, Hannon J, Beach D: A new regulatory motif in cell-cycle control causing specific inhibition of cyclin D/CDK4, *Nature* 366:704, 1993.

64. Marx J: A challenge to p16 gene as a major tumor suppressor, *Science* 264:1846, 1994.

65. Hussussian CJ et al: Germline p16 mutations in familial melanoma, *Nature Genet* 8:15, 1994.

66. Marx J: New tumor suppressor may rival p53, *Science* 264:344, 1994.

67. Trent JM: Cytogenetics of human melanoma. In Balch C et al, editors: *Cutaneous melanoma,* Philadelphia, 1992, JB Lippincott.

68. Fishel R et al: The human mutator gene homolog MSH2 and its association with hereditary nonpolyposis colon cancer, *Cell* 75:1027, 1993.

69. King MC, Rowell S, Love S: Inherited breast and ovarian cancer: what are the risks? what are the choices? *JAMA* 269:1975, 1993.

70. Wells S: The 50/50 chance, Presidential address, Society of Surgical Oncology, 1994.

71. National Advisory Council for Human Genome Research: Statement on use of DNA testing for presymptomatic identification of cancer risk, *JAMA* 271:785, 1994.

9

MISCELLANEOUS TUMORS

Douglas S. Reintgen
John Albertini

BLADDER CANCER

ORAL CANCER

ENDOMETRIAL CANCER

STOMACH CANCER

NASOPHARYNGEAL CANCER

NEUROBLASTOMA

TESTICULAR CANCER

LIVER CANCER

ESOPHAGEAL CANCER

Three basic methods are available to reduce the morbidity and mortality of cancer. Prevention of tumors is in its infancy, with the first trials of chemopreventive agents only beginning. Trials of behavioral interventions remain daunting in their scope and time commitment, and the incidence figures for many cancers continue to increase. These trials are costly and time consuming. The treatment of cancers has been ongoing, but despite advances made in the basic science arena, little has been translated into a clinical effect, and mortality for many cancers has either increased or remained stable during the last decade.

> *Cancer screening holds the greatest promise for public health impact, but similar to prevention trials, these studies are both costly and time consuming.*

Because of practical and organizational difficulties, the potential of cancer screening may not be realized.

The benefits of cancer screening are obvious. Various studies have shown that cancer screening can detect tumors at a lower stage and decrease the mortality in the screened population. The costs associated with doing so are less well defined. For instance, what is the cost of a false positive screen, both in terms of diagnostic tests needed for the workup of a positive screen and the psychologic trauma imparted on the person.

> *How does one begin to factor the price of psychologic trauma or productive life in equations that attempt to calculate the cost-benefit of screening programs?*

Certainly, other potential benefits are possible, such as the possibility of receiving less radial treatment for earlier stage cancers, a reassurance for persons who have a negative screen, and other possible resource savings in treating people early in their disease as compared with the costly treatment that can be associated with caring for patients with stage 4 disease.

Disadvantages of cancer screening are also apparent and, in many people's minds, outnumber the advantages. If cancer screening just provides lead time to diagnosis, quality of life is affected negatively, with earlier detection making no impact on their ultimate survival. A second disadvantage is the overtreatment of borderline cases, since many abnormalities discovered by screening might never have become clinically apparent. For instance, melanoma in situ may have been discovered on a screening skin examination, but the natural history of this histologic diagnosis has not been defined. It is possible that patients with these abnormal moles would do fine without any intervention. Overtreatment of these borderline lesions or tumors in which the natural history is not defined could increase the cost of care.

The false sense of security associated with a negative screen and the stress and trauma associated with a positive screen are often hard to document. Another disadvantage is the potential complications of the screening and diagnostic tests themselves. Because of these potential disadvantages, it is important to evaluate the effectiveness of screening.

> *The gold standard is the prospective randomized study to avoid any bias of screening, but because of cost and contamination of possible control groups, many times these trials are impossible to perform.*

The auditing and monitoring of screening are important to ensure that a program is achieving the benefit expected. Screening programs should not be instituted unless facilities and physicians are available to handle the fallouts of the screening examination.

This chapter reviews the available evidence for the screening of miscellaneous tumors. Most of the evidence for efficacy of screening for these tumors does not come from prospective randomized trials. Indirect evidence of screening effectiveness will be sought to provide guidelines for programs.

BLADDER CANCER

Urinary cytology is capable of detecting urinary bladder cancer in persons in high-risk occupations or those living in areas where urinary schistosomiasis is endemic.[1] Improved survival has been documented with screening in these high-risk groups. Bladder cancer cases detected with screening are often earlier stage cancers and have the potential of requiring less extensive therapy.

Hubert Humphrey's case illustrates the controversies surrounding screening for bladder cancer.[2] In May 1967, while Hubert Humphrey was Vice-President of the United States, he was admitted to Bethesda Naval Hospital for hematuria. Voided urine specimens were obtained for cytologic examination and cystoscopy was performed. Grossly the bladder had the appearance of chronic proliferative cystitis, and a biopsy revealed a focus of dysplasia in the transitional epithelium. No cancer was identified. Humphrey was followed with cystoscopy every 6 months, and a biopsy revealed carcinoma in situ (CIS) in 1969. He remained asymptomatic without any treatment until 1973, when a biopsy revealed CIS with a focus of microinvasion. At that time he was treated with radiation therapy and thiotepa. In August 1976 recurrent hematuria developed and a biopsy showed invasive carcinoma of the bladder. He was treated with a radical cystectomy at the time, and pathology showed a widespread transitional cell carcinoma with lymph node metastases. Humphrey eventually died of his bladder cancer on January 13, 1978.

In this case report urinary cytologies, tumor, and normal tissue were obtained from archival material and analyzed by polymerase chain reaction (PCR) for mutations in the tumor suppressor gene, p53. With this technology a number of cells in Humphrey's urine cytology from 1967 harbored the same p53 mutation that was present in the resected primary carcinoma in 1976.

> *The cells harboring the p53 mutation were detected 9 years before Humphrey underwent cystectomy, 6 years before he received any therapy for bladder cancer, 2 years before the diagnosis of CIS was established and at a time when the cancer could not be detected grossly.[3]*

This finding had a number of implications. The presence of the mutation in 1967 suggests that the neoplasm was already present then. Second, p53-mutated cancers are associated with progressive or high-grade advanced tumors.[4,5] It is possible that the tumor was in a phase of aggressive growth in 1967. Had Humphrey known that he had aggressive bladder cancer in 1967, he might have withdrawn from the presidential race.[6] Just as important, he and his physicians may have elected to pursue a more aggressive, potentially life-saving surgery years earlier.

Disagreements in the interpretation of the case quickly surfaced.[7] It was suggested that the case could just as easily be interpreted to show the limited importance of such techniques. The initial diagnosis of cancer was fully substantiated with the diagnosis of CIS in 1969. It was unlikely that the delay between 1967 and 1969 would have made any clinical difference, particularly when one considers that no treatment was given despite the diagnosis. Determining the clinical importance of early detection also depends on the therapeutic options available at the time and the natural history of the disease.[7] However, it could be argued that it was unclear at what point Humphrey or his physicians accepted the fact that he had bladder cancer that required treatment. With a definitive diagnosis, Humphrey may have elected to undergo a radical cystectomy, a potentially curative surgery.[8] In addition, Humphrey did eventually die of his bladder cancer, not a good outcome for conventional diagnosis and treatment.

The role of urinary cytology in reducing mortality from bladder cancer in high-risk populations must be evaluated in controlled trials. An initial step may be to evaluate treatment trials of early lesions found by screening.[9]

ORAL CANCER

> *The visual oral examination is capable of identifying pre-symptomatic oral cancers.*

Exfoliative cytology is less sensitive than visual examination.[1] There have been no trials to demonstrate a declining mortality with either test. In developing countries programs have been proposed for oral cancer detection based on the inspection of the oral mucosa for epithelial dysplasia by allied health care providers.[10]

> *Primary prevention could be combined with an oral cancer screen or dental examination. An oral examination as part of the routine physical is recommended by the National Cancer Institute (NCI).[11]*

This would be particularly recommended for high-risk groups, such as those with an alcohol or tobacco addiction.

ENDOMETRIAL CANCER

> *Although endometrial cancer is relatively common in Western countries, the person-years saved by screening may be limited, because it is largely a disease of elderly women.[12]*

The screening examination consists of taking endometrial samples for cytologic examination, invasive tests that require good interpretive skills.[13] High-risk populations need to be better defined.

The Food and Drug Administration (FDA) in April 1994 issued a stronger warning for women who take the drug tamoxifen because it poses an increased risk, compared with the normal population, for uterine cancer. A Swedish study that had followed participants for 9 years showed that breast cancer patients who had taken tamoxifen had a higher risk of uterine cancer than the control population. In the latest results of this study 23 of 1372 patients randomized to take tamoxifen, 40 mg/day, developed uterine cancer, compared with four of 1357 patients in the control group (relative risk [RR] = 5.6, $P < .001$).[14] After approximately 6.8 years of follow-up in the ongoing NSABP B-14 trial, 15 of 1419 women randomized to receive tamoxifen, 20 mg/day for 5 years, developed uterine cancer, and two of the 1424 women randomized to receive placebo who subsequently had recurrent breast cancer and were treated with tamoxifen also developed endometrial cancer. Most of the uterine cancers were diagnosed at an early stage, but deaths due to uterine cancer have been reported.[15]

> *It was recommended that patients receiving long-term tamoxifen therapy undergo yearly gynecologic examination, report any vaginal bleeding to their physician, and perhaps undergo a screening intravaginal ultrasound examination.*

These recommendations are applicable to this high-risk population and not necessarily to the normal population.

STOMACH CANCER

The main purpose of mass screening for stomach cancer is early detection at the preclinical stage and prompt treatment with reduction in mortality from cancer at this site in the target population.

> *Data from Japan suggest that stomach cancer screening can reduce mortality, and in areas of high incidence, such as Western Pacific, Central, and South America and Northern Europe, there is a need to develop a cancer control program.*

Mortality from stomach cancer in Japan has been decreasing; however, it is still the leading cause of cancer deaths there, accounting for 24.6% of the deaths in males and 21.6% of the deaths in females.[16]

In Japan gastric cancer mass screening by the barium x-ray method has been conducted nationwide since 1960. The screening test used has gradually been standardized and consists of a photofluorographic barium meal technique with six standard views. Since 1983 the Japanese government established a public policy to try to screen 30% of the people over the age of 40 each year. The number of examinations has been increasing year by year, and the total examined in 1987 exceeded 5 million people, with the number of detected cancers to be 0.13% of the total population. Surgical procedures were performed in 97.2% of the cases, with early-stage cancer being detected in 52.1% of the cases and 60.7% of the resected cases.[17] It was estimated that 21.3% of the target population at risk was screened.

There have been a number of studies in Japan to evaluate the effectiveness of screening for gastric cancer, but none were controlled randomized trials. Other types of analysis, such as time trend analysis, retrospective cohort study, correlation of screening rate, and change in mortality and case-control study have been used to suggest efficacy. In examining trends of incidence and mortality in the Miyagi Prefecture from 1960 to 1988, there has been a steady increase in the number of early-stage cancers diagnosed (Figure 9-1). When examining age-adjusted trends, the incidence in both males and females is shown to be decreasing (Figure 9-2). In addition, since 1970 mortality has also decreased, and the two survival curves have begun to separate. This suggests that the drop in mortality is due not only to a lower incidence of disease, but also to improve techniques for early detection and widespread application of the mass screening, since the surgical approach has not changed and very little advancement has been made with chemotherapy for this disease. The reason given for the reduction in incidence is believed to be the westernization of the Japanese diet. The largest separation of the

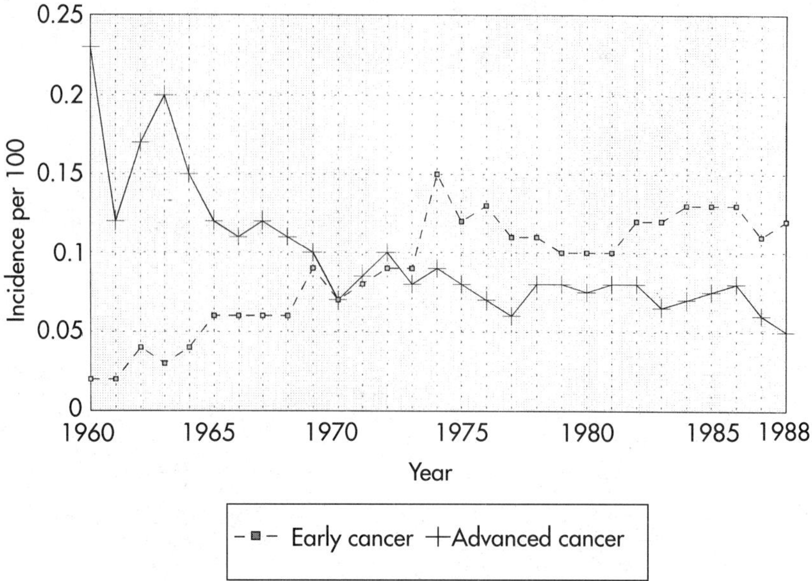

Figure 9-1 Mass screening for stomach cancer in high-incidence areas has resulted in a steady decline in the number of late-stage cancers diagnosed and a corresponding increase in the earlier stage tumors.

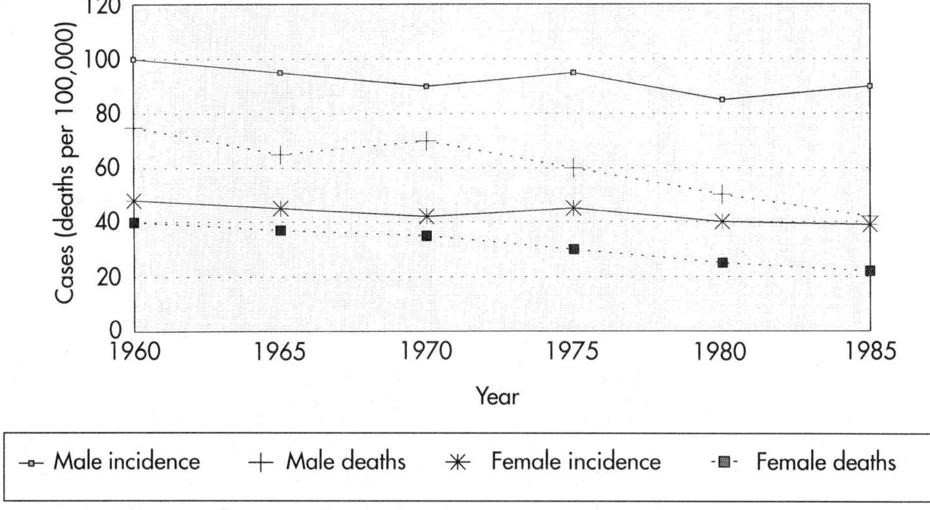

Figure 9-2 With the institution of mass screening of the stomach by barium examination in 1960 in Japan, there has been a steady drop in the incidence and mortality rates for the disease in both sexes.

incidence and mortality curves has occurred in the age group 50 to 70, the exact target population of the screening program.

Fukao et al.[18] conducted a case-control study to evaluate efficacy of screening. Patients with advanced gastric cancer identified by mass screening were compared to age- and sex-matched controls. It was determined that people who were screened every year had approximately three times the chance of not getting advanced cancer in comparison with those who have not been screened at all or not screened within 5 years. The relative protection was the highest among the population screened every year. The trend of relative protection continued until the last negative screen was performed 3 years before diagnosis, suggesting the following:

> *The screening intervals for gastric cancer should not be greater than 3 years.*

A cost-effectiveness analysis was performed of gastric mass screening with the barium examination. The sensitivity was 85%, specificity was 90%, the rate of positive tests was 10%, and the positive predictive value was 1.7%.

> *The 5-year relative survival of 554 patients with stomach cancer detected by mass screening was approximately 70%, whereas that among the 3375 patients with stomach cancer presenting at the various outpatient centers was 25%.*

A mathematical model predicted that, for a population of 100,000 people, with mass screening, 119 cancers could be cured at a cost of $7.6 million. For a similar population of unscreened individuals, only 50 cancers could be cured at a cost of $3.4 million. For every life saved with the mass screen, $55,000 would have to be spent. In today's Japan the insurance value of a life of a 55-year-old is estimated to be $250,000, and from the standpoint of cost effectiveness, screening for stomach cancer is thought to be appropriate in the high-risk Japanese population.[16]

Other groups have added upper endoscopy to the screening program, but the standard has been the barium examination. The yield in these screened populations is substantial, with as many as 40% of the cancers being early-stage gastric cancer and as many as 60% of the population participating in the mass screening program.[19]

At present there is a randomized control trial evaluating gastric screening in Miyagi prefecture in Japan. This has been difficult to establish because many municipalities in Japan have been conducting voluntarily gastric mass screening for a long time. Allocation to the trial is by group randomization. Thirty-nine municipalities agreed to join the trial and were randomized into screened and nonscreened populations. In the screened populations 50- and 60-year-old people were invited to attend mass screening by means of a direct postal invitation written by the head of the local government. The intervention in the study group was performed just once; otherwise the population was exposed to baseline screening activities. This trial is ongoing and the results are as yet unavailable. It was apparent from an initial analysis that there was a difference in compliance with the screen in those age 50 as compared with those age 60, with more 50-year-olds taking advantage of the intervention.

These studies have suggested efficacy, but several biases need to be mentioned. The reduction in the incidence of the disease in Japan would suggest that other factors, such as diet, may be influencing the disease. Screening cannot be expected to reduce the incidence of stomach cancer unless premalignant lesions found with the screening test are being removed. A compliance of 40% of the targeted population would not be expected to have a major effect on the mortality of the disease. The drop in the mortality rate of gastric cancer in Japan cannot be explained by just a decrease in incidence, however. Lesser falls in incidence than mortality rates may be caused by the detection and effective treatment of tumors that would not have been clinically relevant and cause no effect on mortality. Correlation studies do show that the degree of reduction in mortality is related to the extent of screening. Dietary changes need to be controlled for in the screened population to eliminate this potential source of bias. These studies are clinically important because early stomach cancer has a high cure rate if treated surgically. However, the fact that gastric cancer remains the number one cause of death in Japan may reflect the limitations of mass screening if the entire population at risk is not screened.

In one area of Finland, screening using an immunologic test on gastric juice was conducted, but the results of this program are pending.[20] The evidence of the association between *Helicobacter pylori* gastritis and gastric carcinoma has been strengthened by studies showing that patients with gastric cancer are more likely to have had an infection in the years before the diagnosis of cancer. The relative risk for gastric cancer when infected with *H. pylori* is 3.6 to 6 times the normal population, and this factor could be used to identify the population to screen.[21]

NASOPHARYNGEAL CANCER

Nasopharyngeal carcinoma (NPC) is a rare cancer in most parts of the world, with reported incidence around 1 case per 100,000 person-years. The highest reported incidences are in Hong Kong, with a rate of 30 per 100,000 person-years, and Southern China, at a rate of 10 per 100,000 person-years.

The etiology of NPC is thought to be due to 3 factors: the Epstein-Barr virus (EBV), diet, and genetics.

The presence of EBV DNA in malignant cells argues for a close link between the cancer and the virus, and this association is used for screening, early detection, and follow-up of NPC cases.

Old et al.[22] first demonstrated the presence of anti-EBV antibodies in the sera of NPC patients. EBV genomes are found in almost all biopsies of NPC from all parts of the world. The genome exists in the epithelial cells of the tumor. The EBV genome is transcriptionally active in these genomes and is the same as that expressed in latently infected lymphocytes. The fact that patients with NPC have elevated levels of both IgG and IgA antibodies to EBV capsid and early antigens most likely represents the local production of these antigens in the nasopharynx. More recent advances in molecular biology have provided further evidence of the carcinogenic properties of this herpesvirus, including the identification of EBV-related peptides capable of inducing malignant transformation of lymphoblastoid cell lines in vitro.[23] The presence of the immunoglobulin markers provides the opportunity for early serologic identification of patients with NPC.

Genetics also plays a role in the disease, as demonstrated by the association with a specific HLA type[24] and the increased risk for the disease among relatives of patients with NPC. The main environmental risk factor—diet—has been studied, and the consumption of Cantonese salted fish has been linked to the disease.[25] The cooking of such fish results in the release of volatile nitrosamines that distribute over the nasopharyngeal mucosa when carried by steam. Other factors that have been linked to the disease are salt-cured fish and meat, occupational exposure to dust or fumes, nasal oil, and exposure to smoke.[26]

> *NPC has serious consequences, and in specific populations the prevalence of a detectable preclinical phase of the disease is high enough to justify mass screening.*

It is unclear, however, whether early treatment affects survival. Radiotherapy is the treatment of choice, with 5-year survivals reported as high as 84% for stage 1 tumors and a poorer survival noted for more advanced tumors.

Given the association of EBV with the disease, a number of serologic markers have been used as diagnostic aids to follow patients who have been treated for NPC and for early detection.[27] EBV serology was used in screening for the first time in 1978 to 1980 in Zangwu, a rural county in China. No other population besides the Chinese have been subjected to mass screening. The first study used an immunoenzymatic test for the detection of immunoglobulin A to the viral capsid antigen (IgA/VCA). About 33% of the population at risk (450,000) was screened, and 0.3% of the screened population had a titer of greater than or equal to 1:80. These patients were submitted to a clinical examination, and 55 patients with NPC were found on clinical grounds and verified histologically, representing 11.9% of the screened positives or 0.37 prevalent case per 1000 screened.[28]

Another survey of an urban population of Wuzhou City used the IgA/VCA assay. About 5.3% of the screened population were positive with this test, a number that is higher than the positivity rate of the rural population. One prevalent case of NPC per 1000 screened was found. Of the 13 total cases found, nine were in stage 1 and four were stage 2 at diagnosis.[29]

Other studies have reported on the sensitivity and specificity of the screening examination using the IgA/VCA assay. The sensitivity was estimated at 95% and the specificity at 97% with an estimate of the positive predictive value of 0.6%.[30]

With the continued follow-up of the screened population, some of the individuals with positive serology will eventually be diagnosed with NPC. In 1118 individuals who had positive serology but a negative initial screen, 17 additional patients with NPC were found.[31] Thus the incidence rate among IgA/VCA–positive individuals was 7.5% higher than among the remainder of the Wuzhou population. No false negative screens were noted. To date a shift in stage distribution has been documented in Wuzhou and this information has been used as evidence of an effect on mortality.

Critics of these studies state that no valid estimates of the sensitivity and specificity of the screening test are based on populations that are asymptomatic. There has been no strict follow-up of negative screens to identify the rate of false negatives, and the results reported are those from a prevalence screen with no subsequent rescreening of any substantial number of patients. No data on the costs of the tests have been reported, and to date no study has looked at NPC mortality among a screened and control population. At present no strong evidence exists in favor of screening for NPC, but the serologic tests are promising because they may bring about a stage shift at diagnosis. It is important that a randomized study take place in a high-risk population with the hope of demonstrating a difference in mortality between the screened and unscreened population.

> *Serologic tests may identify people at high risk of developing the disease sometime in the future, and these patients would need multiple screens to diagnose the disease early.*

As with all screening examinations, the issue of the proper follow-up for both positive and negative screens needs to be answered. Above all, the mortality rates of the screened and unscreened population should be studied, and inferences from survival rates based on stage shifting should not be the sole evidence of efficacy.

NEUROBLASTOMA

Neuroblastoma (NB) is the second most common malignant tumor of children and accounts for 10% of all childhood malignancies in Japan. Thus most of the impetus for screening for this disease comes from the Japanese experiences. The frequency of diagnosis of NB is approximately 10 cases per million children. In children with a long life expectancy, a one-time screen may be applicable for a rare disease, whereas a rare disease would not justify repeated screenings in adults. The tumor originates from the adrenal glands or sympathetic ganglia and is usually diagnosed with a palpable abdominal mass, leg pains, fever, and diarrhea. Children with the tumor are treated with a multimodality approach, including surgical resection, chemotherapy, and radiation therapy, but the prognosis is unfavorable since the tumor is usually discovered when it is large and palpable.

> *The most important prognostic factors for NB are age and stage at diagnosis. NB patients under the age of 1 have a*

> *good prognosis, but it is difficult to make the diagnosis in infants or at early stages because there are no characteristic symptoms.*

For this reason, other possible screening tests were sought.

> *NB is associated with metabolites that are excreted in the urine, such as vanillylmandelic acid (VMA) and homovanillic acid (HVA). The analysis of the urine for these metabolites forms the basis for massive screening programs.*

The initial programs started in 1972 in Japan with the screening of all 3-year-olds in the province of Kyoto with the VMA spot urine test.[32] This test alone misses 25% of NB—the ones who do not secrete VMA. Only one case of NB was discovered among 42,636 screened children, and this child was detected with stage 2 disease and eventually died.

In 1974 NB mass screening was initiated in a younger population with the hope of identifying earlier disease. Again in Kyoto, mass screening was performed in 6-month-old infants with the VMA spot urine test. Among 78,331 infants screened, four cases of asymptomatic NB were detected during a 6-year period from 1973 to 1979. All were detected at an early stage and considered to have a good prognosis.[33] The spot VMA test was a crude assay and gave over 10,000 false positive tests with this initial screen, most due to the dietary phenolic acid in vanilla and bananas. However, with the encouraging early results, mass screening for NB was instituted in eight other districts of Japan in 1980. Early-stage NB was detected in 16 of the 281,939 screened infants and 15 of the 16 patients were considered cured with therapy.[34]

> *In 1985 nationwide NB screening was initiated throughout Japan with the financial support of the Japanese government, and in 1988 the Ministry of Health recommended that high-performance liquid chromatography (HPLC) for VMA, HVA, and creatinine be used as the screening test instead of the qualitative VMA test to enable the detection on non-VMA–secreting NB.*

It was formerly considered that a 24-hour urine collection was necessary for the accurate quantification of VMA and HVA excretion; however, it has been shown that random specimen collections are adequate provided that the measurements are related to creatinine content. About 90% of all NB have elevations of urinary VMA and/or HVA. In this program all 3-month-olds receive physical examinations at the local health centers under the Child Health Survey Program, at which time the parents are given urine containers and asked to mail back a urine sample at the time the child is 6 months.

> *In 1985 58.6% of all 6-month-old infants in Japan were screened, and this figured increased to 76.9% in 1987, or over 1 million infants.*

During the 5 years that the national program was in effect, 342 cases of NB were diagnosed from over 4 million infants screened. The incidence of NB detected by nationwide screen was 1 in 11,750 infants. By using the HPLC assay the number of discovered NB cases has increased, and 1 NB case is being detected for every 8500 infants screened. With the institution of the HPLC assay, four times the number of NB have been identified and the number of retests and false positives has decreased.

Since mass screening started in Kyoto in 1972, 337 cases of NB have been identified, treated in a standardized fashion, and followed. The majority (85.8%) were diagnosed by the age of 9 months, and only five of the cases (1.5%) were considered symptomatic. Further investigation showed that 86.9% of the cases were located in the abdomen with mediastinal NB accounting for the remainder. Only 52% of the patients had an abdominal mass on physical examination. About 14% of the cases had normal VMA measurements and were detected only with the more sensitive HPLC assay.

> *The stage distribution at diagnosis in the mass screening revealed that 66% of individuals were stages 1 and 2 at diagnosis, and this figure compares favorably with the stage of diagnosis of NB throughout the rest of Japan during the years 1971 to 1976, during which only 20% of the cases were stages 1 and 2 at diagnosis.*

With the institution of the nationwide program, the number of infants with stage 1 or stage 2 NB at diagnosis has increased from the initial value of 20% before mass screening to a value of 38% by the year 1988 in the nationwide registry (Table 9-1). Of the initial 337 cases that were discovered in Kyoto, 97% were still alive.[35]

The frequency of screening is subject to debate. In Japan, as well as other countries, there are two major peaks for incidence of the disease. There is a

---
T A B L E   9 - 1

STAGE DISTRIBUTION OF NEUROBLASTOMA

Stage	Screened (%)	Unscreened (%)
1	32	17
2	34	21
4s	9	11
3	17	20
4	8	39

prominent peak approaching 1 year of age and a later onset of disease at 3 or 4 years. There is a clear association with the early onset of disease and prognosis. Children diagnosed at the age of 3 or 4 have a worse prognosis than those diagnosed earlier. Thus not all NB can be detected by a screening program at the age of 6 months. To detect the second peak of incidence of the disease, a second screen would seem reasonable. Other critics of the program state that perhaps many of these early detected cancers would spontaneously regress and never become clinically relevant, but this is considered a rare phenomenon.

> *Serial examination of all NB deaths in Japan from death certificates shows a decrease in the number of NB deaths and a decreased mortality from NB in Japan since the introduction of screening.*[36,37]

For the Kyoto region of Japan the survival rate improves from a low of 17.1% during the 12-year period from 1962 to 1974 before mass screening, to 71.1% during the 14-year period (1974 to 1988) after mass screening. Although no data are available to compare the death rates in screened and unscreened populations, the inference is made from declining nationwide mortality rates for NB that mass screening is efficacious. The argument that the tumors are just being discovered earlier in their clinical course and lead time bias influences these results will always be present, but the magnitude of the change in the nationwide death rate is impressive and worth studying. The potential discovery of in situ NB that will eventually spontaneously regress and be of no clinical importance could account for the increased number of new cases found with an apparent improvement in the overall survival of the cohort. In this regard, microscopic nodules of primitive neuroblasts, usually larger than 3 mm and occasionally invading blood vessels, referred to as NB in situ, have been observed at autopsy in infants dying before 3 months of age of other causes at 40 to 200 times the expected incidence.

> *Autopsy examination of the adrenal glands of 92 18-week to 20-week fetuses demonstrated NB in situ in all, suggesting that a normal phase of embryogenesis of the adrenal gland, which is histologically similar to NB, may persist into the first year of life.*

Other criticisms of these studies from Japan include the fact that overall compliance with the screen is poor and coverage is at best 65% to 75%. In addition, cancer registration in Japan is very patchy; in some provinces it is less than 5% complete and death certification is unreliable.[38]

Other countries have attempted to perform mass screening for NB, including the north region of England, where the incidence of disease is 1 in 10,580 live births. Mortality rates for NB have been decreasing during the 70s and 80s (Figure 9-3). Data from the European NB study group shows that the 5-year survival for patients diagnosed with NB under the age of 1 is 80%, whereas it is only 38% for patients diagnosed later. Since it costs an estimated 45,000 pounds to treat one patient, and as few as 10% who are diagnosed after the age of 1 live, the estimated cost per life saved is £450,000. Any potential costs of screening can be viewed against this financial background. If all tumors start at stage 1 and eventually progress to stage 4, screening may very well detect disease before it advances to an incurable state. Initial studies were established in the city of North Tyneside in England in 1987. The screening method was by gas chromatography–mass spectrometry for VMA and HVA on urine samples obtained from 6-month-olds. Of the 2470 babies screened in this population seven had abnormal elevations of the two metabolites, but only two babies were subsequently diagnosed with NB. The

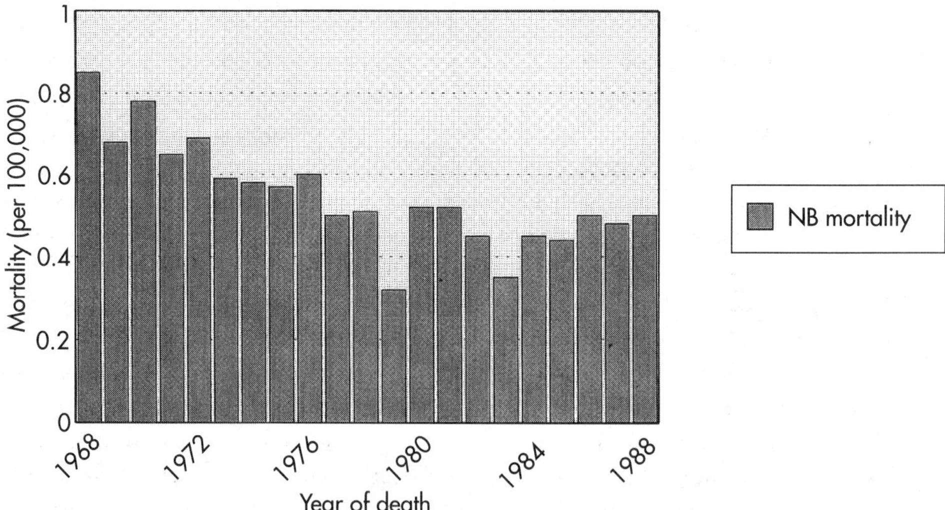

Figure 9-3   Neuroblastoma (NB) mortality rates have been falling throughout England during the last two decades. During this time fledgling screening and education programs have taken place, but a direct relationship is difficult to establish.

other five are being followed serially, and some have had their urine studies return to normal. At the same time, two children who were screened and found to have normal results have subsequently developed NB, and both had stage 4 disease at diagnosis. The specificity of this method was high (99%), with only five false positive results needing clinical workup. A study comparing the incidence and survival rates for five administrative health regions in north England and Scotland with controls from neighboring districts that are not screened is currently under way. A screened population of 561,000 is necessary to detect, at 5% significance, a fall in mortality from 3.27 to 0.96 per 100,000 in the 7 to 72-month age group.

TESTICULAR CANCER

With an incidence of three in 100,000 men per year, testicular cancer represents the most common malignancy in men from the ages of 25 to 40 years.

The last decades have shown a steady increase in the survival of patients with testicular cancer, with a 10% survival noted in the 1970s progressing to over 90% in current series. In a large study of 200 tumors recently reported from France,[39] there was a 5-year survival rate of 92.5% for all stages and histologic types. Testicle cancer is one of the most curable of the solid tumors and is an excellent model for the multimodality treatment of solid cancers.

Progress in decreasing mortality and lessening morbidity of this disease can also be attributed perhaps to the incorporation of the testicular examination in routine physical examinations and to a better understanding of serum tumor markers that allow an earlier intervention in the course of disease after a recurrence.

LeComete, in 1851, was credited with the initial observation of a relationship between cryptorchidism and later testicular tumor formation.[40]

It has been estimated that the relative risk of testicular tumors with undescended testes is 3 to 14 times the normal expected incidence.

In addition, about 5% to 10% of the people with a history of cryptorchidism develop a cancer in the contralateral normally descended testes. This would ordinarily be considered a high-risk population, and certainly a preschool screening for cryptorchism has been suggested and seems reasonable.[41] But there have been no studies to evaluate the efficacy of such an approach.

There is no prospective randomized study to evaluate the efficacy of annual physical examinations, either by oneself or a health care provider in screening for testicular cancer. Primary care physicians have the responsibility to include the testicular examination as part of their routine examination, to educate young males about the frequency of testicular cancer in their age group, and to explain how to perform a self-examination.[42] Early-stage disease (stages 1 and 2a) is associated with low recurrence rates and 5-year survival data approaching 100%, while for bulky stage IIB and more advanced disease; 5 year survival data are much lower. There is a true need for education about the early signs and symptoms of testicular cancer to reduce delay in presentation, but because the testicular self examination is of unproven benefit, the case cannot be made for screening.

LIVER CANCER

Epidemiologic studies of patients with hepatocellular carcinoma (HCC) have shown that hyperepidemic hot spots do occur in such areas as China and sub-Saharan Africa (Table 9-2).

In these countries, the high incidence rates have been associated with high endemic hepatitis B carrier rates and mycotoxin contamination of foodstuffs, stored grains, and drinking water.

TABLE 9-2

AGE-ADJUSTED INCIDENCE FOR HEPATOCELLULAR CARCINOMA

	Number of persons per 100,000 per year	
Country	Male	Female
Mozambique	112.9	30.8
China	34.4	11.6
Gambia	33.1	12.6
South Africa, Bantu	26.3	8.4
Senegal	25.6	9.0
Burma	25.5	8.8
Philippines	19.9	6.2
Nigeria	15.4	3.2
Korea	13.8	3.2
Japan	7.2	2.2
Israel	7.4	1.5

Probably the most studied natural chemical carcinogen is aflatoxin B_1, a product of the *Aspergillus* fungus. This mold has been found in a variety of stored grains, particularly in areas of the world in which rice is stored without refrigeration. In the days following the monsoon season in Southeast Asia, a white mold containing the aflatoxin can be found on the grain and is later eaten. Aflatoxin contamination data correlate with data on the incidence of HCC.[43]

Case-control studies have also shown a strong association between chronic hepatitis B carrier rates and an increased incidence of HCC. In endemic areas such as Taiwan, up to a 200-fold excess of HCC has been reported. Hepatitis C viral infection may act in synergy with hepatitis B infection to cause an even more alarming increase in the incidence of HCC.[44] A large-scale intervention study sponsored by the World Health Organization is under way in Asia and involves the vaccination of newborns against hepatitis B virus. Of this newborn population 10% to 15% have chronic hepatitis B, transmitted at birth. Whether the incidence of HCC can be affected with this intervention may take another 40 years to ascertain.

It has long been recognized that 60% to 80% of the HCC are associated with underlying cirrhosis, but what is not clear is whether the cirrhosis is the causative agent or whether the underlying causes of the cirrhosis are actually the carcinogenic agents.

Tumor markers for the detection of HCC were developed after α-fetoprotein (AFP) was identified in the serum of animals bearing hepatomas and in humans with the cancer.[45] The assay has been improved with the development of a radioimmunoassay, and serum levels have been used to screen high-risk patients as well as follow patients after surgical resection.

> *AFP is elevated in 80% to 90% of Asian individuals bearing a hepatoma, but in the United States this rate drops to 60% to 70%.*

The other assay used to screen populations for HCC is des-γ-carboxy prothrombin (PIVKA-II), a prothrombin induced by vitamin K absence. The serum level of this compound may be elevated in 91% of HCC cases, but other conditions such as vitamin K deficiency, chronic active hepatitis and metastatic carcinoma can be associated with elevations of PIVKA-II. Although elevations in these two tumor markers can be detected early in the clinical course of disease, most clinical studies would suggest that abdominal ultrasound is an even more sensitive study.

Many discrete patient populations are susceptible to HCC, and within high incidence areas screening for the disease has been attempted. Beasely et al.[46] screened a group of Taiwanese male postal carriers who were positive for hepatitis B surface antigen and found an annual incidence of HCC to be 495 per 100,000, a risk 98 times that observed in individuals who were antigen negative. Antigen-positive individuals at greatest risk are men with cirrhosis who have a family history of disease and are older than 45 years.

Mima et al.[47] used abdominal ultrasound and serum AFP levels to screen a high-risk population in Japan, which included hepatitis B antigen carriers, patients with a history or who currently have other liver disease, a history of blood transfusions, a family history of liver cancer or a history of hepatitis C antibody development. Among those judged to be at high risk (5684 people screened), 1.6% were found to have HCC. The 1-, 3-, and 5-year survivals of this screened population were 79%, 43.8%, and 19.3%, respectively, comparable to the control population.

> *The cost per case of HCC detected was $25,000. The authors concluded that the high detection rate made screening worthwhile with reasonable costs, despite the fact that no survival benefit could be demonstrated.*

Pateron[48] used the same two modalities to screen a French population who were considered high risk—those with Child class A or B cirrhosis. There were 118 patients screened every 6 months with abdominal ultrasound, AFP, and PIVKA-II. Fourteen cases of HCC were detected, six by ultrasound alone, four by AFP alone, and none by PIVKA-II alone. Solitary nodules of HCC were detected in nine patients, and three had tumors discovered that were less than 3 cm. However, surgery was performed in only one patient, and it was concluded that, although the incidence of HCC was high in this population, screening did not effectively identify potentially resectable tumors. Martinez[49] from Spain compared the size and treatment of HCC tumors detected in a screened population versus these parameters of patients detected with HCC outside the screening program. Twenty of 43 (46.5%) patients in the screened population had HCC less than 5 cm, whereas only 15.2% of the control population had these smaller size tumors. Significant differences were also noted in the ability of the patients in the screened population to undergo resection versus the controls, but no survival comparisons were performed. Finally, Unoura et al.[50] studied the characteristics of high-risk groups for the development of HCC in Japan. An analysis of factors among 120 patients with chronic hepatitis revealed that only age and histologic findings were independent risk factors. A multivariate analysis of 239 patients with liver cirrhosis showed that age, hepatitis B surface antigen, or hepatitis C antibody level positivity, a family history of liver disease, hepatic reserve, and a history of radical resection were independent risk factors for the subsequent development of HCC. A screening strategy was implemented based on these results with ultrasound every 3 months and tumor markers every 2 months. It was thought that this strategy resulted in the diagnosis of HCC at an earlier stage with an improved prognosis.

> *There is a survival differential per stage of disease for HCC. T_1 and T_2 lesions that are solitary and less than 2 cm with negative nodes have a 3-year survival of 75%; stage 3 and stage 4 persons have a 50% and 10% 5-year*

> *survival, respectively. The screening efforts for HCC in endemic high-risk populations would seem to be straightforward, but despite the finding of smaller lesions that are more often resectable, an impact on survival has not been demonstrated.*

It is reasonable to continue and refine screening efforts in endemic areas of the world and in high-risk population groups because of the availability of noninvasive screening tests with acceptable sensitivities and the mortality differential between early- and late-stage disease. To be more widely incorporated into practice, an eventual survival difference needs to be shown in screened populations.

ESOPHAGEAL CANCER

Esophageal cancer is a substantial cause of mortality in the world, and recent data would indicate that the incidence may be increasing. Despite better understanding in the pathogenesis and the surgical management of the disease, little improvement in survival rates has been achieved anywhere in the world, especially because screening for detection of premalignant lesions cannot, at present, be adequately applied to populations at risk.

Cancer of the esophagus has one of the highest variations in geographic distributions and sex ratios of any solid malignancy. The reason for these extreme geographic distributions (17-fold difference in age-adjusted mortality for males exists between high- and low-incidence countries) is unknown, but environmental and nutritional factors are suspected. If these risk factors or predisposing conditions can be identified, then high-risk populations can be screened for the disease.

Linxian, China, has one of the highest rates of esophageal cancer in the world. In 1983 esophageal balloon cytology screening was performed in three communes in this province. Of the participants, 10,066 with no evidence of cancer were followed prospectively for 7.5 years to evaluate the ability of the initial cytologic diagnosis to identify patients at an increased risk for developing esophageal cancer. A total of 747 incident cases were discovered, and 322 deaths from this malignancy were recorded in the follow-up period. The risks for the development of cancer increased in relation to the severity of the cytologic diagnosis. Relative risks for the development of esophageal cancer by initial cytologic diagnosis were normal (1), hyperplasia (1.25), mild dysplasia (2.2), severe dysplasia (4.22), and near cancer (5.96).

> *These results suggest that esophageal balloon cytology could be used to successfully identify a high-risk population that could then be screened regularly.[51]*

In a later study 12,649 people from the same province were screened with esophageal balloon cytology. Of the population, 65% showed some degree of squamous hyperplasia or dysplasia. Another 2% showed a near cancer cytology, and 2% had overt malignancies.[52] Both of these groups were followed for 15 years in an attempt to identify other risk factors for the disease. A total of 1162 subjects from a total cohort of 12,693 (9.1%) were determined to have developed esophageal cancer over the 15 years. Statistical analysis suggests that increased age, male gender, family history, low education level, drinking water source, and pork consumption were the strongest risk factors for esophageal cancer in this cohort, whereas the use of corn as the primary dietary staple and infrequent consumption of fresh vegetables were weakly associated risk factors. The classic risk factors for the development of esophageal cancer—smoking, alcohol use, and eating pickled vegetables and moldy food—were not significant in this analysis.[53] Dietary factors play a role in this disease, but other constitutional factors such as age, gender, and family history are equally important.

Barrett's esophagus occurs when the normal stratified squamous epithelium of the esophagus becomes replaced with columnar epithelium, usually developing as a complication of gastroesophageal reflux and predisposing the patient to the development of adenocarcinoma. The frequency of the development of adenocarcinoma from Barrett's esophagus averages 10%, and the estimated risk is 30- to 125-fold excess in comparison with the normal population. Dysplasia precedes the development of adenocarcinoma in Barrett's esophagus, and dysplasia has been proposed for a marker to identify a high-risk population for screening. There is some interpathologic variation in classifying dysplasia. An alternative to the histologic classification of dysplasia may be flow cytometric analysis of DNA content. The prevalence of an elevated S phase fraction and tetraploid fractions of the aneuploid population of cells increases with histologic progression from dysplasia to cancer and identifies a patient population at high risk for the disease.[54] A screening series from the United Kingdom in patients with Barrett's esophagus identified four adenocarcinomas at a cost similar to that for the detection of breast cancer by mammography.[55]

Another high-risk population comprises male patients with a previous history of oral or oropharyngeal cancer. Lugol dye–aided endoscopy was used in 127 of these patients, and eight (6.3%) clinically asymptomatic esophageal cancers were detected. Five of the eight superficial lesions could not be detected by ordinary endoscopy, and it was concluded that Lugol dye endoscopy is needed to diagnose these early lesions.[56]

The lack of any efficacy study and the lack of survival data from these trials does not support widespread screening for this disease. In endemic areas it is reasonable to continue to perform trials of screening to generate, in long-term follow-up, survival data that can be compared to current control populations. Because screening may not be widely applicable, preventive measures and dietary interventions may be needed.

REFERENCES

1. Prorok PC et al: UICC workshop on the evaluation of screening programs for cancer, *Int J Cancer* 34:1, 1984.
2. Hruban RH et al: Brief report: molecular biology and the early detection of carcinoma of the bladder—the case of Hubert Humphrey, *N Engl J Med* 330:1276, 1994.

3. Berman E: *Hubert: the triumph and tragedy of the Humphrey I knew,* New York, 1979, GP Putnam.
4. Olumi AF et al: Allelic loss of chromosome 17p distinguished high grade from low grade transitional cell carcinomas of the bladder, *Cancer Res* 50:7081, 1990.
5. Sarkis AK et al: Nuclear overexpression of p53 protein in transitional cell carcinoma: a marker for disease progression, *J Natl Cancer Inst* 85:53, 1993.
6. Cohn V: We must know about our leaders' health, *Washington Post,* March 26, 1978.
7. Homer RJ: Hubert Humphrey's bladder cancer, *N Engl J Med* 331:880, 1994 (letter).
8. Hruban RH, van der Riet P, Sidransky D: Hubert Humphrey's bladder cancer, *N Engl J Med* 331:880, 1994 (letter).
9. Cartwright RA: Screening for bladder cancer with particular reference to individual groups. In Prorok PC et al, editors: UICC workshop on the evaluation of screening programs for cancer, *Int J Cancer* 34:1, 1984.
10. Warnakulasuria KAAS et al: Utilization of primary health care providers for the early detection of oral cancer and precancer cases in Sri Lanki, *Bull World Health Org* 62:243, 1984.
11. Early Detection Branch: *Working guidelines for early cancer detection,* Bethesda, 1987, Division of Cancer Prevention and Control, National Cancer Institute.
12. Miller AB: Cancer screening. In Devita VT, Hellman S, Rosenberg SA, editors: *Cancer principles and practice of oncology,* ed 4, Philadelphia, 1993, JB Lippincott.
13. Hakama M et al: Evaluation of screening programs for gynecologic cancers, *Br J Cancer* 52:669, 1985.
14. Porter KT: Personal communication, April 8, 1994.
15. Fisher B et al: Endometrial cancer in tamoxifen-treated breast cancer patients: findings from the NSABP B-14, *J Natl Cancer Inst* 86:527, 1994.
16. Hisamichi S et al: Evaluation of mass screening program for stomach cancer in Japan. In Miller AB et al, editors: *Cancer screening,* 1990, Cambridge University Press.
17. Hisamichi S: Screening for gastric cancer, *World J Surg* 13:31, 1989.
18. Fukao A, Hisamichi S, Sugawara N: A case-control study to evaluate the effect of mass screening on decreasing advanced stomach cancer, *J Jpn Soc Gastroenterol Mass Survey* 75:112, 1987.
19. Kaneko E et al: A longer term follow-up study of patients with gastric cancer detected by mass screening, *Cancer* 63:613, 1989.
20. Hakama M, Pukkala E: Evaluation of an immunologic screening for stomach cancer. In Chamberlain J, Miller AB, editors: *Screening for gastrointestinal cancer,* Toronto, 1988, Hans Huber.
21. Young GP, Demediuk BH: The genetics, epidemiology and early detection of gastrointestinal cancers, *Curr Opin Oncol* 4:728, 1992.
22. Old LJ et al: Precipitating antibody in human serum to an antigen present in cultured Burkitt's lymphoma cells, *Proc Natl Acad Sci USA* 56:1699, 1966.
23. Fahraeus R et al: Expression of EB virus encoded proteins in nasopharyngeal carcinoma, *Int J Cancer* 42:329, 1988.
24. Chan SH et al: HLA and nasopharyngeal carcinoma in Malays, *Br J Cancer* 51:389, 1985.
25. Yan L, XI Z, Drettner B: Epidemiological studies of nasopharyngeal cancer in Guanzhou area, China: preliminary report, *Acta Otolaryngol* 107:424, 1989.
26. Sasco AJ: Screening for nasopharyngeal carcinoma. In Miller AB et al, editors: *Cancer screening,* New York, 1990, Cambridge University Press.
27. Levine PH et al: Epstein-Barr virus serology in the control of nasopharyngeal carcinoma, *Cancer Detect Prev* 12:357, 1988.
28. Zeng Y et al: Application of an immunoenzymatic method and immunoautoradiographic method for mass survey of nasopharyngeal carcinoma, *Intervirology* 13:162, 1980.
29. Zeng Y et al: Epstein-Barr virus seroepidemiology in China, *AIDS Res* 2:S7, 1986.
30. Chan SH: Screening for NPC, *Ann Acad Med Singapore* 18:80, 1989.

31. Zeng Y et al: Prospective studies on nasopharyngeal carcinoma in Epstein-Barr virus IgA/VCA antibody-positive persons in Wuzhou City, China, *Int J Cancer* 36:545, 1985.

32. Sawada T et al: Mass screening for the early and immediate detection of neuroblastoma in childhood, *Acta Pediatr Jpn* 20:55, 1978.

33. Sawada T et al: Mass screening for neuroblastoma in infancy, *Am J Dis Child* 136:710, 1982.

34. Sawada T et al: Outcome of 25 neuroblastomas revealed by mass screening in Japan, *Lancet:* 1:377, 1986.

35. Sawada T et al: Neuroblastoma: studies from Japan. In Miller AB et al, editors: *Cancer screening,* New York, 1990, Cambridge University Press.

36. Sawada T: Past and future of neuroblastoma screening in Japan, *Am J Pediatr Hematol Oncol* 14:320, 1992.

37. Nishi M et al: Effects of mass screening of NB in Sapporo City, *Cancer* 60:433, 1987.

38. Parker L, Craft AW, Dale G: Screening for neuroblastoma. In Miller AB et al, editors: *Cancer screening,* 1990, Cambridge University Press.

39. Mandron E, Schill H: Epidemiology of testicular cancer, *Ann Urol* 26:71, 1992.

40. Grove JS: The cryptorchid problem, *J Urol* 71:735, 1954.

41. Morecroft JA, Brereton RJ: Preschool screening for cryptorchidism, *Br Med J* 305:424, 1992.

42. Vogt HB, McHale MS: Testicular cancer: role of primary care physicians in screening and education, *Postgrad Med* 92:93, 1992.

43. Linsell CA: Environmental chemical carcinogens and liver cancer. In Lapis K, Johannessen JV, editors: *Liver carcinogenesis,* New York, 1979, Hemisphere Publishing.

44. Okuda K et al: Changing incidence of hepatocellular carcinoma in Japan, *Cancer Res* 47:4967, 1987.

45. Tatarinov YS: Detection of embryospecific α-globulin in the blood sera of patients with primary liver tumor, *Vopr Med Khim* 10:90, 1964.

46. Beasley RP: Hepatitis B virus: the major etiology of hepatocellular carcinoma, *Cancer* 61:1942, 1988.

47. Mima S et al: Mass screening for hepatocellular carcinoma: experience in Hokkaido, Japan, *J Gastroenterol Hepatol* 9:361, 1994.

48. Pateron D et al: Prospective study for screening for hepatocellular carcinoma in caucasian patients with cirrhosis, *J Hepatol* 20:65, 1994.

49. Martinez FJ et al: Value of ultrasound in the early diagnosis of hepatocellular carcinoma, *Rev Esp Enferm Dig* 84:311, 1993.

50. Unoura M et al: High-risk groups and screening strategies for the early detection of hepatocellular carcinoma in patients with chronic liver disease, *Hepatogastroenterology* 40:305, 1993.

51. Liu SF et al: Esophageal balloon cytology and subsequent risk of esophageal and gastric cardia cancer in the high risk Chinese population, *Int J Cancer* 57:775, 1994.

52. Shen O et al: Cytologic screening for esophageal cancer: results from 12,877 subjects from a high-risk population, *Int J Cancer* 54:185, 1991.

53. Yu Y et al: Retrospective cohort study of risk factors for the development of esophageal cancer in Linxian, People's Republic of China, *Cancer Causes Control* 4:195, 1993.

54. Haggitt RC: Barrett's esophagus, dysplasia and adenocarcinoma, *Hum Pathol* 25:982, 1994.

55. Atkinson M et al: The early diagnosis of esophageal adenocarcinoma by endoscopic screening, *Eur J Cancer Prev* 4:327, 1992.

56. Ina H et al: The frequency of a concomitant early esophageal cancer in male patients with oral or oropharyngeal carcinoma: screening results using Lugol's dye endoscopy, *Cancer* 73:2038, 1994.

GENERAL CONSIDERATIONS IN CANCER SCREENING

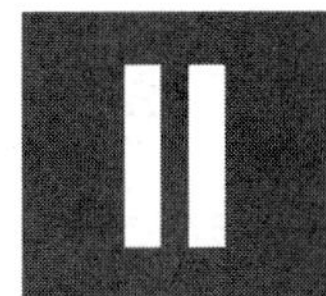

MOLECULAR SCREENING AND PREVENTION OF COLON CANCER

10

Richard C. Karl
Timothy J. Yeatman

Colon cancer is clonal in nature. All colon cancers examined so far have had a monoclonal composition, implying that these tumors arise from a single pocket of cells rather than from various parts of the normal polyclonal colonic epithelium. This finding, with the recognition that colon cancer occurs in families and the observation that societies with diets low in fiber and high in saturated fats have a high incidence of colon cancer, has led to the following hypothesis:

> *Colorectal cancer results from inherited or acquired genetic alterations in the mucosal lining of the gut.*

Inherited genetic changes are evident in familial colon cancer syndromes, whereas sporadic gene mutations appear to be caused or promoted by exposure to carcinogens. There is optimism that the sequence of genetic changes seen in colon cancers as they develop may allow for molecular screening of populations for early detection of these often fatal malignancies. Similarly, an understanding of inherited predisposition to colon malignancy should allow for early intervention in the course of these diseases in individuals at high risk. If the precise mechanism of carcinogen interaction with the genetic material in colon mucosal cells can be understood, the opportunity for behavior modification and chemoprevention may prove useful in the effort to reduce mortality from colorectal cancer. This chapter summarizes the current understanding of the molecular events associated with the development of sporadic and familial colorectal cancer, describes the screening strategies that may take advantage of these molecular markers of cancer development, and surveys the theoretical and practical considerations of current and proposed prevention efforts.

GENETIC ISSUES IN COLORECTAL CANCER

Approximately 150,000 new colorectal cancers will be diagnosed in the United States in 1996. About 94% of these cancers will develop in patients with no known familial predisposition to colon cancer. One percent and 5%, respectively, will be found in patients with familial adenomatous polyposis coli (FAP) and hereditary nonpolyposis colorectal cancer (HNPCC). Taken together, these conditions make colorectal cancer the third most common type of malignancy found in the United States.

Sporadic Colon Cancers

The association of high dietary fat intake (which causes high fecal excretion of neutral sterols and bile acids, compounds that may be metabolized by bacteria to carcinogens), low fiber intake (which causes reduced stool bulk and reduced transit times, leading to the concentration of carcinogenic agents), and colorectal cancer has been noted for some time. What was not clear was why larger numbers of the general population with these dietary habits did not develop malignancy. The clue lay in an understanding of the genetics of colon cancer, even in those patients whose cancers were sporadic. Although some family clusters of sporadic colon cancer were described, no inheritance pattern could be detected because each family had a relatively low incidence of colon cancer, and the number of individuals in these families was too small to allow for sufficient statistical power to prove an inherited predisposition.

> *Recently studies examining the familial incidence of much more common adenomas, known to be precursors of colorectal cancers, have concluded that genetic susceptibility is present in most, if not all, sporadic colon cancers.*[1,2]

The gene predisposing to colon cancer (susceptibility allele) was found in about 19% of the study group and was estimated to have increasing penetrance as an individual ages, that is, penetrance was estimated to be 41% by age 50 and 63% by age 80. These studies make the interaction between genetic and environmental factors more understandable.

Familial Colon Cancers

Familial colon cancers have provided geneticists with a rich supply of clinical material to help identify the precise gene alterations associated with these syndromes. In particular, studies involving families with the FAP syndrome and HNPCC syndrome have been instrumental in the development of a genetic model of inheritance for this process. FAP is a dominantly inherited syndrome characterized by the progressive development of hundreds of adenomatous polyps, a few of which inevitably progress to malignancy. The diagnosis of the syndrome and its variants (Turcot syndrome and Gardner's syndrome) has historically been made by detecting numerous colonic polyps in the second and third decade of life. An associated phenotypic finding that might be useful in screening for affected individuals is congenital hypertrophy of the retinal pigment epithelium (which can be detected by routine ophthalmologic examination). Although these patients represent only 1% of all colon cancers, the number of individuals at risk in the United States alone is estimated to be 50,000.

HNPCC is sometimes referred to as the Lynch syndromes I and II. Lynch syndrome I is characterized by colon cancer development at an early age (mean, 44 years), proximal colon involvement predominantly (70% are proximal to the splenic flexure), and a high frequency of synchronous and metachronous colorectal cancers (40% within 10 years of diagnosis of first cancer). Lynch syndrome II includes all the features of Lynch syndrome I plus a coinherited increased risk for the development of other cancers, most notably of the ovary and endometrium.[3-5] Recently an increased risk for integral malignancies (ureter, renal pelvis transitional cell, stomach, small bowel, and pancreas) has been found in Lynch syndrome II patients.[3] HNPCC was first recognized in 1895 when Aldred Warthin's seamstress sadly predicted to him that she would die young of a cancer, because "most of my family members die of . . . cancers." She died of endometrial cancer. Her family, known as family G, was the first recorded example of aggregated cases of colon, stomach, and endometrial cancer.[4]

IDENTIFIED GENETIC CHANGES IN COLON CANCER

The identification of the genetic loci responsible for the inherited colon cancer syndromes has led to the discovery of several gene alterations that may have a role in the development of sporadic colon cancers as well. Colorectal cancer provides an especially useful model for the study of genetic changes associated with the development of cancer.

> *It appears that all cancers (carcinomas) arise from preexisting benign lesions (adenomas).*[6] *Not all adenomas become carcinomas; one third regress, one third stop growing, and one third become cancers.*

This sequence of events allows for investigation of various stages of tumor formation, from normal mucosa, to small adenomas, to large adenomas, to carcinomas, and on to metastatic disease. Furthermore, clinical material may be obtained by colonoscopic retrieval over time. A succinct and compelling description of a genetic model for colorectal tumorigenesis has been published by Fearon and Vogelstein.[7] The predominant genetic changes found in colon cancer are depicted in Figure 10-1.

Genetic Alterations in Sporadic Colorectal Cancers

Oncogenes

There are three closely related *ras* genes in humans: K-*ras,* H-*ras,* and N-*ras.* These genes code for G proteins integral to signal transduction pathways. Antibodies to the gene products of the three *ras* genes block the ability of cells to synthesize DNA, implying a central role for these genes in cell division.[8,9] Activation of the *ras* gene is the most frequent protooncogene activation seen in human tumors (it occurs in about 20% of all cancers).[8,10] Mutation of *ras* genes

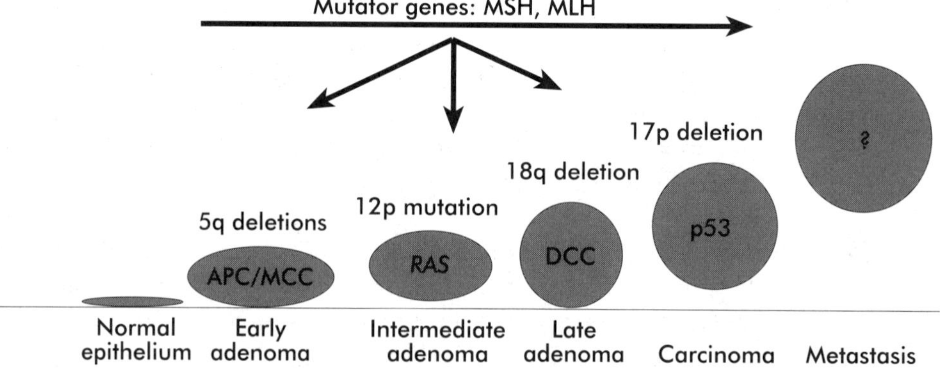

Figure 10-1 Colorectal carcinogenesis: a multistep process. Known genetic changes found in the adenoma to carcinoma sequence. *APC,* Adenomatous polyposis coli; *MCC,* mutated in colon cancer; *DCC,* deleted colon cancer.

may result in G proteins that are always activated and constitutively activate downstream factors involved in cell growth.

> *ras Gene mutations are found in about 50% of colorectal cancers and adenomas greater than 1 cm in diameter, but only in fewer than 10% of adenomas smaller than 1 cm, implying that genetic alterations of this oncogene may be important in the adenoma-to-carcinoma sequence.*[11,12]

These observations were made with equal frequency in both sporadic and inherited tumors.[13,14]

> *Using polymerase chain reaction techniques, K-ras mutations can be detected in the colonic effluent of patients at high risk for the development of colon cancer before the cancer develops.*[15]

These findings may be a basis of molecular screening for colorectal cancer (see further).

Another protooncogene associated with both familial and sporadic colon cancer is c-*myc*.[8,16] Products of the *c-myc* gene act to increase transcription. Almost 70% of human colon cancers have elevated c-*myc* RNA or proteins.[8,17-19] c-*myc* Expression in cancers does not correlate with recurrence or survival.[8,20] Elevated c-*myc* products may interact with other genetic changes such as those that occur with the adenomatous polyposis coli (APC) gene.[8]

Tumor Suppressor Genes

The loss of specific chromosomal regions is common in colon cancers, and this observation has been interpreted as evidence that these regions contain tumor suppressor genes, which code for products that regulate growth and differentiation.[21] Tumor suppressor genes are thought to be recessive; therefore both alleles must be altered for the suppressive function to be deleted and for uncontrolled growth to occur. The most clearly understood tumor suppressor gene model has been developed in studies of retinoblastoma.[22] In this disease an inherited deletion of one gene must be accompanied by a subsequent loss or mutation of the remaining wild type gene for the phenotypic expression of retinoblastoma to occur. This sequence of events has been called the two hit hypothesis of Knudson.[21]

> *More than 75% of colon cancers exhibit a loss of a large segment of chromosome 17p, although this finding is uncommon in adenomas. This finding implies that the genetic alteration occurs late in the adenoma-to-carcinoma sequence.[13,23]*

This region has been shown to contain the p53 gene, and in several colorectal cancers changes in the remaining p53 allele have been identified.[24,25] Thus it appears that the p53 gene functions as a tumor suppressor gene, and these observations are compatible with the Knudson hypothesis. When one allele is lost along with a portion of chromosome 17p, then a mutation in the remaining wild type allele leads to interruption of tumor suppression. The p53 gene product acts as a transcription factor. It binds to other genes and controls their expression; p53 has been called the "guardian of the genome."[26]

Another common region of genetic loss seen in colorectal cancers is chromosome 18q.[13,23] A candidate tumor suppressor gene from this region has been named deleted colon cancer (DCC) and appears to code for a protein that functions as a cell adhesion molecule.[27,28] The loss of a protein or proteins that control the adhesion of colon epithelial cells to one another could account for a decrease in the growth-restraining signals associated with cell-to-cell adhesion. Recently loss of chromosome 18q has been associated with a poorer prognosis for patients with lymph node–negative colon cancer.[29]

Tyrosine kinase activity, controlled by *C-src* gene in some tissues, has been reported to be increased in primary colonic tumors when compared with normal adjacent mucosa.[8,30,31] Tyrosine kinase has been implicated in a number of signal transduction pathways. Larger, more villous polyps are more likely to have increased tyrosine kinase activity than smaller ones, implying some role in malignant transformation.[8] The tyrosine kinase inhibitor, herbimycin A, inhibits growth in colonic tumor cell lines and may be useful as a chemoprevention agent.[8,32]

There is now evidence that cancer results from genetic mutations that allow cells to reproduce with genetic instability, thus increasing the chances of uncontrolled growth.[33] Cell cycle progression is carefully controlled in normal cells at cell cycle checkpoints, which allow for accurate replication and segregation of the genome for DNA repair. Loss of normal cell cycle checkpoints can result in genetic instability and the replication of genetically damaged and potentially malignant cells.

Genetic Alterations in Familial Colon Cancer Syndromes

The family cancer syndromes have provided a rich source of information about genetic changes in colon cancer.

The locus for familial polyposis has been mapped to chromosome 5q.[34,35]

Paradoxically, although 20% to 50% of sporadic colon cancers and 30% of adenomas have allelic losses of chromosome 5q, adenomas from patients with familial polyposis syndromes rarely have this deletion. This observation, that the failure of tumors of patients with inherited cancers to exhibit a loss of the chromosome to which the gene for the inherited disease has been mapped, is in agreement with those observations made in multiple endocrine neoplasia but not with findings made in material gathered from patients with retinoblastoma.[13,22] This tumor suppressor gene on the short arm of chromosome 5 has been called the APC gene.

Similarities between APC and the GTPase activating protein (GAP), which regulates ras gene products, have been detected. This implies a signal transduction, or gatekeeper, role for this gene.

Identical mutations have been identified in the FAP syndrome and Gardner syndrome, an FAP variant characterized by extracolonic tumors in addition to colonic polyps. This observation of similar mutations in the APC gene in both syndromes implies that the different phenotypes must be due to additional genetic alterations.

The APC gene product appears to bind to catenins, proteins that bridge the cytoskeleton to E-cadherin, an intercellular adhesion molecule. The interruption of E-cadherin to catenin binding might alter intercellular adhesion and contribute to tissue invasion, a characteristic of malignancies.

APC gene alterations are the earliest primary genetic changes detected in adenomas, occurring in tumors as small as 5 mm.[8,36] Because the APC gene is altered so early in the development of colorectal cancer, it may be a useful marker for screening populations at risk.

In addition to the APC gene, other genes in the chromosomal 5q21 region are frequently missing in colon cancer, including the mutated in colon cancer (MCC) gene. The relationship between APC and MCC is not clear, but it is known that the latter is not associated with polyp development in FAP syndrome, although it is located close to the APC gene on chromosome 5 and has a similar structure.

It appears that the genetic alterations responsible for HNPCC are different from those found in FAP syndromes. Because the Lynch syndromes are not associated with preneoplastic polyps and because they are three to five times more common than the FAP syndromes, the elucidation of the genes associated with these inherited disorders is important for screening individuals potentially affected by them.

APC, p53, and DCC genes do not display loss of heterozygosity in HNPCC, but a microsatellite marker has been found on chromosome 2p that may be associated with HNPCC in some kindreds but not in others.[8,37,38] Microsatellites are portions of the human genome that contain 50,000 to 100,000 highly repetitive dinucleotide, trinucleotide, and tetranucleotide segments of DNA that display length polymorphisms. These microsatellite DNA markers may be altered in HNPCC and, it turns out, in some right-sided sporadic colon cancers.[8,39] Alterations in these microsatellite DNA repeats probably indicate an increase in DNA instability. Another gene, called *hMSH 2,* has been located on chromosome 2 near the microsatellite marker described above. This gene appears to code for proteins that bind to mispaired DNA bases. DNA repair is now recognized as a critical function of normal cells. Mismatch repair molecules scan newly made DNA for mispaired bases, cut out the mistakes, and fill in the appropriate bases. A DNA repair gene product was designated the molecule of the year in 1994 by *Science.*[40] This gene is mutated in some HNPCC tumors and in some sporadic tumors. Three additional mismatch repair genes (hMLH 1, hPMS 1, and hPMS 2) have been identified as altered in HNPCC.

Phenotypic Markers and the Progression from Adenoma to Carcinoma

Three phenotypic markers may be useful in following the progression of adenoma to carcinoma: sucrase-isomaltose, MAC-2, and DF-3 antigen. Sucrase-isomaltose is a disaccharidase present in the fetal colon that disappears at birth.[8] It is reexpressed in adenomas, particularly those with other characteristics that make them likely to progress to cancer.

MAC-2 is a galactose-binding lectin that is normally found in the nuclei of normal columnar epithelial cells but in the cytoplasm of adenoma cells.

Monoclonal antibodies to DF-3 antigen identify a sialmucin (the peptide core of which is called *MUC-1*) found in neoplastic transformed colon cells. These three phenotypic markers are seen as adenomas progress to carcinoma. When combined with the genetic alterations found in both the FAP and HNPCC models of neoplastic transformation, they establish an elaborate model for colorectal carcinogenesis.

MOLECULAR SCREENING FOR COLORECTAL CANCER

Which, if any, of these laboratory observations may be useful in identifying individuals with sporadic or familial colon cancers or the propensity to develop such malignancies?

Individuals at High Risk for the Development of Colorectal Cancer

A recent study[15] has examined the colonic effluent from persons at high risk for the development of colorectal cancer (those with adenomatous polyps, a previous history of a colorectal cancer, or inflammatory bowel disease) and found that enough tumor cell DNA was present to perform a polymerase chain reaction–based assay for K-*ras* mutations.

> *Approximately 40% of high-risk patients had a mutation in codon 12 of the K-ras gene. It is significant that no evidence of such mutations was found in patients without risk factors. Most important of all is that these changes were observed in the effluent of patients before the development of malignancy.*

This test is possibly a powerful tool for the detection of individuals at risk for colorectal cancers.

There are several potential difficulties with the use of PCR K-*ras* mutation assays. First, only 30% to 50% of colorectal cancers exhibit a *ras* gene mutation. The addition of testing for APC gene mutations might increase the usefulness of molecular screening for colorectal cancer, but tumor suppressor gene mutations are often found in many different parts of the gene as opposed to a specific codon, making the logistics of detecting such a mutation much more difficult than detecting the *ras* mutations.[41] Despite these difficulties, it appears that it is now time to collect colonic effluent from persons at high risk for the development of colorectal cancer so that the specificity and sensitivity of molecular screening can be determined.

> *The ultimate goal is to screen the general population for genetic evidence of a predisposition to colorectal cancer and then to follow it with careful molecular screening of the colonic effluent.*

Individuals with Familial Colon Cancer Syndromes

Both FAP and HNPCC are autosomal dominant inherited disorders and are therefore prime candidates for molecular genetic screening. The HNPCC syndromes (Lynch I and II) are more common than FAP, but the lack of multiple polyps makes colonoscopic screening more difficult. In addition, the genetic alterations seen in sporadic cancers and FAP do not seem to be present in HNPCC. This makes genetic screening difficult. Some of the phenotypic changes seen in HNPCC cancers may lead to the understanding of genetic alterations, which will make screening more practicable, but at the moment no systematic molecular screening rationale for HNPCC has been devised.

FAP syndromes, on the other hand, may be now amenable to molecular screening. A combination of molecular carrier testing and examination for biomarkers has been reported to successfully segregate high-risk from low-risk individuals in FAP kindreds.[42] Using restriction fragment length polymorphism (RFLP) linkage analysis, the inheritance pattern of a DNA probe closely linked to the APC gene can provide carrier risk estimates with 95% to 99% probability.

The familial adenomatous polyposis variant, Gardner's disease, is characterized by osteomas, epidermoid cysts, desmoid tumors, extra dentition, and congenital hypertrophy of retinal pigment epithelium (CHRPE). Ophthalmologic examination for CHRPE complements the RFLP linkage analysis for several reasons. It is suggested that the combination of CHRPE and RFLP studies can distinguish low- from high-risk individuals and that screening guidelines can be tailored to risk assessment.[42] All patients at risk for an FAP syndrome should be given baseline colonoscopy at age 10 to 12 years. High-risk patients should undergo annual or biennial screening for the development of polyps at least until the age of 40 (to detect late-developing FAP). In patients assessed to have low risk, colonoscopic monitoring can be reduced to every 3 to 5 years.

CHEMOPREVENTION OF COLORECTAL CANCER

An understanding of the molecular basis for the progression of normal colon mucosa to adenoma to carcinoma and the influence of dietary factors on the development of sporadic colorectal cancers suggests that chemical intervention in this process may prove useful in an effort to decrease the incidence of new colorectal cancers. A variety of compounds has been advocated as agents effective in interrupting the mucosa to adenoma to carcinoma sequence. There are now data to suggest the mechanisms of action of some of these agents and, in some instances, to pinpoint the site of interaction in the sequence. Chemical agents can block malignant progression at any point along the sequence of the development of colorectal cancer or even cause regression of changes.

Diet and Colorectal Cancer

As mentioned above, the interaction of diet with the genetic material found in the mucosal cells of the intestine is emerging as a fundamental explanation for colorectal cancer in humans. The association of high dietary fat and excess calories with cancer and the inverse relationship between the intake of fiber, calcium, and other micronutrients and malignancy had prompted numerous hypotheses about mechanisms of action and the initiation of some clinical prevention trials.[43]

Because the progression of normal mucosa to adenoma to carcinoma occurs over many years, strategies have been devised to identify early alterations in the sequence, so that various chemoprevention studies can be conducted more quickly. One method widely used to evaluate proliferative activity is the tritiated thymidine labeling index, which has been shown to correlate with risk for colon cancer.[43-46] In addition, the site of cellular proliferation in normal mucosa is in the base of the colonic epithelial crypts, but in patients with precancerous changes, the zone of proliferation has been shown to migrate upward.[43,47,48]

Fat Intake

The two dietary factors most commonly proposed as risk factors for colorectal cancer are fat and fiber. Dietary fat intake correlates closely with colorectal cancer incidence in most epidemiologic studies, is associated with an increase of induced colon cancer in laboratory animals, and has been shown to increase bile acid excretion in humans and laboratory animals.[43,49-58] The metabolites of bile acids produced by normal gut bacteria are thought to be carcinogenic. The epidemiology studies are confounded by associated high intake of protein and low intake of dietary fiber frequently noted in populations consuming a Western diet. Unfortunately, programs designed to change long-established dietary habits have a high attrition rate.[43,59]

Fiber Intake

The association of high dietary fiber intake and lowered risk for colorectal cancer is thought to be attributable to the decrease in gut transit time and decrease in colonic secondary bile acid concentration caused by fiber.[43,60,61] Not all dietary fiber has the same effect on colon carcinogenesis; however[43,60,62-66] dietary cellulose and wheat bran are most protective against chemically induced colon cancer, whereas corn and oat brans are ineffective.[43,60,62-66] Trials are now in progress to examine the effectiveness of dietary fiber intake as a chemopreventive agent in colorectal cancer.

Calcium Intake

There is both experimental and epidemiologic evidence that high calcium intake and the development of colorectal cancer are inversely related. An excess of 1250 mg/day of dietary calcium has been shown to decrease the thymidine labeling index in patients with familial colon cancer.[43,45] A decrease in labeling index was also seen in patients with sporadic adenomas after 10 weeks of calcium gluconate supplementation.[43,67] In experimental animals, increasing calcium intake decreased epithelial cell proliferation in response to exposure to 0.5% cholic acid.[43,68] Calcium's effect may depend on binding the cation to carcinogenic bile acid metabolism.

Epidemiologic studies in Utah (including Mormons and Seventh-Day Adventists, groups with high dietary calcium intake in the form of milk and milk products and low smoking and alcohol consumption) have shown a lower incidence of colorectal cancer when compared with the general population.[43,69] Most epidemiologic studies are seriously flawed by the dietary association of calcium with fiber intake and fat intake.

Antioxidant Vitamins and Lactulose

Antioxidant vitamins appear to have anticancer effect in some experimental models. Retinoids are potent inhibitors of carcinogenesis in skin, liver, and mammary gland tumors in mice and rats.[70-72] Ascorbic acid can cause neoplastic cell lines to revert to normal phenotype.[70,73] The precise mechanism of these effects is not known.

Lactulose has been proposed as a possible chemoprevention agent in colorectal carcinoma. This unabsorbable disaccharide is degraded to lactic acid by intestinal bacteria and effectively lowers ambient pH. Bacterial 7-α-dehydroxylase, the rate-limiting enzyme of bile acid degradation to carcinogenic metabolites, is inactivated at pH levels less than 6.[70]

In a trial conducted in Italy to test the effectiveness of antioxidant vitamins and lactulose on the recurrence of adenomas in patients followed by colonoscopy, both chemoprevention agents had lower adenoma recurrence rates than a control population.[70] In this study participants were treated with a combination of vitamins A, C, and E, or lactulose, or nothing. Adenomas recurred in 5.7%, 14.7%, and 35.9%, respectively.

Nonsteroidal Antiinflammatory Agents

Since 1983, when the regression of colon polyps in familial adenomatous polyposis patients treated with sulindac was first reported, nonsteroidal antiinflammatory agents (NSAIDs) have been proposed as practical chemoprevention agents.[74,75]

There are several additional lines of evidence suggesting that NSAIDs may be useful for the prevention of colorectal cancer. Experimental studies have shown that indomethacin, sulindac, and piroxicam protect the colonic mucosa of mice and rats from the effects of chemical carcinogens.[76-84]

In addition, three large epidemiologic studies have shown that regular aspirin use decreases the risk of dying of colorectal cancer.[76,85-87]

Furthermore, at least two controlled studies have shown *regression* of polyps in FAP patients treated with sulindac. Finally, sulindac and piroxicam have been associated with the regression of *sporadic* colon polyps as well.[76,84]

The protective mechanism of action exhibited by NSAIDs on the colonic mucosa is not clear, but an effect on arachidonic acid metabolism and prostaglandin synthesis has been proposed. These substances have been associated with tumor initiation, promotion, growth, and spread. The mechanism of action of aspirin may be different from that of other NSAIDs. Aspirin causes the acetylation of prostaglandin H synthetase, which inactivates its cyclooxygenase activity irreversibly, whereas other NSAIDs inhibit the enzyme in a concentration-dependent and reversible manner.[78,88-90] The effect of aspirin appears to be related to the cumulative days of administration and not to total dosage.[78] Its effect is seen at dosages currently prescribed for the prevention of stroke or myocardial infarction. Acetaminophen, a commonly prescribed analgesic, has no effect on colon polyps.[78]

It should be noted that some studies have not shown an effect of NSAIDs on colorectal cancer incidence[78,91] and that other studies may harbor inherent biases. For instance, studies evaluating death from colorectal cancer as an outcome may be affected by a higher incidence of bleeding from early cancers or even premalignant lesions in the NSAIDs group when compared with controls. This herald bleeding might lead to earlier intervention in a colon cancer and hence better survival.[78]

Other Possible Chemoprevention Molecules

As mentioned above, activation of *ras* gene expression by point mutation is the most frequent protooncogene activation observed in human cancers. Because *ras* gene expression requires membrane association, an event mediated by farneslyation, inhibitors of farnesyl protein transferase may prevent malignant transformation. Studies with lovastatin (Mevacor), which blocks farnesyl pyrophosphate, show that it inhibits *ras* function in mouse tumorigenesis models.[8,92,93] This molecule, if it proves to have selective effect, may be useful in colon cancer prevention.

As described above, tyrosine kinase (controlled in part by C-*src* gene) is active in signal transduction. There is abundant evidence that C-*src* activation is important in the malignant transformation of colonic cells.[8,94-96] Interestingly, the tyrosine kinase inhibitor, herbimycin A, has inhibited the growth of every malignant colonic cell line tested, but not normal colon epithelial cells.[8,76] These findings imply a potential usefulness for herbimycin A in the prevention of colon cancer.

Chemoprevention Strategies

For several reasons, the strategies necessary for chemoprevention trials are more complex than cancer treatment trials. First, the individuals assigned to drug intervention are without symptoms or known disease. Therefore the toxicity of the chemoprevention agent must approach zero. Second, although in most cancer treatment trials recurrence of cancer is likely, in chemoprevention trials in the general population the risk of disease is low (an average person 50 years old has a 5% risk of developing colon cancer by age 80).[76] This low incidence implies trials including thousands of persons over many years must be conducted to obtain sufficient statistical power to detect an effect of a prevention agent.

There are two ways that trials could be designed to increase the chances of detecting a salutary effect of a chemoprevention agent. First, high-risk groups (FAP, HNPCC, inflammatory bowel disease, history of adenoma) could be studied.

> *Second, intermediate points along the normal mucosa to adenoma to carcinoma sequence could be used as end points of the study, rather than occurrence of an actual cancer. Shorter follow-up trials may be possible if biomarkers such as histology (aberrant crypts), proliferation, differentiation, and genetic characteristics (aneuploidy, DNA methylation, oncogenes, tumor suppression genes) are used as end points.*[76]

A less elegant but less expensive trial might use adenoma incidence rather than carcinoma incidence as an end point.

Trials are now being conducted to evaluate the efficacy of dietary modification (low-fat, high-fiber, high-vegetable diet), specific nutrients (fiber, calcium, vitamins C and E, β-carotene), and xenobiotics (NSAIDs, polyamine synthesis inhibitor, difluoromethyl ornithine) in the prevention of colorectal cancer.

It has been suggested that chemoprevention trials will be conducted in phases like cancer treatment trials. In prevention studies phase I will evaluate agents for lack of toxicity, phase II will evaluate an intermediate end point (biomarker, adenomas), and phase III will test the most promising agents for their ability to prevent the development of colorectal cancer.[76]

REFERENCES

1. Burt RW et al: Dominant inheritance of adenomatous colonic polyps and colorectal cancer, *N Engl J Med* 312:1540, 1985.
2. Cannon-Albright LA et al: Common inheritance of susceptibility to adenomatous polyps and associated colorectal cancers, *N Engl J Med* 319:533, 1988.
3. Lynch HT et al: Cancer control problems in the Lynch syndromes, *Dis Colon Rectum* 36:254, 1993.
4. Lynch HT et al: Genetics, natural history, tumor spectrum, and pathology of hereditary nonpolyposis colorectal cancer: an updated review, *Gastroenterology* 104:1535, 1993.
5. Powell SM et al: Molecular diagnosis and familial adenomatous polyposis, *N Engl J Med* 329:1982, 1993.
6. Sugarbaker JP, Gunderson LL, Wittes RE: Colorectal cancer. In DeVita VT, Hellman S, Rosenberg SA, editors: *Cancer: principles and practices of oncology,* Philadelphia, 1985, JB Lippincott.
7. Fearon ER, Vogelstein B: A genetic model for colorectal tumorigenesis, *Cell* 61:759, 1990.
8. Jessup JM: Molecular biology of neoplastic transformation of the large bowel, *Surg Oncol Clin North Am* 3:449, 1994.
9. Stacey DW et al: Critical role of *ras* proteins in proliferative signal transduction, *Cold Spring Harbor Symp Quant Biol* 53:871, 1988.
10. Bos JL: *ras* Oncogenes in human cancer: a review, *Cancer Res* 49:4682, 1989.
11. Bos JL et al: Prevalence of *ras* gene mutations in human colorectal cancers, *Nature* 327:293, 1987.
12. Forrester K et al: Detection of high incidence of K-*ras* oncogenes during human colon tumorigenesis, *Nature* 327:298, 1987.

13. Vogelstein B et al: Genetic alterations during colorectal tumor development, *N Engl J Med* 319:525, 1988.

14. Farr CJ et al: A study of *ras* gene mutations in colonic adenomas from familial polyposis coli patients, *Oncogene* 3:673, 1988.

15. Tobi M, Luo FC, Ronai Z: Detection of K-*ras* mutation in colonic effluent samples from patients without evidence of colorectal carcinoma, *J Natl Cancer Inst* 86:1007, 1994.

16. Erisman MD, Scott JK, Astrin SM: Evidence that the familial adenomatous polyposis gene is involved in a subset of colon cancer with a complementable defect in c-*myc* regulation, *Proc Natl Acad Sci USA* 86:4262, 1989.

17. Alitalo K et al: Homogeneously staining chromosomal regions contain amplified copies of an abundantly expressed cellular oncogene (c-*myc*) in malignant neuroendocrine cells from a human colon cancer, *Proc Natl Acad Sci USA* 80:1707, 1983.

18. Erisman MD et al: Deregulation of c-*myc* gene expression in human colon cancer is not accompanied by amplification or rearrangement of the gene, *Mol Cell Biol* 5:1969, 1985.

19. Erisman MD et al: The c-*myc* protein is constituitively expressed at elevated levels in colorectal carcinoma cell lines, *Oncogene* 2:367, 1988.

20. Erisman MD et al: Noncorrelation of the expression of the c-*myc* oncogene in colorectal carcinoma with recurrence of disease or patient survival, *Cancer Res* 48:1350, 1988.

21. Knudson AG: Hereditary cancer, oncogenes, and anti-oncogenes, *Cancer Res* 45:1437, 1985.

22. Hansen MF, Cavenee WK: Genetics of cancer predisposition, *Cancer Res* 47:5518, 1987.

23. Delattre P et al: Multiple genetic alterations distinguish distal from proximal colorectal cancer, *Lancet* 2:353, 1989.

24. Baker SJ et al: Chromosome 17 deletions and p53 gene mutations in colorectal carcinomas, *Science* 244:217, 1989.

25. Nigro JM et al: Mutations in the p53 gene occur in diverse human tumour types, *Nature* 342:705, 1989.

26. Culotta E, Koshland DE: Molecule of the year: p53 sweeps through cancer research, *Science* 262:1958, 1993.

27. Fearon ER, Hamilton SR, Vogelstein B: Clonal analysis of human colorectal tumors, *Science* 238:193, 1987.

28. Edelman GM: Morphoregulatory molecules, *Biochemistry* 27:3533, 1988.

29. Jen J et al: Allelic loss of chromosome 18q and prognosis in colorectal cancer, *N Engl J Med* 331:213, 1994.

30. Hunter T: A thousand and one protein kinases, *Cell* 50:823, 1987.

31. Bolen JB et al: Activation of pp60[c-src] protein kinase activity in human colon carcinoma, *Proc Natl Acad Sci USA* 84:2251, 1987.

32. Garcia RA et al: The antimycin antibiotic herbimycin A inhibits colon tumor cell lines by interaction with pp60[c-src], *Oncogene* 6:1983, 1991.

33. Hartwell LH, Kastan MB: Cell cycle control and cancer, *Science* 266:1821, 1994.

34. Bodmer WF et al: Localization of the gene for familial adenomatous polyposis on chromosome 5, *Nature* 328:614, 1987.

35. Leppert M et al: The gene for familial polyposis coli maps to the long arm of chromosome 5, *Science* 238:1411, 1987.

36. Powell SM et al: APC mutations occur in early colorectal tumorigenesis, *Nature* 359:235, 1992.

37. Aaltonon LA et al: Clues to the pathogenesis of familial colorectal cancer, *Science* 260:812, 1993.

38. Peltomaki P et al: Genetic mapping of a locus predisposing to human colorectal cancer, *Science* 260:810, 1993.

39. Thibodeau SN, Bren G, Schnaid D: Microsatellite instability in cancer of the proximal colon, *Science* 260:816, 1993.

40. Culotta E, Koshland DE: Molecule of the year: DNA repair works its way to the top, *Science* 266:1926, 1994.

41. Sidransky D: Molecular screening—how long can we afford to wait? *J Natl Cancer Inst* 86:955, 1994.

42. Bapat BV et al: Combined use of molecular and biomarkers for presymptomatic carrier risk assessment in familial adenomatous polyposis: implications for screening guidelines, *Dis Colon Rectum* 37:165, 1994.

43. Vargas PA, Alberts DS: Primary prevention of colorectal cancer through dietary modification, *Cancer Suppl* 70:1229, 1992.

44. Lipkin M et al: Tritiated thymidine labeling distribution as a marker for hereditary predisposition to colon cancer, *Cancer Res* 43:1899, 1983.

45. Lipkin M: Effect of added dietary calcium on colonic epithelial cells' proliferation in subjects at high risk for familial colonic cancer, *N Engl J Med* 313:1381, 1985.

46. Deschner EE, Maskens AP: Proliferation patterns in colonic mucosa in familial polyposis, *Cancer* 35:413, 1975.

47. Cole JW, McKalen A: Studies on the morphogenesis of adenomatous polyps in the human colon, *Cancer* 8:998, 1963.

48. Deschner EE, Maskens AP: Significance of the labeling index and the labeling distribution as kinetic parameters in colonic mucosa of cancer patients and DMH treated animals, *Cancer* 50:1136, 1982.

49. Gastrointestinal Tumor Study Group: Adjuvant therapy of colon cancer: results of prospectively randomized trial, *N Engl J Med* 310:737, 1984.

50. Willet WC et al: Relation of meat, fat, and fiber intake to the risk of colon cancer in a prospective study among women, *N Engl J Med* 323:1664, 1990.

51. Armstrong B, Doll R: Environmental factors and cancer incidence and mortality in different countries, with special reference to dietary practices, *Int J Cancer* 15:617, 1975.

52. Rose DP, Boyar AP, Wynder EL: International comparisons of mortality rates for cancer of the breast, ovary, prostate, and colon, and per capita food consumption, *Cancer* 58:2363, 1986.

53. Kune GA, Kune S: The nutritional causes of colorectal cancer: an introduction to the Melbourne study, *Nutr Cancer* 9:1, 1987.

54. Knox EG: Foods and diseases, *Br J Prev Soc Med* 31:71, 1977.

55. Reddy BS et al: Effect of quality and quanity of dietary fat and dimethylhydrazine in colon carcinogenesis in rats, *Proc Soc Exp Biol Med* 151:237, 1976.

56. Reddy BS et al: Effect of type and amount of dietary fat and 1,2-dimethylhydrazine on biliary bile acids and neutra sterols in rats, *Cancer Res* 37:2132, 1977.

57. Hill MJ: The role of unsaturated bile acids in the etiology of large bowel cancer. In Hiatt HH, Watson JD, Winsten JA, editors: *Origins of human cancer,* New York, 1977, Cold Spring Harbor Laboratories.

58. Reddy BS: Diet and excretion of bile acids, *Cancer Res* 41:3766, 1981.

59. Stunkard AJ: Biological and psychological factors in obesity. In Goldstein RK, editor: *Eating and weight disorders: advances in treatment and research,* New York, 1983, Springer.

60. Reddy BS et al: Biochemical epidemiology of colon cancer: effect of types of dietary fiber on fecal mutagens, acid and neutral sterols in healthy subjects, *Cancer Res* 49:4629, 1989.

61. Reddy BS et al: Metabolic epidemiology of colon cancer: effect of dietary fiber on fecal mutagens and bile acids in healthy subjects, *Cancer Res* 47:644, 1987.

62. Freeman HJ, Spiller GA, Kim YS: A double blind study on the effect of purified cellulose dietary fiber on 1,2-dimethylhydrazine–induced rat colonic neoplasia, *Cancer Res* 38:2912, 1978.

63. Freeman HJ: Effects of dietary fiber on fecal β-glucuronidase in colon carcinogen treated rats, *Clin Res* 29:32A, 1981.

64. Freeman HJ, Spiller GA, Kim YS: A double blind study of the effect of differing purified cellulose dietary fiber and pectin fiber diets on 1,2-dimethylhydrazine-induced rat colonic neoplasia, *Cancer Res* 40:2661, 1980.

65. Reddy BS, Mori H: Effect of dietary wheat bran and dehydrated citrus fiber on 3,2'-di-

methyl-4-aminobiphenyl–induced intestinal carcinogenesis in F344 rats, *Carcinogenesis* 2:21, 1981.

66. Smith-Barbaro P, Hansen D, Reddy BS: Carcinogen binding to various types of dietary fiber, *J Natl Cancer Inst* 67:495, 1981.

67. Rozen P et al: Oral calcium suppresses increased rectal epithelial proliferation of persons at risk of colorectal cancer, *Gut* 30:650, 1989.

68. Bird RP, Stamp D: Effect of high fat diet on the murine colonic epithelium, *Cancer Lett* 31:61, 1986.

69. Slattery ML, Sorenson AW, Ford MH: Dietary calcium intake as a mitigating factor in colon cancer, *Am J Epidemiol* 128:504, 1988.

70. Roncucci L et al: Antioxidant vitamins or lactulose for the prevention of the recurrence of colorectal adenomas, *Dis Colon Rectum* 36:227, 1993.

71. Thompson HJ et al: Effect of the duration of retinyl acetate feeding on inhibition of 1-methyl-1-nitrosourea–induced mammary carcinogenesis in the rat, *Cancer Res* 39:3977, 1979.

72. Newberne PM, Rogeres AE: Rat colon carcinomas associated with aflatoxin and vitamin A, *J Natl Cancer Inst* 50:439, 1973.

73. Benedict WF, Wheatley WL, Jones PA: Inhibition of chemically induced morhpological transformation and reversion of the transformed phenotype by ascorbic acid in C3H/10T1/2 cells, *Cancer Res* 40:2796, 1980.

74. Labayle D et al: Sulindac causes regression of rectal polyps in familial adenomatous polyposis, *Gastroenterology* 101:635, 1991.

75. Waddell WR, Longhry RW: Sulindac for polyposis of the colon, *J Surg Oncol* 24:83, 1983.

76. Ahnen DJ: Multiphase chemoprevention of large bowel carcinogenesis, *Am J Gastroenterol* 88:1647, 1993 (editorial).

77. Reddy BS et al: Inhibition of colon carcinogenesis by prostaglandin synthesis inhibitors and related compounds, *Carcinogenesis* 13:1019, 1992.

78. Peleg II: Aspirin and nonsteroidal anti-inflammatory drug use and the risk of subsequent colorectal cancer, *Arch Intern Med* 154:394, 1994.

79. Narisawa T et al: Inhibition of development of methylnitrosourea-induced rat colon tumors by indomethacin treatment, *Cancer Res* 41:1954, 1981.

80. Sato M et al: Growth inhibition of transplantable murine colon adenocarcinoma 38 by indomethacin, *J Cancer Res Clin Oncol* 106:21, 1983.

81. Pollard M, Luckert PH: Prolonged antitumor effect of indomethacin on autochronous intestinal tumors in rats, *J Natl Cancer Inst* 70:1103, 1983.

82. Olson NO: Effect of indomethacin on the growth of colon cancer cells in syngeneic rats, *Int J Immunopharmacol* 6:329, 1984.

83. Reddy BS, Maruyama H, Kelloff G: Dose-related inhibition of colon carcinogenesis by dietary piroxicam, a nonsteroidal anti-inflammatory drug, during different stages of colon tumor development, *Cancer Res* 47:5340, 1987.

84. Skinner SA, Penney AG, O'Brien PE: Sulindac inhibits the rate of growth and appearance of colon tumors in the rat, *Arch Surg* 126:1094, 1991.

85. Rosenberg L et al: A hypothesis: nonsteroidal anti-inflammatory drugs reduce the incidence of large bowel cancer, *J Natl Cancer Inst* 83:355, 1991.

86. Kune GA, Kune S, Watson LF: Colorectal cancer risk, chronic illness, operations, and medications: case control results from the Melbourne colorectal cancer study, *Cancer Res* 48:4399, 1988.

87. Thun MJ, Namboodiri MM, Heath CW: Aspirin use and reduced risk of fatal colon cancer, *N Engl J Med* 325:1593, 1991.

88. Weisman G: Aspirin and aspirin-like drugs. In Wyngaarden JB, Smith LH Jr, Bennett JT, editors: *Cecil textbook of medicine*, Philadelphia, 1992, WB Saunders.

89. Vane JR, Botting RM: The mode of action of anti-inflammatory drugs, *Postgrad Med J* 66:2, 1990.

90. Cyrer B, Feldman M: Effects of nonsteroidal anti-inflammatory drugs on endogenous gastrointestinal prostaglandins and therapeutic strategies for prevention and treatment of nonsteroidal anti-inflammatory drug-induced damage, *Arch Intern Med* 152:1145, 1992.

91. Gann PH et al: Low-dose aspirin and incidence of colorectal tumors in a randomized trial, *J Natl Cancer Inst* 85:1220, 1993.

92. Miller AC et al: Increased radioresistance of EJ*ras*-transformed human osteosarcoma cells and its modulation by lovastatin, an inhibitor of p21*ras* isoprenylation, *Int J Cancer* 53:302, 1993.

93. Rilling HC et al: Differential prenylation of proteins as a function of mevalonate concentration in CHO cells, *Arch Biochem Biophys* 301:210, 1993.

94. Cartwright CA et al: pp60$^{c\text{-}src}$ activation in human colon carcinoma, *J Clin Invest* 83:2025, 1989.

95. Weber TK et al: Differential pp60c-src activity in well and poorly differentiated human colon carcinoma and cell lines, *J Clin Invest* 90:815, 1992.

96. Talamonti MS et al: The c-*src* oncogene participates in the development of human colorectal liver metastases, *Surg Forum* 42:422, 1991.

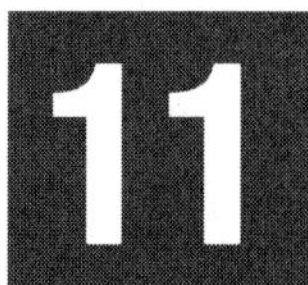

BREAST CANCER GENETICS

Sofia D. Merajver
Judy E. Garber
Barbara L. Weber

CLINICAL SIGNIFICANCE

In Western society, breast cancer is the most common malignancy in women, with a lifetime risk of 1 in 8.[1] In the United States it is the second most common cause of death by cancer in women, accounting for approximately

This work was supported, in part, by grant GCRC-MCAP 3MO11RR 00042-3451 TOSDM from the National Institutes of Health.

48,000 fatalities each year.[2,3] The incidence of breast cancer has been increasing at a rate ranging from 1.2% to 4% a year in the second half of this century.[4] Mammography, an aging population, late age at first birth,[5] early menarche,[6,7] and increased body weight[8] have all been implicated as potential causes of this steady increase in incidence.

> *However, the mortality rate that remained stable for several years is now showing a decrease, most likely as a result of increased awareness of and compliance with early-detection guidelines.[3,9-12]*

Therapeutic advances in systemic therapy are also thought to play an important role in limiting mortality.

In the last 15 years exciting advances in molecular and cellular biology have started to unravel the events leading to the development of cancers.[13,14] Oncogenes have been implicated in the establishment of uncontrolled growth in cancers. For example, the HER2/neu oncogene is amplified in 21% of breast cancers, and this amplification is positively correlated with nodal status.[15] Novel therapeutic modalities emanating from this knowledge have already entered clinical trials, such as anti-HER2/neu antibody and other growth factor antagonists. The recognition[16] and isolation of genes termed *tumor suppressors,*[17-21] whose loss of function[18,22-25] leads to cancer, have been a focus of molecular genetics research. Tumor suppressor genes appear to be important in cellular functions designed to regulate growth and to prevent the replication or propagation of damaged DNA. They are involved in cell cycle regulation *(TP53),* in DNA repair *(MSH, MSH2, MLH1, PMS1, PMS2),*[26-28] and in the regulation of expression of other genes *(WT1).*[29] Tumor suppressor genes, which are inactivated by mutations or deletions, lose these regulatory functions, potentially leading to malignant transformation.[29-31] Many of the genes responsible for familial cancer syndromes appear to be tumor suppressor genes.

The recognition of other adult-onset diseases for which a single locus has been implicated—such as Huntington's disease[32] (HD) and adult polycystic kidney disease (APKD),[33] has led to pioneering research on the clinical and ethical aspects of genetic screening and testing.

> *Advances in the discipline of genetic counseling combined with the knowledge of cancer susceptibility genes will likely lead to the unprecedented situation in which a significant proportion of the population may seek risk assessment and/or predictive testing for cancer susceptibility genes in the near future.[9,34-40]*

Although only 5% to 8% of all breast cancer cases are caused by germline mutations in susceptibility genes, their high penetrance (90%) warrants efforts to identify this at-risk population and offer early detection and preventive options.[41-46] In addition, these single-gene disorders will afford new opportunities to study in vitro and animal models of mammary epithelial carcinogenesis, which may closely resemble human mammary and ovarian carcinogenesis.

The information derived from molecular genetics research, combined with rational predictive testing and counseling, has the potential for preventing cancers, averting unnecessary prophylactic surgery in women not at increased risk, and detecting cancer at an early stage through heightened awareness and rational surveillance protocols.[47] Risk assessment information has the potential for negatively affecting the individual tested and her family through breach of confidentiality and discrimination in employability and insurability, loss of autonomy because of passive or active cohersion, and the psychologic and emotional burden of knowing one's cancer risk.[34,48]

FAMILIAL BREAST CANCER CHARACTERISTICS

Familial aggregation of breast cancer was first described over 2000 years ago.[49] However, the scientific study of the frequency and possible causes of this phenomenon has developed rapidly only in the last 15 years. Although single-gene disorders have recently received considerable attention, other causes for familial clustering of breast cancer cases must also be considered. In general, familial clustering of breast cancer cases can be attributed to the following factors (Table 11-1): (1) rare, highly penetrant single-gene defects transmitted through a lineage with a predictable pattern of mendelian inheritance (such as *BRCA1*, *BRCA2*,[50] *TP53*), (2) common single-gene defects of low penetrance or variable expressivity, (3) complex polygenic interactions, (4) shared exposures to environmental[51] and dietary risk factors, (5) culturally influenced risk factors associ-

---

TABLE 11-1

CAUSES OF FAMILIAL AGGREGATION OF BREAST CANCER

Phenomenon	Family Characteristics	Examples
Single-gene disorder	Rare, high penetrance	*BRCA1, BRCA2*
	Common, low penetrance	Unknown
Polygenic defects	Inherited factors modulate expressivity and penetrance of other genes	Unknown
Environmental exposures	Unknown; familial cluster	Pesticides, radiation,[53-55] HRT,[52] diet[56-60]
Cultural influences	Unknown; familial cluster	Reproductive habits: age at first birth, contraceptive use, diet
Common modulating influences	Familial clustering ≥ 1 generation with multiple cases of common tumors	Breast, ovarian, and prostate cancers may be modulated by common hormonal milieu

---

TABLE 11-2

CHARACTERISTICS OF INHERITED BREAST CANCER

* Younger age of onset
* Bilaterality
* Multiple primary cancers in one individual
* Clustering of different tumor types in family members

---

ated with lifestyle patterns such as age at first birth, number of pregnancies, exercise, body weight, contraceptive practices,[52] socioeconomic status, and (6) coincidental occurrence of sporadic cases of a prevalent disease within a family. Although considerable progress has been achieved in recent years in the localization and identification of highly penetrant cancer susceptibility genes, research on the complex molecular interactions that give rise to cancer in a given individual still lies ahead. Increasing knowledge about the identity and function of genes responsible for hereditary breast cancer syndromes will lead to a better understanding of the interactions among all these factors in the pathways leading to carcinogenesis.

> *Inherited breast cancer has several clinical characteristics that are, on the average, different from those of sporadic breast cancer: the age of onset is younger, bilaterality is more common, and the presence of associated tumors at other sites in affected individuals is noted in some families.[61-66]*

Associated tumors may include ovarian, colon, prostate, and endometrial cancers and sarcomas.[24,66-70] However, inherited and sporadic breast cancers are otherwise indistinguishable by histologic type, grade, metastatic behavior, detectability by clinical or radiographic means, or response to therapy (Table 11-2).[71]

EPIDEMIOLOGIC AND GENETIC LINKAGE STUDIES

Family history is, after age, the most important predictor of breast cancer risk.[72-76] About 38% of persons with breast cancer have a family history of some kind.[43] A very strong association between family history and the risk of breast cancer has been observed in a small subgroup of the population for a long time.[49,75] In the last 20 years epidemiologic methodology has elucidated that there is a population of individuals who belong to families with apparent autosomal dominant transmission of breast cancers associated with highly penetrant susceptibility alleles; they account for approximately 5% to 8% of all breast cancer cases.[43,73] Typically three or more relatives in a given lineage (maternal or paternal) are affected with breast cancer. Other cancers such as ovarian, colon, and prostate may also be present. Although it has long been known that breast cancer in first-degree relatives is a major contributor to the risk of developing the disease, in most studies this link is especially significant in the presence of early-onset (premenopausal) and bilateral breast cancer in the family.[43,62,63]

Several population-based studies in the United States and Sweden have attempted to estimate the contribution of a positive family history to breast cancer risk.[61,62,74,75,77] They found a standardized relative risk of 2.0 to 3.0 for women with a first-degree relative with breast cancer compared with controls without a family history. Higher risks were reported in studies involving large cohorts of volunteers, who may have been more inclined to participate if they had a family history of breast cancer, thereby biasing the studies. The relative risk measure is useful for a variety of public health applications, but it is not amenable to the risk assessment of individual patients. The lifetime risk and the risks at 5, 10, and 20 years are more helpful in this regard.[43] These empiric risks are estimates that can be deduced from a number of studies; it is unavoidable, however, that they be subject to the limitations of the study from which they derive.

The Cancer and Steroid Hormone (CASH) Study determined that the risk of developing breast cancer for a woman with a sister and mother affected was 14-fold greater than the risk of women with no family history of breast cancer (background risk).[74] The CASH study was retrospective and questionnaire based. The risks are likely to be exaggerated primarily due to classic recall bias because patients with breast cancer may be more likely to be aware of affected family members than normal controls.[78]

Prospective studies such as the Nurses' Health Study (NHS)[72] and the Utah Population Database (UPD),[75] a case control study, are not subject to this bias. Both studies concluded that the risk of developing breast cancer approximately doubles if the proband has a sister or a mother affected, and it is over three times higher if more than one first-degree relative is affected. However, these studies significantly disagree on the total risk of breast cancer attributable to familial factors: 2.5% and 17% to 19% for the NHS and the UPD, respectively. The NHS probably underestimates the family history contribution to breast cancer risk because small families predominate and the paternal family history was not included in the analysis. In contrast, the UPD is influenced by large families, which were common in its study population, and affected distant relatives were included in the calculations of risk.

> *If both studies are analyzed taking into account only first- and second-degree relatives, the proportion of the total breast cancer risk ascribed to heredity is 7% to 10% in their respective populations.*

This may be a more realistic estimate of the breast cancer risk attributable to family history.[79]

Studies in which the population under investigation is enriched with high-risk families proved especially useful for the detection of a strong association between family history and breast cancer.[73,75] Factors that were shown to increase risk within families were premenopausal status at diagnosis and bilateral disease. Additionally, first-degree relatives of probands were found to be at higher risk than second-degree relatives.

> *More strikingly, calculation of risk in individuals with two affected first-degree relatives (such as mother-daughter or sister-sister) with premenopausal, bilateral disease yielded almost a 50% lifetime risk of breast cancer. These data suggested the presence of an autosomal dominant susceptibility gene, with nearly complete penetrance, responsible for the development of breast cancer in this subgroup of families.*[61,73]

In contrast, the calculated lifetime risk of 7% to 9% in first-degree relatives of women with postmenopausal diagnosis and unilateral disease hardly differs from the general population risk.[2] Table 11-3 summarizes the empiric risks for different relative pairs.

TABLE 11-3

EMPIRIC RISK OF DEVELOPING BREAST CANCER AS A RESULT OF FAMILY HISTORY

Affected relatives	Clinical characteristics	Lifetime empiric risk (%)
Mother or sister	Both premenopausal	13-21
	Both postmenopausal	9-11
Mother and sister	Both premenopausal	24-48
	Both postmenopausal	11-25
Mother and maternal aunt	Both premenopausal	20-45
	Both postmenopausal	11-37
	Mother premenopausal and aunt postmenopausal	20-39
	Mother postmenopausal and aunt premenopausal	18-37
Mother and paternal aunt	Both premenopausal	15-26
	Both postmenopausal	10-12
	Mother premenopausal and aunt postmenopausal	13-22
	Mother postmenopausal and aunt premenopausal	15-19
One maternal and one paternal second-degree relative	Both premenopausal	13-20
	One premenopausal	11-16

From Claus EB, Risch N, Thompson WD: *Cancer* 73:643, 1994.

Genetic linkage and positional cloning studies leading to the ascertainment of the highly penetrant tumor suppressor genes *BRCA1, BRCA2,* and *TP53* have led to the isolation of genes that can now be studied in detail in at-risk populations. Hall et al.[80] first identified 17q21 as the chromosomal location for *BRCA1.* Coincident transmission of the susceptibility to breast and ovarian cancer was shown by Narod et al.[81] on a different cohort of families whose genetic linkage analyses confirmed the close linkage to chromosome 17q.

Initial estimates suggest that up to 67% of families with apparent autosomal dominant transmission of breast cancer and average age of onset below 45 years show linkage to genetic markers in this region.[45]

> *For familial early-onset breast and ovarian cancer, 90% of such families appear to be linked to BRCA1. The lifetime risks of developing breast and ovarian cancer for BRCA1 mutation carriers who are part of large kindreds are different. There is estimated to be an 85% lifetime risk of developing breast cancer by age 80. The distribution of risk as a function of age is skewed toward younger ages, with a 60% risk by age 50.*

For ovarian cancer, the lifetime risk is estimated to be 35% to 63%, although this figure is less well established than for breast cancer secondary to the lower and more variable incidence of ovarian cancer in the *BRCA1*-linked families.[44,68]

> *Based on susceptibility allele frequency estimates and the overall incidence of breast cancer, BRCA1 germline mutations are likely to be responsible for approximately 3% to 5% of all breast cancers and approximately half of all inherited breast cancers.*

TUMOR BIOLOGY

One definition of cancer that agrees with decades of research is that of the clonal expansion of a single cell which has acquired alterations in its DNA that are heritable by its progeny. Most human cancers exhibit diverse genetic changes such as point mutations, translocations, amplifications, and deletions, which occur during the malignant transformation and progression to an invasive phenotype. When these alterations upregulate genes that stimulate cellular proliferation or downregulate genes involved in limiting growth by promoting differentiation, cancers may arise and progress.

Oncogenes can induce cellular transformation and deregulated proliferation when activated by a genetic alteration in the tissues. They encode protein products that function as growth modulators, growth factor receptors, second messengers, and transcription regulators. Oncogenes are involved in the early transformation events in certain cancers such as colon cancer and in the progression toward the malignant phenotype in most kinds of cancers, including breast. To date, no hereditary cancer syndromes have been ascribed to mutated oncogenes.

Recently attention has been focused on genes that are believed to play a role in the suppression of malignant transformation. Using somatic cell hybrids, several groups showed that tumorigenicity can be suppressed by the presence of normal chromosomes.[82,83] The first evidence for the role of tumor suppressor genes in the pathogenesis of human cancers was provided by pioneering work on the retinoblastoma gene *(Rb)*. It is now known that all patients with hereditary retinoblastoma carry a germline mutation in one allele of the *Rb* gene.[19,24] Knudson's two hit hypothesis postulated a defect or mutation in the wild-type allele arising in the tumor; this has proven to be the case with the *Rb* gene.[16] Loss of the wild-type allele results in the inactivation of both *Rb* alleles: the first one by the inherited germline mutation, the second one by a somatic event. This second deletion or inactivation event can often be detected in tumor samples by the loss of the wild-type allele for informative markers in the region of interest; this phenomenon is termed loss of heterozygosity (LOH). Other examples of tumor suppressor genes have now been described, including those responsible for neurofibromatoses *(NF1* and *NF2)*, the Li-Fraumeni syndrome *(TP53)*, adenomatous polyposis coli *(APC)*, Wilms' tumor *(WT1)*, and the breast/ovarian cancer syndrome *(BRCA1)*, all of which exhibit high frequency of LOH when tumor samples are analyzed with genetic markers flanking the gene. Breast cancer is present in excess of the predicted rate in several familial cancer syndromes (Table 11-4). Several of the genes implicated in these syndromes have been identified, and that knowledge is contributing to the emerging field of genetic screening and counseling for increased cancer susceptibility risk.

TABLE 11-4

HEREDITARY SYNDROMES ASSOCIATED WITH BREAST AND OVARIAN CANCER

Tumor	Syndrome or gene (if known)	Other malignancies or characteristics
Breast	Ataxia-telangectasia[92,93]/*AT*	Telangiectasia, spinocerebellar degeneration
	Li-Fraumeni[70,94-97]/*TP53*	Sarcomas, brain tumors, leukemia
	Cowden's disease[98,99]	Trichilemmomas, gastrointestinal polyposis, uterine leiomyomata
	Muir-Torre[100,101]/*MSH*	Basal cell carcinoma, gastrointestinal tumors
Ovary	Lynch II[66]/*MSH2*	Uterine, colon, genitourinary cancers
	Gonadal dysgenesis	46,XY
	Peutz-Jeghers[102]/*APC*	Oral pigmented lesions, gastrointestinal polyposis
	Ollier's disease[103]	Enchondromatosis
	Basal nevus syndrome[104]	Basal cell carcinomas, jaw cysts
	Familial ovarian fibromatosis	Ovarian hyperplasia

LOH observed in tumors from breast/ovarian cancer families with a high likelihood of being linked to BRCA1 has led to the hypothesis that BRCA1 is a tumor suppressor gene.

Although the disease is inherited in an autosomal dominant pattern, inactivation of both alleles at the tissue level is required for carcinogenesis.[84-90] Women who harbor a *BRCA1* germline mutation are thus poised for developing breast and/or ovarian tumors in adult life. The role of *BRCA1* in sporadic carcinogenesis is being investigated at this time. Initial studies[31] of 12 ovarian and 35 breast sporadic tumors failed to identify somatic mutations. Only germline alterations were revealed in this study. A recent study[91] of 47 sporadic ovarian tumors revealed four distinct somatic mutations present only in the tumor DNA; LOH was observed at a *BRCA1* intragenic marker in the tumors with somatic mutations. These data strengthen the tumor suppressor hypothesis for *BRCA1* and suggest that inactivation of *BRCA1* may play a role in a fraction of sporadic ovarian tumors.

BRCA1

Since 1990 it has been known that a single locus on chromosome 17q21, termed *BRCA1,* is responsible for most cases of hereditary early-onset breast/ovarian cancer.[80] The data cooperatively contributed to the Breast Cancer Linkage Consortium (BCLC)[44-46,68,105] have helped define the risks of cancer associated with *BRCA1* mutations. Approximately 67% of families with members with breast cancer diagnosed before age 45 and 95% of families with members with breast and ovarian cancer appear to be linked to *BRCA1.* Easton et al. have recently reported that the penetrance, by age 70, is 87% (95% confidence interval (CI) = 72% to 95%) for breast cancer and 44% (95% CI = 28% to 56%) for ovarian cancer. The ovarian cancer risk may be an overestimate, however, because of a bias favoring ascertainment of families with both breast and ovarian cancer. In addition, Ford et al. have reported a significant increase in the relative risks for colon (RR = 4.11; 95% CI = 2.36-7 to 15) and prostate cancer (RR = 3.33; 95% CI 1.78-6.20) in *BRCA1* mutation carriers.[68,106]

In contrast to the general population in which only 10% of breast cancers occur in women under 60 years of age, for BRCA1 mutation carriers, 60% of the risk of breast cancer occurs by age 50.[4]

A widely recognized feature of families linked to *BRCA1* has been the apparent segregation of families into two types: those with a high incidence of ovarian cancer and those with little or no excess of ovarian cancer. Based on this observation, the BCLC data have been analyzed assuming genetic heterogeneity in the form of a 2-allele system. A strikingly improved fit of the epidemiologic data is achieved by a model in which allele 1 (representing 71% of mutations) confers 62% and 11% lifetime risk by age 60 of breast and ovarian cancer, respectively, whereas the risks by age 60 of allele 2 (representing 29% of the mutations) are 39% for breast and 42% for ovarian cancer.[45,105] Detailed analyses of the spectrum of mutations are underway to elucidate the potential molecular basis for this model. However, at this time no clear phenotype-genotype correlations have been found. One possible exception is the increased incidence of the 185 delAG mutation in women of Ashkenazi Jewish origin.

The *BRCA1* gene has recently been isolated, and disease-associated mutations in its coding and regulatory regions have been found in approximately 60% of breast and breast/ovarian kindreds with a high likelihood of linkage to markers flanking the *BRCA1* locus.[22,23,25,106a] One technique employed so far in mutation searches has been the single-strand conformation polymorphism (SSCP), which is known to have a sensitivity of approximately 60% to 80%.[107] In addition, most of the intronic sequence and portions of the 5′ and 3′ untranslated regions have not been analyzed so far. It is likely that in the next 1 to 2 years the disease-associated *BRCA1* mutations will be elucidated in over 90% of breast and ovarian families.

> *The* BRCA1 *protein comprises 1863 amino acids and is a putative transcription factor. About 70% of the mutations encountered so far give rise to a truncated and/or qualitatively altered protein product that may, in the future, prove to be an appropriate target for a specific and sensitive diagnostic screening test.*

However, approximately 10% to 15% of the disease-related mutations produce missense changes at codons interspersed throughout the gene; at the present time these alterations can be detected only by detailed analyses of the germline DNA coding sequence, which spans 7.8 kilobase.[20] Given these complicating factors, it is unlikely that a thorough and reliable mutation test will be available or warranted for the general population at mildly increased risk. However, individuals from breast/ovarian cancer families interested in risk assessment or in participating in research related to *BRCA1* may be referred to specialized centers where research protocols are being conducted. Innovative methods of screening and counseling high-risk women and of training genetic counselors and nurse practitioners for the assessment and long-term follow-up of these individuals are being developed at some of these centers.

BRCA2, Familial Male Breast Cancer, and Other Breast Cancer Genes

> *Germline mutations in* BRCA2 *localized to chromosome 13q12-13 are likely to account for approximately 40% to*

> *70% of the site-specific breast cancer families not linked to BRCA1.[108] BRCA2 confers a 90% lifetime risk of breast cancer and a 6% risk of male breast cancer.*

Preliminary data seem to point to an elevated risk of prostate cancer in male *BRCA2* mutation carriers.[108a] Ovarian cancer also appears to cosegregate with breast cancer in *BRCA2*-linked families. Site-specific breast cancer families, especially those who also have cases of male breast cancer, are actively being sought for research at the present time.

Familial male breast cancer is extremely rare in the context of an already rare form of cancer; only 16 families with two or more cases of male breast cancer were reported in a 100-year period in a single-institution review.[109-111] More than half of these families show that first-degree relatives of male breast cancer cases have other types of cancers, including oropharyngeal, ovarian, and female breast cancer, suggesting an inherited component to familial clustering of male breast cancer. *BRCA2* is thought to be responsible for the increased susceptibility observed in some of these families.

An interesting association between germline mutations in the androgen receptor gene and familial male breast cancer may provide the molecular basis for the increased susceptibility to breast cancer in males with relative androgen deficiency or estrogen excess manifested by gynecomastia, orchitis, testicular atrophy, and Klinefelter's syndrome.[108,112]

Other genes that are being actively sought on chromosomes 17p, 17q distal to the *BRCA1* locus on 17q23 and 17q25 and proximal to the *BRCA1* locus between markers known as *D17S776* and *D17S846*,[84] 18q, 3p, and 8p, may be responsible for most of the remaining autosomal dominant breast cancer families.[90,113,114] It is not entirely clear that other highly penetrant genes, in addition to *BRCA1* and *BRCA2*, are involved in familial breast cancer.

TP53

The *TP53* gene is localized to chromosome 17p13.1 and encodes for a 393-amino acid nuclear phosphoprotein. This gene is mutated in 50% to 60% of a wide variety of human cancers in a nonrandom pattern, which preferentially involves regions of highly conserved sequence motifs.[18,70,96,97,115] Intriguing phenotype-genotype correlations have arisen from comparison of the patterns and types of mutations present in different kinds of cancers. Hot spots of missense mutations are observed in sporadic tumors of many organs and in certain viral- or toxin-associated cancers, leading to the production of faulty *TP53* protein and to uncontrolled growth. In contrast, virtually all the alterations seen in osteosarcomas and chronic myelogenous leukemias involve rearrangements and homologous deletions resulting in the absence of *TP53* protein. *TP53* mutations are also found in the germline of about 50% of families affected with the Li-Fraumeni syndrome.[96,115a] These families have several close relatives affected with diverse cancers at younger ages, including sarcomas, leukemias, brain tumors, and other carcinomas. Although early-onset breast cancer does occur in these kindreds, they are distinguished from the *BRCA1* and *BRCA2* families by the striking preponderance of a wide variety of other types of cancer. These families are rare, and the diverse clinical concerns they elicit warrant early referral to a specialized clinic. Mutation testing is available for families at risk; genetic testing and counseling are used to guide individuals into appropriate surveillance protocols for early-detection.

OTHER SYNDROMES ASSOCIATED WITH INCREASED RISK OF BREAST CANCER AND OVARIAN CANCER

The Mendelian inheritance of a germline mutation plays a major role in the development of breast and ovarian cancers in other familial syndromes listed in Table 11-1. In some cases the genes affected are known, such as *MSH2* and *MLH1* in Muir-Torre syndrome, which is characterized by skin tumors and multiple benign and malignant tumors of the upper and lower gastrointestinal and genitourinary tracts.[100,101] Cowden's disease (multiple hamartoma syndrome) is a rare autosomal dominant syndrome with variable expressivity.[26,98,99] Patients are affected by various mucocutaneous lesions, including multiple facial trichilemmomas, papillomatosis of the lips and oral mucosa, acral keratoses, vitiligo, and angiomata. Other benign proliferations affect a variety of epithelial tissues and include breast fibroadenomas, fibrocystic lesions, areolar and nipple malformations, ductal epithelial hyperplasia, thyroid goiter and adenomata, gastrointestinal polyps, and uterine leiomyomata.

Ataxia-telangiectasia (AT) is an autosomal recessive disorder characterized by cerebellar ataxia, oculocutaneous telangiectasias, radiation hypersensitivity, and an increased incidence of malignancies.[92,93,116,117] The genetic defect that underlies the clinical syndrome of ataxia-telangiectasia has recently been elucidated. It is anticipated that, similar to *BRCA1*, many distinct mutations will account for the AT syndrome, making a test challenging. AT homozygotes have a risk of cancer 60 to 180 times greater than the general population, manifested by a nearly 100% lifetime risk of non-Hodgkin's lymphoma and lower risks of developing breast and ovarian cancer, lymphocytic leukemia, head and neck, stomach, pancreas and bladder cancer.[93] The breast cancer risk in *AT* mutation carriers (heterozygotes) is much lower than the risk observed in women with germline mutations in *TP53* or *BRCA1*. AT heterozygotes do not demonstrate the neurologic symptoms but may have a fivefold increased incidence of breast cancer. Radiosensitivity in AT heterozygotes has been observed; the coincidental aggregation of excess breast cancer in these individuals has raised concerns about mammographic screening in the general population with a relative high frequency of AT heterozygotes.[93,118] Basic research is under way to provide answers to these important questions.

The recognition of the features and distribution of lesions associated with these syndromes will expedite referral to a specialized cancer genetics clinic for recommendations on a surveillance program that can often be implemented in the patient's community.

PREDICTIVE TESTING
What Variables Affect Cancer Risk Assessment?

The accumulation of genetic alterations in individual cells gives rise to cancers.

> *The understanding that the increased cancer susceptibility in individuals harboring a* BRCA1 *germline mutation stems primarily from their having been born with "one hit" (of the two required for carcinogenesis by the Knudson model) has led to the concept of testing cancer-free individuals who are part of breast/ovarian families in the hope of decreasing the morbidity and mortality of mutation carriers by prophylactic or surveillance measures.*

If the penetrance of the disease (that is, the probability that a carrier of a given mutation will develop cancer in her lifetime) and the disease-predisposing mutations are known, an unaffected individual may be tested for the presence of one or more specific mutations in *BRCA1* in his or her germ-line (lymphocytes, skin fibroblasts) in a minimally invasive manner. An estimate of the lifetime risk of developing breast and/or ovarian cancer (colon and/or prostate cancer in male carriers) can be provided to the individual tested. This constitutes predictive testing for a tumor suppressor cancer susceptibility gene.

Another challenge is presented by cases of sporadic tumors arising in germ-line mutation carriers. If all of the excess breast cancer seen in individuals who harbor a germ-line mutation is ascribed to *BRCA1,* the penetrance will be overestimated to an unknown, but presumed small, extent, as, even in mutation carriers, some cancers may have arisen by mechanisms unrelated to inactivation of the *BRCA1* wild-type allele in the target tissues. Of more concern is the difference in penetrance that a given mutation may have in a less affected family, perhaps because of interactions with other heritable factors. The isolation and molecular characterization of *BRCA1* have fostered research on these important questions, as we strive to understand the principles and practice of genetic screening.

Ethical Principles

The availability of predictive testing for cancer susceptibility genes raises important ethical issues that warrant assessment. In this regard considerable insight can be derived from the experience with other adult-onset autosomal dominant disorders.

Huntington's disease (HD) provides the most relevant example, although it differs most notably from the familial cancer disorders in the lack of pre-symptomatic interventions (which in the case of breast and ovarian cancer have not yet been definitely proven to increase survival or prevent a diagnosis of cancer). Huggins et al.[32] have clearly delineated some of the ethical dilemmas and principles that govern predictive testing for adult-onset diseases. The principles put forth for HD are widely applicable and relevant to breast/ovarian cancer. However, because of the different nature of the disease itself and because prophylactic (albeit controversial) and heightened surveillance interventions do exist for these cancers, we will outline these ethical principles in a manner that should help the practitioner evaluate the design of protocols for predictive testing. These considerations may be helpful to guide those seeking referrals for predictive testing and risk assessment.

The following four ethical principles constitute the foundation of the informed consent for genetic testing: autonomy, confidentiality, beneficence, and justice.[32] Each principle has several parts, and only a subset of these is within the control of the physician, nurse, or genetic counselor caring for the patient. These principles set the stage for specific recommendations regarding the management of high-risk individuals and their families in cancer susceptibility testing.

Autonomy

The principle of autonomy takes precedence in Western medicine over all others.

> *A person's right to an informed decision based solely on her perception of what is best for her health or any other set of criteria she chooses to employ, must be upheld.*

In the context of genetic screening, however, some specific aspects of this principle are worth emphasizing.

The informed consent process must be a dynamic one. New information about the risk of breast, ovarian, and other cancers in families linked to *BRCA1*, or who are known to have *BRCA1* mutations, is becoming available at a fast rate. Likewise, novel options for treatment, prevention, and surveillance are reaching the clinic. The individual must be made aware of the rapidly evolving nature of the data on which the risk assessment or test is based. Therefore the informed consent should specifically address the manner in which new information will be conveyed. The provision of new information should also afford the opportunity for further counseling, if warranted.

The informed consent process includes the initial authorization for testing.

> *However, the consent for testing to proceed should not be construed to also imply consent to be informed of one's risk after the test has been performed.*

Autonomy must be preserved at every step of the testing and counseling process, and a woman's right to not be informed of her cancer risk is protected by providing her with the opportunity to refuse to receive information on the results of testing.

The risks and benefits of testing should be discussed in a pretest session and in the informed consent. The risks are divided into two major categories: intrinsic and extrinsic to the individual. Examples of intrinsic risks after learning of a positive result include depression and anxiety, marital distress, difficulty with reproductive decisions, and the fear of having passed the defective gene to one's offspring. Knowledge of a negative test result can give rise to survival guilt, which may interfere with the ability of the proband to assist affected family members in dealing with their positive results.

The extrinsic risks are those which are caused by third parties who gain access to the test results and may adversely affect the person's (and her family's) insurability and employability, and may make the person subject to coercion. The extrinsic risks are in general not under the control of the individual or her physician, are difficult to predict, and have the potential to result in severe psychologic and economic loss.

Confidentiality

This component of the informed consent has special relevance to genetic screening. In addition to the extrinsic risks described above, violations of confidentiality within the family may also have untoward repercussions for the screened person.

> *The ability to make decisions that are free from coercion implies that the individual chooses who she wants to share the results of her testing with.*

An important corollary of this principle is that the individual being tested should not interfere with the decisions about testing made by parents, children, or any other family member. In this regard, recent work by Lerman et al.[10,38] appears to point to the ability to gain knowledge about one's offspring risk as a very important motivation to seek testing in 75% of first-degree relatives of ovarian cancer patients.

For the case of a *BRCA1* family with a known mutation, whereas a negative test in the parent indicates she could not have passed the defective gene on to her offspring, a positive test indicates a 50% chance of having passed on the gene.

> *Although parents often request to know their children's risk more specifically, there are at present no guidelines or medical reasons to test minors for an adult-onset disease for which no surveillance or other interventions are indicated before adulthood.*

Beneficence

For this principle to be upheld, the following components need to be in place: (1) an accurate and reliable test, (2) conveyance of results to the individual by knowledgeable and caring health care professionals, (3) availability of reasonable prophylactic surgery and/or heightened surveillance options the individual can freely choose from, (4) the opportunity for long-term care, and (5) no harm is incurred in the process (the risks do not outweigh the benefits). The components of this principle are largely within the control of the health care delivery system to which the proband presents for testing or risk assessment.

Justice

The most general meaning of this principle is that predictive testing and counseling are equally accessible to all persons. Equality is, however, much more complex to define in detail, especially in a culturally and economically diverse society. Unfortunately, most of the risk assessment data for breast cancer have been derived from overwhelmingly white populations, with very little information, outside of a few small studies, being available for other ethnic populations.

As heightened surveillance procedures and prophylactic surgery reach the clinic with increasing frequency, the costs associated with these activities also rise. Unless there are mechanisms for the cost of these interventions to be paid for all persons, they are not likely to be equally accessible to all persons.

Practical Aspects of Risk Assessment for Breast Cancer

Dissemination of information by advocacy groups, the media, medical professional organizations, and the government has increased public awareness of the high incidence of breast cancer in the United States. Recent advances in the genetics of breast cancer have received considerable attention. As a result, women are more informed about issues surrounding risk factors and are concerned about their individual risk of developing breast cancer.[119] These women are bringing their concerns to primary care practitioners and requesting specific risk assessment. Recognition of the contribution of heritable factors to the development of breast cancer has resulted in an important role for genetic counseling when available in the care of women with a family history of the disease.[35,120,121] The task of risk assessment for women and families concerned about breast cancer consists of the collection of a detailed medical history of the extended family, interpretation of this history in light of current information to assess individual risk, clear communication of this information to the woman and her family, and discussion of options for minimizing the risk.

Family history information constitutes the main focus around which all subsequent tasks revolve. It is initially collected in the community by concerned practitioners.

A thorough history should include the characteristics (organ of origin, laterality, histologic type, age of onset) of all cancers in relatives as well as the positions of these

> *relatives within the family pedigree. The positions of un-affected relatives within the family are essential to the assessment of inheritance patterns.*

Whenever possible, family history data should be confirmed by medical and pathology records to ensure accuracy. Patients have been shown to correctly identify the sites of primary cancer in first-degree relatives 83% of the time, with significant declines in accuracy as the distance of relationship increases.

Following the isolation of *BRCA1*, families can be studied for mutations in this gene, and estimates of breast cancer risk can be made with a level of accuracy that is yet to be fully determined. Mutation carriers appear to have an 85% lifetime risk of developing breast cancer; individuals with two normal copies of *BRCA1* have a breast cancer risk equivalent to the general population. The estimation of the risk of ovarian cancer is more difficult due to variability in the penetrance of this disease. *BRCA1* families are being studied and counseled at several centers under approved protocols.[77,121,122]

A daunting challenge is presented by the large number of families with apparent autosomal dominant inheritance of breast cancer where *BRCA1* mutations are not detected in affected family members, or where linkage to *BRCA1* cannot be determined.[121] Although issues related to autosomal dominant inheritance of breast cancer susceptibility are discussed, little individual information can be given to the individuals. Research is under way on the contribution of *BRCA1, BRCA2,* and other breast cancer genes to the risk of breast cancer in families with apparent autosomal dominant transmission (but fewer cases of breast cancer).

Most persons seeking risk assessment do not have a family history consistent with a highly penetrant breast cancer susceptibility gene.[122a] The breast cancer risk of an individual in this situation can be estimated from empiric data[43,77] on the frequency of breast cancer in a large population of women with an equivalent family history (Table 11-3).[43,77] This method of risk assessment makes no assumptions regarding the mode of transmission of breast cancer among the relatives. It is important to remember and share with the woman that these estimates are subject to the design limitations of the study from which they derive and will likely be altered by future studies.

An alternative approach, termed analytic, is based on a specific model of transmission to estimate risk of breast cancer in these small families. Although the estimation of analytic risk is used in genetic counseling for many inherited disorders, it has not been routinely employed for breast cancer because of the absence of a widely accepted model of disease transmission. Two analytic models are in use in limited settings. The Gail model[123] is being employed in the calculation of risk for the NSABP Breast Cancer Prevention Trial. These models appear appropriate for breast cancer because they take into account influences of genetic and environmental factors. In general, for a given individual the analytic breast cancer risk estimates are lower than are the empiric risks. As more genetic information becomes available, it is expected that the analytic models will be refined and may prove useful in the assessment of individual risk.

The information derived from risk assessment (by any method) for breast cancer is of great importance for the patient and her family.[25,36,40,124] Whether an actual blood test is involved or not, the individual usually receives this information in a medical setting. This environment inspires in individuals assumptions of high accuracy and sound scientific backing that might not be entirely justified by the present state of knowledge, which is evolving rapidly. Therefore, in addition to advances in the understanding of the molecular basis for breast cancer, equally important studies are being conducted on the methods and ethics of risk assessment procedures. Interested persons should be encouraged to participate in approved protocols conducive to acquiring this important knowledge.

REFERENCES

1. American Cancer Society: *Cancer facts and figures,* Atlanta, 1994, The Society.
2. American Cancer Society: Cancer statistics, *CA Cancer J Clin* 42:30, 1992.
3. Chu K, Smart C, Tarone R: Breast cancer mortality and stage distribution by age for the health insurance plan clinical trial, *J Natl Cancer Inst* 80:1125, 1988.
4. National Cancer Institute: *Cancer statistics review 1973-1989,* Bethesda, Md, 1992, The Institute.
5. Ewertz M et al: Age at first birth, parity and risk of breast cancer: a meta-analysis of 8 studies from the Nordic countries, *Int J Cancer* 46:597, 1990.
6. Henderson BE et al: Do regular ovulatory cycles increase breast risk? *Cancer* 56:1206, 1985.
7. Irwin KL et al: Hysterectomy, tubal sterilization, and the risk of breast cancer, *Am J Epidemiol* 127:1192, 1988.
8. London SJ et al: Prospective study of relative weight, height and risk of breast cancer, *JAMA* 262:2853, 1989.
9. Becker MH, editor: *The health belief model and personal health behavior,* Thorofare, NJ, 1974, Charles B. Slack.
10. Lerman C et al: Factors associated with repeat adherence to breast cancer screening, *Prev Med* 19:279, 1990.
11. Skinner CS, Strecher VJ, Hospers H: Physicians' recommendations for mammography: do tailored messages make a difference? *Am J Public Health* 84:43, 1994.
12. Wender RC: Cancer screening and prevention in primary care: obstacles for physicians, *Cancer Suppl* 72:1093, 1993.
13. Klein G: The approaching era of tumor suppressor genes, *Science* 238:1539, 1987.
14. Knudson AG: All in the (cancer) family, *Nature (Genetics)* 5:103, 1993.
15. Slamon DJ et al: Studies of the HER-2/NEU proto-oncogene in human breast and ovarian cancer, *Science* 244:707, 1989.
16. Knudson AG: Mutation and cancer: statistical study of retinoblastoma, *Proc Natl Acad Sci USA* 68:820, 1971.
17. Fishel R et al: The human mutator gene homolog MSH2 and its association with hereditary nonpolyposis colon cancer, *Cell* 75:1027, 1993.
18. Frebourg T et al: Germline mutations of the p53 tumor suppressor gene in patients with high risk for cancer inactivate the p53 protein, *Proc Natl Acad Sci* 89:6413, 1992.
19. Reference deleted in proofs.
20. Miki Y et al: A strong candidate for the breast and ovarian cancer susceptibility gene BRCA1, *Science* 266:66, 1994.
21. Srivastava S et al: Germ-line transmission of a mutated p53 gene in a cancer-prone family with Li-Fraumeni syndrome, *Nature* 348:747, 1990.
22. Castilla LH et al: Mutations in the *BRCA1* gene in families with early-onset breast and ovarian cancer, *Nature (Genetics)* 8:387, 1994.

23. Friedman LS et al: Confirmation of *BRCA1* by analysis of germline mutations linked to breast and ovarian cancer in 10 families, *Nature (Genetics)* 8:399, 1994.

24. Friend SH et al: A human DNA segment with properties of the gene that predisposes to retinoblastoma and osteosarcoma, *Nature* 323:643, 1986.

25. Simard J et al: Common origins of *BRCA1* mutations in Canadian breast and ovarian cancer families, *Nature (Genetics)* 8:392, 1994.

26. Bronner EC et al: Mutation in the DNA mismatch repair gene homologue hMLH1 is associated with hereditary non-polyposis colon cancer, *Nature* 368:258, 1994.

27. Leach FS et al: Mutations of a mutS homolog in hereditary nonpolyposis colon cancer, *Cell* 75:1215, 1993.

28. Papadopoulos N et al: Mutation of mutL homolog in hereditary colon cancer, *Science* 263:1625, 1994.

29. Akasaka Y et al: A point mutation found in the *WT-1* gene in a sporadic Wilms tumor without genitourinary abnormalities is identical with the most frequent point mutation in Denys-Drash syndrome, *FEBS Lett* 317:39, 1993.

30. Coppes M et al: Homozygous somatic *WT-1* point mutations in sporadic unilateral Wilms tumor, *Proc Natl Acad Sci USA* 90:1416, 1993.

31. Futreal PA et al: *BRCA1* mutations on primary breast and ovarian carcinomas, *Science* 266:120, 1994.

32. Huggins M et al: Ethical and legal dilemmas arising during predictive testing for adult-onset disease: the experience of Huntington's disease, *Am J Hum Genet* 47:4, 1990.

33. Hanning V et al: Presymptomatic testing for adult-onset polycystic kidney disease in at-risk kidney transplant donors, *Am J Med Genet* 40:425, 1991.

34. Anderson DE, Williams WR: Familial cancer: implications for healthy relatives. In Chaganti RSK, German J, editors: *Genetics in clinical oncology,* New York, 1985, Oxford University Press.

35. Biesecker BB et al: Genetic counseling for families with inherited susceptibility to breast and ovarian cancer, *JAMA* 269:1970-1974, 1993.

36. Kelly PT: Informational needs of individuals and families with hereditary cancers, *Semin Oncol Nurs* 8:288, 1992.

37. Lerman C et al: Attitudes about genetic testing for breast-ovarian cancer susceptibility, *J Clin Oncol* 12:843, 1994.

38. Lerman C et al: Psychological side effects of breast cancer screening, *Health Psychol* 10:259, 1991.

39. Mullvihil JJ: Prospects for cancer control and prevention through genetics, *Clin Genet* 36:313, 1989.

40. Polednak AP, Lane DA, Burg MA: Risk perception, family history, and use of breast cancer screening tools, *Cancer Detect Prev* 15:257, 1991.

41. Anderson DE, Badzioch MD: Risk of familial breast cancer, *Cancer* 56:383, 1985.

42. Anderson DE: A genetic study of human breast cancer, *Cancer* 40:1855, 1977.

43. Claus EB, Risch N, Thompson WD: Autosomal dominant inheritance of early-onset breast cancer, *Cancer* 73:643, 1994.

44. Easton DF et al: Breast and ovarian cancer incidence in *BRCA1* mutation carriers, *Lancet* 343:692, 1994.

45. Easton DF et al: *Am J Hum Genet* 56:265, 1995.

46. Easton DF et al: Genetic linkage analysis in familial breast and ovarian cancer: results from 214 families, *Am J Hum Genet* 52:678, 1993.

47. Taplin S, Anderman C, Grothaus L: Breast cancer risk and participation in mammographic screening, *Am J Public Health* 79:1494, 1989.

48. Kash KM et al: Psychological distress and surveillance behaviors of women with a family history of breast cancer, *J Natl Cancer Inst* 84:24, 1992.

49. Lynch HT, editor: *Genetics and breast cancer,* New York, 1992, Van Nostrand Reinhold.

50. Wooster R: Localization of a breast cancer susceptibility gene, *BRCA2,* to chromosome 13q12-13, *Science* 265:2088, 1994.

51. Wolff MS et al: Blood levels of organochlorine residues and risk of breast cancer, *J Natl Cancer Inst* 85:648, 1993.

52. White E et al: Breast cancer among young U.S. women in relation to oral contraceptive use, *J Natl Cancer Inst* 86:505, 1994.

53. Hildreth NG, Shore RE, Dvoretsky PM: The risk of breast cancer after irradiation of the thymus in infancy, *N Engl J Med* 321:1281, 1989.

54. Land CE: Temporal distributions of risk for radiation-induced cancers, *J Chronic Ids* 40(suppl 2):45S, 1987.

55. Tokunaga M et al: Incidence of female breast cancer among atomic bomb survivors, Hiroshima and Nagasaki, 1950-1980, *Radiat Res* 112:243, 1987.

56. Rosenberg L, Metzger LS, Palmer JR: Alcohol consumption and risk of breast cancer: a review of the epidemiologic evidence, *Epidemiol Rev* 15:133, 1993.

57. Roth AD et al: Alcoholic beverages and breast cancer: some observations on published case-control studies, *J Clin Epidemiol* 47:207, 1994.

58. Simon MS et al: Alcohol consumption and the risk of breast cancer: a report from the Tecumseh community health study, *J Clin Epidemiol* 44:755, 1991.

59. Willet WC et al: Dietary fat and fiber in relation to risk of breast cancer: an 8-year follow-up, *JAMA* 268:2037, 1992.

60. Young TB: A case-control study of breast cancer and alcohol consumption habits, *Cancer* 64:552, 1989.

61. Claus EB, Risch N, Thompson WD: Genetic analysis of breast cancer in the cancer and steroid hormone study, *Am J Hum Genet* 48:232, 1991.

62. Adami HO et al: Characteristics of familial breast cancer in Sweden: absence of relation to age and unilateral versus bilateral disease, *Cancer* 48:1688, 1981.

63. Anderson DE, Badzioch MD: Bilaterality in familial breast cancer patients, *Cancer* 56:2092, 1985.

64. Kelsey JL, Gammon MD: The epidemiology of breast cancer, *CA Cancer J Clin* 41:147, 1991.

65. Malkin D et al: Germ line p53 mutations in a familial syndrome of breast cancer, sarcomas, and other neoplasms, *Science* 250:1233, 1990.

66. Nelson CL et al: Familial clustering of colon, breast, uterine and ovarian cancers as assessed by family history, *Genet Epidemiol* 10:235, 1993.

67. Lynch HT, Bewtra C, Lynch JF: Familial ovarian carcinoma: clinical nuances, *Am J Med* 81:1073, 1986.

68. Ford D et al: Risks of cancer in *BRCA1* mutation carriers, *Lancet* 343:692, 1994.

69. Anderson DE, Badzioch MD: Familial breast cancer risks: effects of prostate and other cancers, *Cancer* 72:114, 1993.

70. Li FP et al: A cancer family syndrome in twenty-four kindreds, *Cancer Res* 48:5358, 1988.

71. Young RH, Scully RE: Pathology of epithelial tumors, *Hematol Oncol Clin North Am* 6:739, 1992.

72. Colditz GA et al: Family history, age and risk of breast cancer, *JAMA* 270:338, 1993.

73. Newman B et al: Inheritance of breast cancer: evidence for autosomal dominant transmission in high-risk families, *Proc Natl Acad Sci USA* 85:3044, 1988.

74. Sattin RW et al: Family history and the risk of breast cancer, *JAMA* 253:1908, 1985.

75. Slattery M, Kerber R: A comprehensive evaluation of family history and breast cancer: the Utah population database, *JAMA* 270:1563, 1993.

76. Williams WR, Anderson DE: Genetic epidemiology of breast cancer: segregation analysis of 200 Danish pedigrees, *Genet Epidemiol* 1:7, 1984.

77. Offit K, Brown K: Quantitation familial cancer risk: a resource for clinical oncologists, *J Clin Oncol* 12:1724, 1994.

78. Floderus B, Barlow L, Mack T: Recall bias in subjective reports of familial cancer, *Epidemiology* 1:318, 1990.

79. Weber BL, Garber JE: Family history and breast cancer: probabilities and possibilities, *JAMA* 270:1602, 1993.

80. Hall JM et al: Linkage of early onset breast cancer to chromosome 17q21, *Science* 250:1684, 1990.

81. Narod SA et al: Familial breast-ovarian cancer locus on chromosome 17q12-23, *Lancet* 338:82, 1991.

82. Harris H: Suppression of malignancy by cell fusion, *Nature* 223:363, 1969.

83. Stanbridge EJ et al: Human cell hybrids: analysis of transformation and tumor genicity, *Science* 215:252, 1982.

84. Cropp CS et al: Evidence for involvement of *BRCA1* in sporadic breast carcinomas, *Cancer Res* 5:2548, 1994.

85. Eccles DM et al: Allele losses on chromosome 17 in human epithelial ovarian carcinomas, *Oncogene* 5:1599, 1990.

86. Merajver SD et al: Germline mutations and loss of the wild-type allele in *BRCA1* in tumors from families with early-onset breast and ovarian cancer, *Clin Cancer Res* 1:539, 1995.

87. Sato T et al: Allelotype of human ovarian cancer, *Cancer Res* 51:5118, 1991.

88. Smith S et al: Allele losses in the region 17q12-21 in familial breast and ovarian cancer involve the wild-type chromosome, *Nature (Genetics)* 2:128, 1992.

89. Kelsell DP et al: Human genetic analysis of the *BRCA1* region in a large breast/ovarian family refinement of the minimal region containing *BRCA1*, *Hum Molec Genet* 2:1823, 1993.

90. Jacobs IJ et al: A deletion unit on chromosome 17q in epithelial ovarian tumors distal to the familial breast/ovarian cancer locus, *Cancer Res* 53:1218, 1993.

91. Merajver SD et al: Somatic mutations in the *BRCA1* gene in sporadic ovarian tumors, *Nature (Genetics)* 9:439, 1995.

92. Cortessis V et al: Linkage analysis of DRD2, a marker linked to the ataxia-telangectasia gene, in 64 families with premenopausal bilateral breast cancer, *Cancer Res* 53:5083, 1993.

93. Swift M et al: Incidence of cancer in 161 families affected by ataxia-telangectasia, *N Engl J Med* 325:1831, 1987.

94. Coles C et al: p53 Mutations in breast cancer, *Cancer Res* 52:5291, 1992.

95. Hartley AL et al: Breast cancer risk in mothers of children with osteosarcoma and chondrosarcoma, *Br J Cancer* 54:819, 1986.

96. Santibanez-Koref MF et al: p53 Germline mutations in Li-Fraumeni syndrome, *Lancet* 338:1490, 1991.

97. Toguchida J et al: Prevalence and spectrum of germline mutations of the p53 gene among patients with sarcoma, *N Engl J Med* 326:1301, 1992.

98. Brownstein MH, Wolf M, Bikowski JB: Cowden's disease: a cutaneous marker of breast cancer, *Cancer* 41:2393, 1978.

99. Starink TM: Cowden's disease: analysis of fourteen new cases, *J Am Acad Dermatol* 11:1127, 1984.

100. Hall NR et al: Muir-Torre syndrome: a variant of the cancer family syndrome, *J Med Genet* 31:627, 1994.

101. Muir EG, Yates-Bell AJ, Barlow KA: Multiple primary carcinomata of the colon, duodenum, and larynx associated with keratoacanthomata of the face, *Br J Surg* 54:191, 1967.

102. Spigelman AD, Murray V, Phillips RKS: Cancer and the Puetz-Jeghers syndrome, *Gut* 30:1588, 1989.

103. Weyl-Ben AM, Oslander L: Ollier's disease associated with ovarian Sertoli-Leydig cell tumor and breast adenoma, *Am J Pediatr Hematol Oncol* 13:49, 1991.

104. Raggio M, Kaplan AL, Harberg JF: Recurrent ovarian fibromas with basal cell nevus syndrome (Gorlin syndrome), *Obstet Gynecol* 61(suppl):95S, 1983.

105. Narod SA et al: An evaluation of genetic heterogeneity in 145 breast-ovarian cancer families: Breast Cancer Linkage Consortium, *Am J Hum Genet* 56:254, 1995.

106. Arason A, Barkardottir RB, Egilsson V: Linkage analysis of chromosome 17 markers and breast-ovarian cancer in Icelandic families and possible relationship to prostatic cancer, *Am J Hum Genet* 52:711, 1993.

106a. Lynch HT et al: DNA screening for breast/ovarian cancer susceptibility based on linked markers, *Arch Intern Med* 153:1979, 1993.

107. Orita M et al: Rapid and sensitive detection of point mutations and DNA polymorphisms using the polymerase chain reaction, *Genomics* 5:874, 1989.

108. Wooster R et al: A germline mutation in the androgen receptor in two brothers with breast cancer and Reifenstein syndrome, *Nature (Genetics)* 2:132, 1992.

108a. Goldgar D: Private communication, p 249.

109. Demeter J, Waterman N, Verdi G: Familial male breast carcinoma, *Cancer* 65:2342, 1990.

110. Hauser AR, Lerner IJ, King RA: Familial male breast cancer, *Am J Med Genet* 44:839, 1992.

111. Kozak FK, Hall JG, Baird PA: Familial breast cancer in males: a case report and a review of the literature, *Cancer* 12:2736, 1986.

112. Lobaccaro J-M et al: Male breast cancer and the androgen receptor gene, *Nature (Genetics)* 5:109, 1993.

113. Kirchweger R et al: Patterns of allele loss suggest the existence of five distinct regions of LOH on chromosome 17 in breast cancer, *Int J Cancer* 56:193, 1994.

114. Lee JH et al: Frequent loss of heterozygosity on chromosomes 6q, 11, and 17 in human ovarian carcinomas, *Cancer Res* 50:2724, 1990.

115. Frank TS et al: Loss of heterozygosity and overexpression of the p53 gene in ovarian carcinoma, *Modern Pathol* 7:3, 1994.

115a. Borresen A-L et al: Screening for germ type *TP53* mutations in breast cancer patients, *Cancer Res* 52:3234, 1992.

116. McConville CM et al: Fine mapping of the chromosome 11q22-23 region using PFGE, linkage and haplotype analysis: localization of the gene for ataxia telangiectasia to a 5cM region flanked by NCAM/DRD2 and STMY/CJ52.75, *Nuclear Acids Res* 18:4335, 1990.

117. Morrell D, Cromartie E, Swift M: Mortality and cancer incidence in 263 patients with ataxia-telangectasia, *J Natl Cancer Inst* 77:89, 1986.

118. Swift M et al: The incidence and gene frequency of ataxia-telangiectasia in the United States, *Am J Hum Genet* 39:573, 1986.

119. Shapiro DE et al: The effect of varied physician affect on recall, anxiety, and perceptions in women at risk for breast cancer: an analogue study, *Health Psychol* 11:61, 1992.

120. Li FP et al: Recommendations on predictive testing for germ line p53 mutations among cancer-prone individuals, *J Natl Cancer Inst* 84:1156, 1992.

121. Stopfer et al: Assessment and counseling for breast cancer risk: a guide for clinicians, *JAMA* 273:577, 1995.

122. National Advisory Council for Human Genome Research: Statement on the use of DNA testing for presymptomatic identification of cancer risk, *JAMA* 271:785, 1994.

122a. Evans DL et al: Perception of risk in women with a family history of breast cancer, *Br J Cancer* 67:612, 1992.

123. Gail MH et al: Projecting individualized probabilities of developing breast cancer for white females who are being examined annually, *J Natl Cancer Inst* 81:1879, 1989.

124. Wellisch DK et al: Psychosocial functioning of daughters of breast cancer patients. Part II. Characterizing the distressed daughter of the breast cancer patient, *Psychosomatics* 33:171, 1992.

ADHERENCE TO CANCER SCREENING

12

Barbara K. Rimer

> Track how well you are doing
> Consider adjuncts to improve counseling
> Participate in low-cost community-based screening activities

---

International trials have shown that routine breast cancer screening can reduce mortality from breast cancer by about 30% to 35%. Regular Pap tests can decrease mortality from cervical cancer dramatically. And skin cancer screening could decrease deaths from melanoma. The National Cancer Institute (NCI) and the Department of Health and Human Services have issued Year 2000 goals that include increasing the proportion of women who get regular mammograms to 80%.[1] Similar goals have been issued for Pap tests. Yet most women still are not being screened for breast cancer regularly, and there are subgroups of women who are not being screened for cervical cancer. Most people also do not have checks of their skin for cancer regularly. This section reviews the status of cancer screening, summarizes the barriers and facilitators to adherence, and suggests strategies that clinicians and others can use in facilitating adherence to regular screening.

Adherence in this context means that a person follows recommended screening procedures. In the case of breast cancer and cervical cancer, unlike many other cancers, such as lung cancer, there are proven, acceptable, and cost-effective techniques for reducing cancer mortality through screening. In the case of skin cancer screening there is a large volume of indirect evidence from lay and professional education programs that skin screening can reduce the incidence and mortality of malignant melanoma. Yet screening falls short of the ideal. Nonadherence reduces the potential of screening to lower the risk of death and disability from these diseases. Clinicians can play an important role in encouraging women to be screened for breast and cervical cancer and men and women to be screened for skin cancer. They can do this through their office systems, through counseling patients, and responding to patient barriers. In addition, larger scale scientific efforts are required to overcome other barriers. Although this chapter focuses primarily on breast and cervical screening and briefly on skin cancer, the barriers are similar for other types of screening, such as colorectal cancer screening,[2] and the potential solutions also are similar. Thus breast, cervical, and skin cancer are used to illustrate the larger issues related to adherence.

RECOMMENDATIONS FOR BREAST CANCER SCREENING

There is considerable debate about the appropriate age for screening women for breast cancer. The NCI, the American College of Physicians, American College of Family Medicine, and the U.S. Preventive Services Task Force recommend mammograms every 1 to 2 years for women age 50 to 69. The American Cancer Society (ACS), the American College of Radiology, and the American College of Obstetrics and Gynecology recommend that women in their 40s be screened every 1 to 2 years. In 1993 the NCI withdrew its guidelines recommending regular mammograms for women in their 40s and instead issued a statement of evidence because mammography has not been shown in randomized clinical trials to reduce mortality for women in their 40s.[3,4] NCI continues to recommend mammograms every 1 to 2 years for women in their 50s. Too little is known about the efficacy of mammography for women over age 70. But in view of the increased risk of breast cancer with advancing age, prudence dictates regular mammograms for older women who are otherwise healthy.[5]

> *The most rigorous efforts to encourage women to obtain mammograms should occur among women age 50 to 79.*

Routine mammograms *may not be* indicated for women in their 40s, but some women in this age group may require mammograms. These include women with a strong family history, women who have a personal history of breast cancer or atypical ductal hyperplasia from previous breast biopsies, and perhaps women who are extremely anxious about breast cancer, although this is open to question. Women also should practice breast self-examination monthly and obtain yearly clinical breast examinations from a health care provider.

RECOMMENDATIONS FOR CERVICAL CANCER SCREENING

There also are controversies related to screening for cervical cancer. The NCI and many other organizations recommend screening every 3 years once a history of negative tests has been established.[6] Pap tests decrease mortality from cervical cancer among women age 20 to 79, but many clinicians stop at age 65.[7,8] This is unfortunate, since too many other women are dying of cervical cancer.

WAYS OF THINKING ABOUT THE ADHERENCE PROBLEM

A number of theoretical approaches have been advanced to explain why women do or do not get screened for cancer and why men and women do not get screened for skin cancer. One of the most widely used theoretical models of the past is the health belief model (HBM).[9] The HBM postulates that, for a person to be screened, he or she must believe the problem is serious, that he or she is susceptible to the problem, that there is an effective action, and he or she must receive some sort of a cue to action. The HBM has been useful but has limitations. Notable, the HBM explains only a small amount of the variance in health behavior.

The transtheoretical model is becoming the dominant theoretical approach in cancer screening as it has in smoking cessation.[10] This model posits that behavior change is a circular process (Figure 12-1). As an example, some women are not even thinking about mammograms, and they are called precontemplators. Other women are thinking about getting a mammogram, but have not yet decided to take action (they are called contemplators). Some women have had one mammogram, and they are defined as in the action stage. A small proportion of women are in maintenance—they are getting regular mammo-

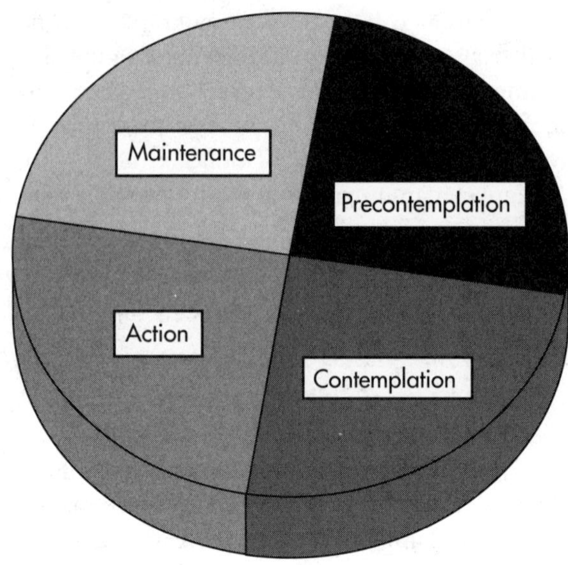

Figure 12-1 Transtheoretical model. (Modified from Prochaska JO, Goldstein MG: *Clin Chest Med* 12:727, 1991.)

grams. Some women have gotten mammograms in the past but are not planning to do so in the future.

The usefulness of the transtheoretical model is that it can help to plan interventions to increase mammography use on a macro level. But it can be equally valuable in counseling a person about mammography, Pap tests, skin cancer screening, or smoking cessation. What is known is that people in different stages have different barriers and beliefs about mammography and different information and education needs. Precontemplators need to be convinced that they need mammograms, whereas women in action may need a referral. People in maintenance may require only reinforcement and reminders. The clinician's time can be used most effectively when it is known where a person is in the cycle and can then match the message to the woman's needs.

STATUS OF MAMMOGRAPHY

In 1995, 182,000 women were diagnosed with breast cancer and 46,000 women died of the disease. There have been dramatic increases since 1987 in the proportion of U.S. women who are getting regular mammograms. In 1987 only about 33% of women had ever had a mammogram, and only about 17% had one in the previous year.[11] By the 1990 Mammography Attitudes and Usage Study nearly 66% of women age 40 and over reported having had at least one mammogram, although only 31% were following guidelines.[12]

> *The 1990 National Health Interview Survey (NHIS), the best source of national data about health behaviors, found that 63% of women over age 40 reported having had a mammogram—use had almost doubled since 1987.*

T A B L E   1 2 - 1

**SUMMARY OF CHARACTERISTICS OF SCREENING UNDERUTILIZERS
FOR BREAST AND CERVICAL CANCER SCREENING**

- Smoker
- No regular exercise
- Do not know breast self-examination
- Don't live in a standard metropolitan statistical area
- Minority
- Low income
- Older
- Less than a high school education
- No regular source of care

Only 39.8% of women reported having had both a clinical breast examination (CBE) and a mammogram in the preceding year, and 38% of women had never had mammograms.[13] Rakowski et al.[14] concluded that only 29% of women are getting regular mammograms, according to data from the 1990 NHIS.

> *Thus, whereas dramatic increases have occurred in use of screening, the majority of women still are not on a program of regular mammograms and Pap tests.*

Along with the increase in mammography use, an important demographic shift has occurred. In 1987 the NHIS had shown that most underusers were those with less education, minorities, and those in nonmetropolitan areas. By 1990 the racial gap had been reduced on a national level, although it was still strong in many regions of the United States.

> *Most important now is the effect of lower income and education. These are the demographic characteristics of most relevance in predicting mammography use.*

They transcend the impact of race alone.[13]

BARRIERS AND FACILITATORS TO MAMMOGRAPHY USE

A number of studies now have been done to characterize women who do and do not have regular mammograms. The barriers are reasonably consistent from study to study (Table 12-1) and are similar to those for Pap tests. The most important barrier is the lack of a recommendation by a woman's physician.[15-18] Older women, black women, and Hispanic women are less likely than middle-age white women to report such a recommendation. The other most common reasons women do not get mammograms, according to their self-report, is that they believe there is no need in the absence of symptoms.

There are other barriers, but they account for much less of the variance in explaining the behavior. These include concern about radiation, anxiety about what might be found, and concern about pain. However, they may be important for individual women or subgroups of women. For example, black and Hispanic women seem to be more concerned about pain and seem to report more anxiety about the mammography experience. There is some evidence that older, black women are more fatalistic about cancer in general, so this also should be addressed.[19] Calle[20] also found that unmarried women were less likely to have had mammograms.

In addition, smokers are less likely to get mammograms.[21,22] This may have more to do with their avoidance of health care in general. But it does make these women a special concern.

There also is evidence that access and environmental barriers may be important. In a study conducted in an HMO, McBride[22] found that nonparticipants in mammography had more trouble getting to the facility, would have to travel farther, and were more likely to rate the facility as inconvenient. Women without health insurance are less likely to get mammograms or Pap tests.[13] Cost is not one of the major barriers reported by women, although it certainly is a barrier for some women, such as those in their 50s and Hispanic women.[16] However, studies show that even when the cost barrier is removed, other important psychologic barriers remain.[15] If these barriers are not addressed, women still may not get regular mammograms.

In some ways the facilitators to mammography are the obverse of the barriers.

> *Women who are advised by their physicians to get mammograms are indeed more likely to get them.[11,15]*

Women who know the recommended screening interval for their age and who know the relationship between age and breast cancer screening also are more likely to get regular mammograms.[23,24] There also is recent evidence that women with more social ties are more likely to get mammograms.[25]

The role of family history has been inconsistent as a predictor of screening. Some studies show it increases the likelihood that women will get regular mammograms, but others do not.[26,27] In a review of the data, Lerman and Schwartz[28] showed that different studies found different kinds of relationships between family risk and screening behavior, ranging from negative effect to no effect to positive effect. However, many of the studies have used self-selected groups of women who volunteered to participate in high-risk programs. Perceptions of personal risk and levels of distress may mediate actual risk in determining screening behavior. When Curry[29] reinforced family history as a risk factor, women were more likely to participate in a screening program.

Physicians' barriers and facilitators are quite different from those reported by women.

> *Physicians are more likely to be deterred by cost or to say that they think women will reject a referral. Physicians also cite the daily demands of acute and chronic care, failure to remember to recommend prevention and early detection, and concern about equivocal radiology reports.*[30-34]

In fact, as discussed previously, cost is not the major barrier for women, and most women get mammograms when their physicians recommend that they do so. This is especially important for older, minority women.

STATUS OF CERVICAL CANCER SCREENING

In 1995, 15,800 women were told they had cervical cancer, and 4400 died of the disease.[35] There are less comprehensive current data about the use of cervical screening among U.S. women. According to the 1987 NHIS, about 11% of women overall reported never having a Pap test: 10% of white women, 11.9% of black women, and 24.7% of Hispanic women. As age increased, the proportion of women who reported having had a Pap test declined.[36] Black women were more likely to be screened regularly from age 30 to 49, but in women age 70 and older, white women were more likely to have had a Pap test in the last 3 years, showing that Pap test use is negatively related to age and positively associated with income.[37]

BARRIERS AND FACILITATORS TO CERVICAL CANCER SCREENING

There are many similarities between the barriers and facilitators for Pap testing and mammography for cervical and breast cancer screening, respectively.

> *Knowledge barriers are important for older women, and women past childbearing age may not recognize that they need Pap tests.*[38]

Knowledge and beliefs vary by age and ethnicity. For example, Hispanic women are less likely to be aware of Pap tests, so messages for them may require some background information. Most studies have shown a relationship between believing in the benefits of Pap tests and getting screened on a regular basis.[39]

Women who feel embarrassed about getting a Pap test and women who say they are too busy also are less likely to be screened.[40] Women who have not been screened are most likely to cite procrastination or believing the test not necessary as the reasons for not being screened.[41] As with mammograms, women who do not get other preventive services are less likely to get Pap tests.[39,42] Minority women seem to be more embarrassed than white women about getting Pap tests.[20]

Older, Hispanic women are especially at risk for underutilizing both mammograms and Pap tests. Some studies have shown that women who are more knowledgeable about Pap tests, including the recommended screening interval, are more likely to have had them.[43]

STATUS OF SKIN CANCER SCREENING

Skin cancer is increasing dramatically in the United States. There has been a 120% increase in male melanoma cases since 1958 and a 48% increase in women.[44] In 1995 there were 34,100 new cases of melanoma in the United States and 7200 deaths. Each year there are also over 700,000 nonmelanoma skin cancers. Screening for skin cancer is quick, painless, inexpensive and requires no special technology. Thus it should be acceptable to most patients and clinicians. The ACS advises that adults age 20 to 40 have a skin examination every 3 years and annually after age 40. Because the skin is accessible, patients also should be trained to observe their own skin and to be aware of changes.

Koh et al.[45] and others have suggested that skin cancer screening should focus on persons at high risk: those with dysplastic nevi, white or light skin, a family history, or a propensity for sunburns. Because the risk of skin cancer increases with age, older people require special attention.

BARRIERS AND FACILITATORS TO SKIN CANCER SCREENING

Little is known about the extent to which barriers that have been identified in breast and cervical screening, such as patient embarrassment and lack of provider time, may apply to skin cancer screening. Lay public and community physician education may be the primary reasons why delays occur. In a study by Cassileth et al.[46] the sequence of events leading ultimately to the diagnosis and treatment of melanoma was investigated. In a population of 275 patients ultimately diagnosed with melanoma, an average of 1 year elapsed between the time the patient first noticed a new or changed lesion and the eventual diagnosis of melanoma. This delay in diagnosis was attributed to both patients and physicians. An average of 6 months elapsed between a patient's recognition of new or changed lesion and their realization that the lesion was suspicious and needed medical attention. For 21% of the cases at least 2 months elapsed between the physician's observation of the lesion and the definitive diagnosis of melanoma, and 13% were diagnosed with a minimum of a 4-month delay. It was concluded that patients cannot distinguish between melanomas and moles and that physicians do not always diagnose melanoma accurately or act promptly in response to suspicious lesions. Education barriers may have to be overcome to take advantage of the unique opportunity for the early detection and cure of melanoma. With this in mind, the Queensland Melanoma Project was established in 1969, a massive lay and professional education project for the prevention and early detection of melanoma. It was argued that this mass education would be much more cost-effective than mass screening of the population. Over the ensuing two decades this approach has resulted in a decreasing tumor thickness at diagnosis and a corresponding increase survival in this population.[47]

FOLLOW-UP OF ABNORMAL TEST RESULTS

It is beyond the scope of this chapter to review the issues associated with adherence to follow-up procedures among those with abnormal test results. However, there is extensive evidence that a significant proportion of people who are screened for breast cancer, cervical cancer and skin cancer do not receive appropriate evaluation.[7,46]

The ideal intervention strategy varies according to the population. Marcus et al.[48] demonstrated that transportation incentives were highly effective in increasing adherence of low-income women to follow-up after an abnormal Pap test. However, personalized approaches and a slide tape program were more effective among other women.

Letters and reminder calls should be the first step. But some people require more intensive methods of follow-up.

Lerman et al.[49] and others have shown that the psychologic consequences of abnormal test results can be profound. Adequate support should be provided to such patients.

INTERVENTIONS TO INCREASE BREAST AND CERVICAL SCREENING

Many more intervention studies have been conducted to test interventions to increase breast cancer screening compared with other cancers. The literature shows that the best approach to screening is to use multiple interventions, directed at patients, physicians, the system, and, if possible, the community. In some cases single approaches have been successful. But in general there has been less impact with single-strategy then multiple-strategy interventions. A few studies are exceptions. Mandelblatt[7] reorganized a hospital clinic and gave a nurse practitioner responsibility for identifying the names of older, poor black women who were due for mammograms and then calling them. This resulted in a significant increase in the proportion of these women who received mammograms. Rothman[50] created a video in which he heightened women's awareness about their responsibility for getting mammograms, and this tool increased use of mammography, according to self-reports.

A number of strategies have been found to increase physicians' referrals for mammography and performance of Pap tests. These have included audits with periodic feedback, detailing strategies, and computerized reminders. Unfortunately these strategies have not been used widely outside academic medical centers. Recently Costanza[26] found that a hospital-based in-service program significantly improved mammography referrals in their intervention community.

> *The most effective behavior change studies have been those in which multiple interventions have been used. Most all of these studies used a mix of intervention strategies directed at physicians, patients and, in some cases, the community.*[26,51-53]

The physician-directed strategies included traditional CME programs at community hospitals as well as office-based strategies based on the academic detailing model.[54] Most of these studies used reminder systems as integral to the interventions. But all of these successful studies also developed and tested special interventions for women.

Rimer et al[51] invited women in an independent practice association (IPA)-model HMO to participate in breast cancer screening. Nonadherent women were sent reminders, and this dramatically decreased nonadherence. For women who remained nonadherent, telephone counseling tripled the odds that a woman would get a mammogram. During the brief counseling session (average 5 minutes), the counselor's goal was to identify and overcome a woman's personal barriers to mammography. Costanza et al.[26] conducted patient education in a community health center, and Fletcher et al.[53] implemented a community-wide media campaign. Lane et al.[52] used community health education strategies, including a game.[18] All these studies also included free or low-cost mammograms as part of the intervention package. Thus these programs included patient-directed, physician-directed, system-directed, and sometimes community-based strategies as well.

Although there has been less research on cervical cancer screening compared with breast screening, many of the same approaches appear to work. Ansell et al.[55] and Lacey et al.[56] showed that the use of community health workers can increase the use of cervical cancer screening. They also showed that in-reach interventions within community health centers can be effective.

In addition, attempts to streamline the process of appointments and waiting time contribute to improved adherence.[57] Invitations from providers also increase cervical cancer screening.[58] In addition, there is some evidence that screening of emergency hospital patients can be a useful component of case finding.[59,60]

The lessons from the literature are that usually more than one intervention strategy is required, and that those interventions should be directed not only at patients but also at physicians, other providers, and the health care system.

INTERVENTIONS TO INCREASE SKIN CANCER SCREENING

The United States lags behind many other countries in the creative application of interventions to reduce the incidence of and mortality from melanoma and other skin cancers. Australia, which has the highest reported incidence of melanoma anywhere, has mounted successful population-based programs that have had dramatic impact.[61,62] Because early sun exposure is a predictor of both skin cancer, generally, and melanoma, in particular, education of children and intervention with their parents is a necessary component of programs. This is different from breast and cervical cancer screening, where the recommended behaviors are generally adult behaviors.

Because a prevention strategy is available, such as using sunscreens and limiting sun exposure, prevention must be a major feature of education programs.

A wide range of intervention strategies has been used to decrease sun exposure.[47] In general, the literature shows that combinations of interventions, including mass-media and community-based education, can increase the proportion of people who practice safe sun behaviors. However, the focus of this chapter is on screening rather than prevention. Fewer concerted efforts have been made in this area. Because skin cancer screening is not technology driven, it can be done almost anywhere. Programs have been conducted at churches, health fairs, county fairs, and in mobile settings.[45] The American Academy of Dermatology and the ACS sponsor an annual free skin cancer demonstration project. As with similar breast and cervical cancer screening events, low-income people are underrepresented.

Because over 90% of the U.S. population has a routine source of medical care and 85% see a physician every 2 years, skin cancer screening should be integrated into routine primary care. Thus use of the same prompting systems that increase breast and cervical cancer screening also can increase skin cancer screening.

WHAT CLINICIANS CAN DO TO INCREASE BREAST, SKIN, AND CERVICAL CANCER SCREENING

Although the use of breast screening lags behind acceptance of Pap testing, it is useful to think of them as integrated behaviors. For one thing, there are women who are not getting either test. In addition, the Pap test is often the gateway to preventive medicine for women. It may be done as a part of a checkup. During that time a breast examination should be done and the woman given a referral for a mammogram. A skin examination could be performed on women at the same time with very little increased time commitment. This all can be done in the context of women's health. But what works? How can an individual clinician increase the use of cancer screening? The following section includes recommendations that can be used in clinical practice (Table 12-2).

Use an Office System

There is now a substantial body of literature asserting that system-wide innovations, such as prompts and manual or computer-generated reminders, can increase use of breast and cervical cancer screening.[57,63-66] There is reason to believe that such systems also could increase the acceptance of skin cancer

---

T A B L E 1 2 - 2

CLINICAL APPROACHES TO IMPROVE ADHERENCE

* Use an office system.
* Take a detailed family history.
* Counsel patients about the importance of screening.
* Take a stage-based approach.
* Use age- and ethnicity-appropriate patient education materials.
* Get feedback from patients.
* Have a system in place for follow-up.
* Track how well you are doing.
* Consider adjuncts to increase counseling.
* Participate in low-cost community-based screening activities.

From Prochaska JO, Goldstein MG: *Clin Chest Med* 12:727, 1991.

screening. Fewer than 33% of physicians report the use of such systems. But without planned systems, recommendations for cancer screening often are left to chance and therefore are sporadic and inconsistent. Ideally, women should be sent yearly reminders regarding when they are due next for Pap tests and breast cancer screening. The evidence is that most women welcome these reminders. Skin cancer screening can be integrated into annual checkups for men and women.

Take a Detailed Family History

Increasingly, there will be genetic information available to characterize the 5% or so of patients who are at increased risk for cancer due to family history. It is important to maintain a detailed family history on all patients. This is the only way to determine if they should be offered genetic screening and counseling and if they should be on more aggressive screening schedules.

Counsel Patients about the Importance of Screening

There is clear evidence that the most important reason women get screened is that their providers have urged them to do so. Brief advice can be highly effective. To increase use of mammographic screening, clinicians should give women a clear, unambiguous recommendation about the importance of screening, and this should be accompanied by a referral. This helps to facilitate the behavior. Even better would be for the receptionist or office nurse to schedule the mammogram appointment while the woman is in the office. Similarly, women should be given a strong message about the importance of regular Pap tests. Ideally, the test would be performed during a routine visit. During an annual checkup, physicians should emphasize the importance of regular, thorough skin examinations.

Counseling should reflect a recognition of personal health behaviors that may affect risk. For example, current or previous smoking, sexual history, and oral contraceptive use affect the risk of cervical cancer and should be considered in counseling patients.

Use Age- and Ethnicity-appropriate Patient Education Materials

The impact of counseling can be enhanced through the provision of carefully selected patient education materials. These should be appropriate to the patient's age and ethnicity. Many excellent, free materials are available through the ACS and the NCI Cancer Information Service.

Take a Stage-based Approach

The clinician's time is a scarce commodity, so it should be used wisely. The most effective approach is to structure the counseling using a stage-based approach.[10] The woman who refuses even to contemplate a mammogram has very different educational needs from one who has been getting regular mammograms. The former may benefit from information about the relationship between age and breast cancer incidence or the ability of mammography to detect early, curable cancers. Older precontemplators may not know that women need to continue to get regular Pap tests. The latter may benefit most from reinforcement for getting screened regularly and a referral. Many people still do not appreciate the value of sun protection or of regular skin examinations. The best place to start is where the patient is.

Get Feedback from Patients

Stay in touch with the women who are referred for mammography or Pap tests. If they complain about waiting time for appointments or how they are treated, it may be time to identify a new facility. Word of mouth is important, and patients can provide important information about mammography facilities and other referral services.

Have a System in Place for Follow-up

Not all the women who are given referrals for mammograms will keep their appointments. And, as surprising as it may seem, not even all the women with abnormal Pap or mammography test results will complete the recommended diagnostic tests. Adherence to recommended skin cancer diagnostic procedures could be expected to be a similar problem. Either the reminder system or some other system should be used to track adherence to recommended follow-up procedures.

Track How Well You are Doing

Most clinicians believe they are doing better than they really are. Chart audits and other procedures can be used to obtain this information regularly. Areas of below-par performance then can be identified and appropriate strategies devised for improvement.

Consider Adjuncts to Improve Counseling

Cost-effective techniques, such as reminder letters, can double the proportion of women who receive cancer screening.[67] Such strategies can be very low cost, less than $1 a letter. Telephone counseling, in which a trained counselor calls a woman to identify and overcome her individual barriers to mammography, can triple the odds that a woman will have a mammogram. Telephone counseling costs $4.93 per *successful* call. Patients also can be referred to the NCI's free telephone information line, the Cancer Information Service (1-800-4-CANCER).

Participate in Low-cost Community-based Screening Activities

Many communities now offer organized approaches to screening for low-income residents. These activities can help to reduce financial barriers for many people. It is critical that the planning for such events also include referral and follow-up for those with abnormal findings.

REFERENCES

1. Greenwald P, Sondik E, editors: Cancer control objectives for the nation: 1985-2000, Monogr 2, Pub No 86-2880, Bethesda, Md, 1986, National Cancer Institute.
2. Myers RE et al: Modeling adherence to colorectal cancer screening, *Prev Med* 23:142, 1994.
3. Elwood JM, Cox B, Richardson AK: The effectiveness of breast cancer screening by mammography in younger women, *Online J Curr Clin Trials* 32:93, 1993.
4. Fletcher SW et al: Report of the international workshop on screening for breast cancer, *J Natl Ca Inst,* 85:1644, 1993.
5. Costanza ME et al: Supporting statements and rationale, *J Gerontol* 47:7, 1992.
6. Sox HC: Preventive health services in adults: current concepts, *N Engl J Med* 330:1589, 1994.
7. Mandelblatt J et al: Breast and cervical cancer screening of poor, elderly, black women: clinical results and implications, Harlem Study Team, *Am J Prev Med* 9:133, 1993.
8. Norman SA et al: The relationship of Pap testing and contacts with the medical care system to stage at diagnosis of cervical cancer, *Arch Intern Med* 151:58, 1991.
9. Rosenstock I: The health belief model. In Glanz K, Lewis F, Rimer B, editors: *Health education theory, research, and practice,* San Francisco, 1990, Jossey Bass.
10. Prochaska JO, Goldstein MG: Process of smoking cessation: implications for clinicians, *Clin Chest Med* 12:727, 1991.
11. Dawson DA, Thompson GB: *Breast cancer risk factors and screening: United States, 1987,* DHHS Pub No 900-1500, Hyattsville, Md, 1990, US Department of Health and Human Services.
12. Marchant DJ, Sutton SM: Use of mammography—United States, *MMWR* 39:621, 1990.
13. Breen N, Kessler L: Changes in the use of screening mammography: evidence from the 1987 and 1990 national health interview surveys, *Am J Public Health* 84:62, 1994.
14. Rakowski W, Rimer BK, Bryant SA: Integrating behavior and intention for the study of mammography data from the 1990 supplement to the national health interview survey, *Public Health Rep* 108:605, 1993.
15. Rimer BK et al: Why women resist screening mammography: patient-related barriers, *Radiology* 172:243, 1989.
16. Fox SA, Murata PF, Stein JA: The impact of physician compliance on screening mammography for older women, *Arch Intern Med* 151:50, 1991.
17. Coleman EA, Feuer EJ, NCI Breast Cancer Screening Consortium members: Breast cancer screening among women from 65 to 74 years of age in 1987-88 and 1991, *Ann Intern Med* 117:961, 1992.
18. Burg M, Lane D, Polednak A: Age group differences in the use of breast cancer screening tests, *J Aging Health* 2:514, 1990.
19. Rimer BK et al: Older women's participation in breast screening, *J Gerontol* 47:85, 1992.
20. Calle EE et al: Demographic predictors of mammography and Pap smear screening in US women, *Am J Public Health* 33:51, 1993.
21. Rimer BK et al: The older smoker: status, challenged and opportunities for intervention, *Chest* 97:547, 1990.
22. McBride CM et al: Exploring environmental barriers to participation in mammography screening in an HMO, *J Cancer Epidemiol Biomarkers Prev* 2:599, 1993.
23. Slenker SE, Grant MC: Attitudes, beliefs, and knowledge about mammography among women over forty years of age, *J Cancer Educ* 4:61, 1989.
24. Champion VL: The relationship of selected variables to breast cancer detection behaviors in women 35 and older, *Oncol Nurs Forum* 18:733, 1991.
25. King E et al: Breast cancer screening practices among retirement community women, *Prev Med* 22:1, 1993.
26. Costanza ME et al: Impact of a physician intervention program to increase breast cancer screening, *J Cancer Epidemiol Biomarkers Prev* 1:581, 1992.

27. Vogel VG, Peters GN, Evans WP: Design and conduct of a low-cost mammographic screening project: experience of the American Cancer Society, Texas division, *Am J Roentgenol* 158:51, 1992.

28. Lerman C, Schwartz M: Adherence and psychological adjustment among women at high risk for breast cancer, *Breast Cancer Res Treat* 28:145, 1993.

29. Curry SJ et al: A randomized trial of the impact of risk assessment and feedback on participation in mammography screening, *Prev Med* 22:350, 1993.

30. American Cancer Society: 1989 survey of physicians' attitudes and practices in early cancer detection, *Cancer* 40:77, 1990.

31. Rimer BK et al: Breast screening practices among primary physicians: reality and potential, *J Am Board Fam Pract* 3:26, 1990.

32. Costanza ME et al: Physician compliance with mammography guidelines: barriers and enhancers, *J Am Board Fam Pract* 5:143, 1992.

33. Burg MA, Lane DS: Mammography referrals for women age 75 and older: is Medicare reimbursement likely to make a difference? *Health Serv Res* 27:505, 1992.

34. Pommerenke FA, Weed DL: Physician compliance: improving skills in preventive medicine practices, *Am Fam Physician* 43:560, 1991.

35. American Cancer Society: *Facts and figures 1993,* New York, 1993, The Society.

36. US Department of Health and Human Services, Public Health Service: *Cervical cancer control: status and directions,* 1991.

37. Boring CC: Cancer statistics for African Americans, *CA Cancer J Clin* 42:7, 1992.

38. Caplan LS, Wells BL, Haynes S: Breast cancer screening among older racial/ethnic minorities and whites: barriers to early detection, *J Gerontol* 47:101, 1992.

39. Rimer BK: Audiences and messages for breast and cervical cancer screening, *Health Educ Q* (in press).

40. Cockburn J et al: Barriers to cervical screening in older women, *Aust Fam Physician* 21:973, 1992.

41. Harlan LC, Bernstein AB, Kessler LG: Cervical cancer screening: who is not screened and why, *Am J Public Health* 81:885, 1991.

42. Rimer BK: Understanding the acceptance of mammography by women, *Ann Behav Med* 14:197, 1992.

43. Howard J: Using mammography for cancer control: an unrealized potential, *CA Cancer J Clin* 37:33, 1987.

44. American Cancer Society: *Facts and figures 1994,* New York, 1994, The Society.

45. Koh HK, Mackie RM, Reintgen DS: The prevention and early detection of melanoma: screening for melanoma, *Cancer Screen* 18:72, 1993.

46. Cassileth BR et al: Patient and physician delay in melanoma diagnosis, *J Am Acad Dermatol* 18:591, 1988.

47. Smith T: The Queensland Melanoma Project—an exercise in health education: aspects of Australian medicine, *Br Med J* 1:253, 1979.

48. Marcus AC et al: Improving adherence to screening follow-up among women with abnormal Pap smears: results from a large clinic-based trial of three intervention strategies, *Med Care* 30:216, 1992.

49. Lerman C et al: The impact of mailed psychoeducational materials to women with abnormal mammograms, *Am J Public Health* 82:1, 1992.

50. Rothman AJ et al: Attributions of responsibility and persuasion: increasing mammography utilization among women over 40 with an internally oriented message, *Health Psychol* 12:39, 1993.

51. Rimer BK et al: The effect of a comprehensive breast screening program on self-reported mammography use by primary care physicians and women in a health maintenance organization, *J Am Board Fam Pract* 6:443, 1993.

52. Lane DS, Polednak AP, Burg MA: Measuring the impact of varied interventions on community-wide breast cancer screening. In Anderson PN, Engstrom PF, Mortenson LE,

editors: *Advances in cancer control: innovations and research,* New York, 1989, Alan R. Liss.

53. Fletcher SW et al: Increasing mammography utilization: a controlled study, *J Natl Cancer Inst* 85:112, 1993.

54. Soumerai SB, Avorn J: Principles of educational outreach (academic detailing) to improve clinical decision making, *JAMA* 263:549, 1990.

55. Ansell D et al: A nurse-delivered intervention to reduce barriers to breast and cervical cancer screening in Chicago inner city clinics, *Public Health Rep* 109:104, 1994.

56. Lacey L et al: Referral adherence in an inner city breast and cervical cancer screening program, *Cancer* 72:950, 1993.

57. Harris RP et al: Prompting physicians for preventive procedures: a five-year study of manual and computer reminders, *Am J Prev Med* 6:145, 1990.

58. Creighton PA, Evans AM: Audit of practice based cervical smear programme: completion of the cycle, *Br Med J* 304:963, 1992.

59. Hogness CG et al: Cervical cancer screening in an urban emergency department, *Ann Emerg Med* 21:933, 1992.

60. Marcus AC et al: Screening for cervical cancer in emergency centers and sexually transmitted disease clinics, *Obstet Gynecol* 75:453, 1990.

61. McCarthy WH: Public response to a television programme on melanoma: The Sydney melanoma unit, Sydney, Australia: Third International Conference on Melanoma, *Melanoma Res* 3:7, 1993 (abstract).

62. Marks R, Hill D: The outcomes of melanoma education programs in Australia: Third International Conference on Melanoma, *Melanoma Res* 3:7, 1993 (abstract).

63. Smith RA, Haynes S: Barriers to screening for breast cancer, *Cancer* 69:1968, 1992.

64. Carney PA et al: Tools, teamwork, and tenacity: an office system for cancer prevention, *J Fam Pract* 35:388, 1992.

65. Garr DR et al: The effect of routine use of computer-generated preventive reminders in a clinical practice, *Am J Prev Med* 9:55, 1993.

66. Yarnall KSH et al: Increasing compliance with mammography recommendations: health assessment forms, *J Fam Pract* 35:59, 1993.

67. King E et al: Promoting mammography use through progressive interventions: is it effective? *Am J Public Health* 84:104, 1994.

OPERATIONAL ISSUES IN DEVELOPING A CANCER SCREENING PROGRAM

13

Stephen L. Luther

Cancer screening services should be high quality, accessible, convenient, and inexpensive.

> *The most logical and efficient way to provide cancer screenings is to include the examinations as part of routine preventive services, provided by primary care practitioners.[1,2]*

However, barriers related to cost and access may limit the likelihood of cancer screening occurring in the primary care setting. Many, if not most, traditional health insurance plans, including Medicare, do not reimburse for common cancer screening procedures, and approximately 15% of the population in the United States have no health insurance.[3] Therefore most individuals incur out-of-pocket expenses if they receive cancer screening examinations, reducing the likelihood of their seeking screening. Moreover, few primary care practices have the volume of eligible patients to efficiently support dedicated mammography or other specialized screening equipment.[4-6]

> *Therefore it is unlikely that all cancer screening services can be delivered during a single clinical visit.*

Because multiple visits to different providers are required, the probability is increased that the screening battery may not be completed.

Even if the reimbursement and logistical issues could be resolved, research indicates that there are additional barriers to cancer screening in the primary care setting. Physicians consistently indicate that lack of time is a significant barrier to providing prevention and screening services in their primary care practices.[4-6] Too often provision of preventive services must compete with management of multiple chronic health problems such as hypertension, diabetes, congestive heart failure, and depression, as well as acute health problems.[7] Other barriers to implementing cancer screening described by primary care physicians include lack of expertise in performing particular screening procedures and failure to remember to recommend or arrange for screening services. The most common reason reported by women for not having a mammogram is that their physician did not recommend the procedure.[4,7-11]

An alternative method for providing cancer screening services in a convenient, efficient manner is to expand the model of the dedicated low-cost, high-volume breast screening center to include all cancer screening procedures. Dedicated breast screening centers use nonphysician staff (radiology technologists and nurse practitioners if breast examination is included in the screen), under the supervision of a physician, to provide high-volume screening services. These facilities can be organized as free-standing offices or clinics, part of a larger radiology facility, or as part of a breast treatment center. Breast screening centers may serve thousands of screenees per year while maintaining high-quality service at low cost.[11,12] Such screening centers supplement rather than replace the primary care practitioner.

This chapter discusses some of the more important operational issues related to developing a comprehensive cancer screening program (CCSP) based on the high-volume screening center model. A CCSP, as described here, is a clinical program in which individuals can receive many, if not all, of the recommended cancer screening examinations based on their age and other risk factors. Such a clinical screening program might be implemented by a hospital, a cancer center, a group of physician providers, or an integrated health care delivery system. The intent of this chapter is not to outline the one and only "correct way" to design a CCSP, but rather to describe some of the important operational issues that should be incorporated into the planning of such services.

This discussion identifies logistic, economic, and political factors that affect the development of a CCSP, fully realizing that the relative importance of these issues depends on the nature of the institution or organization in which the screening program is developed. For example, a community hospital may have a different set of issues and goals when developing a CCSP than may a university-based cancer center or an integrated health care delivery system.

DEFINING A COMPREHENSIVE CANCER SCREENING PROGRAM
Goals of the Program

The primary goal of a CCSP is to provide effective, efficient comprehensive cancer screening services to individuals at a risk for developing cancer.

However, a CCSP may contribute to a wide range of organizational goals beyond clinical service that address the public health needs of the community.

> *A CCSP can be a link to well populations relevant to research initiatives, or it can be an effective health promotion and outreach activity. A CCSP may be used as a public relations vehicle for the sponsoring institution.*

The exact operational design of the CCSP may vary depending on the role the program fills for the parent organization.

Nature of the CCSP

Eddy[13] has defined screening as "the application of a test to detect a potential disease or condition in a person who has no known signs of that disease or treatment." He observes that qualifying adjectives, such as *routine, general,* or *mass,* are often applied to screening with little agreement about the meaning of these terms. He recommends categorizing screening efforts in two levels. The first level differentiates screening as either mass screening, where large numbers of people are screened under fairly impersonal circumstances, or individualized screening, where the decision to screen accommodates the individual's concerns and preferences (such as in a practitioner's office). A second level differentiates between screenings designed for individuals with specific risk factors (such as family history), referred to as selective screening, as opposed to screening that is not dependent on risk factors (other than age and gender criteria), referred to as general screening.

Eddy's categories provide a useful framework to describe the options to be considered in developing the nature of a CCSP. A CCSP may choose between mass and individualized screening and between selective and general screening, or exist as a hybrid that combines elements from both dimensions. A CCSP may have many of the traits of mass screening with high volume, provider-defined examinations at its core, yet allow for elements of individualized screening to be included. Practitioners in a CCSP may incorporate elements of individual prevention and screening services, such as risk assessment and counseling, at a greater efficiency than physicians in an individual office. Although most often a CCSP focuses on screenings that have clear and simple guidelines for participation, selective screenings can be incorporated. For example, risk assessment, counseling, and stool blood tests might be offered as a low-cost, high-volume general screening for colorectal cancer, with the individual having the option to receive screening sigmoidoscopy, based on personal preference.

The CCSP must decide which services to include in its program. One institution might choose to emphasize cancer screenings based on American Cancer Society (ACS) screening guidelines, whereas another might use the guidelines of the American College of Physicians. A community institution might emphasize only women's services as part of a program in general women's health, and a research institution might focus only on familial or genetic high-risk individuals.

Establishing Clinical Guidelines for Screening Examinations

A CCSP should have a physician leader or medical director who is responsible for creating or adopting clinical screening guidelines and for supervising nonphysician staff. The medical director may enlist an advisory committee representing a variety of disciplines to assist in this effort.

There is a great deal of controversy about guidelines for cancer screening. Ideally the CCSP clinical guidelines would only include those screening strategies that have been shown to reduce mortality in randomized clinical trials to high-risk individuals. Unfortunately, only breast cancer screening with mammography has been subjected to such rigorous evaluation, and even for this strategy disagreement exists about the age to begin screening, the age to stop screening, and the intervals to be screened.[11,14,15]

Scientific validation of cancer screening procedures involves large, lengthy, expensive randomized studies. Screening procedures become available based on evidence from nonrandomized studies and are often implemented in primary care settings before conclusive efficacy data have been collected. An example of this phenomenon is screening for prostate cancer with serum prostate-specific antigen (PSA). Randomized clinical trials assessing the efficacy of this procedure are under way but will not be complete until the next century. Yet prostate cancer screening with PSA has been advocated by the ACS and is widely available and utilized in clinical practice.

Although there are many philosophical and policy issues related to establishing guidelines for cancer screening, the discussion here is limited to operational issues. The CCSP should have a set of guidelines that are clear and acceptable to patients and to referring physicians.

For most programs the most appropriate strategy is to adopt guidelines established by national policy bodies. Private, governmental, and voluntary health organizations have been active in developing cancer screening guidelines.

Probably the most widely recognized cancer screening guidelines are those established by the ACS, the American College of Physicians, and the United States Preventive Services Task Force.[1,11,15]

Establishing Referral Policies

A CCSP is not intended to replace the primary care physician, but rather to supplement the physician's interactions with the patient. To this end all CCSP screenees must identify a physician to whom screening results can be delivered.

This is not a difficult issue if the CCSP accepts only physician-referred individuals for screening. However, many individuals who may desire screening do not have a primary care physician; this is especially true if the CCSP targets its services to medically underserved populations. If the CCSP decides to accept self-referred screenees, a system should be established to provide screenees with the name of a physician willing to receive the individual as a patient and provide clinical follow-up. This may be accomplished by establishing a physician referral list or a referral service.

A screening program that limits itself to physician referrals may directly serve the needs of primary care providers and more easily allow individualized or selective screening services.

A program that chooses to accept self-referred patients assumes additional clinical burdens.

It must rely more heavily upon and clearly communicate the clinical guidelines under which the program operates. It must assume responsibility for determining the appropriateness of screening for the individual and for risk assessment, education, and counseling. It must also assume responsibility for clinical follow-up until the screenee is accepted by another practitioner.

Providing CCSP Services

> *A goal of the CCSP is to provide all relevant screening services in a convenient and efficient manner, a "one-stop-shopping model."*

However, some people may not want to receive all the appropriate services offered. An individual may refuse some of the appropriate screening examinations available in the program because of health insurance restrictions or personal choice. The CCSP should decide whether to offer cancer screenings separately only or as a comprehensive package. To this end a menu package of services may be offered by the CCSP. A comprehensive screening examination, including all appropriate tests, may be packaged and priced as the best value choice, but site-specific screenings should also be available for the individual.

FACILITIES
Office or Clinic

Although a rather extensive comprehensive screening program can be operated in modest clinical space, some procedures need special equipment and facilities. Certainly the most expensive and complex of the commonly recommended screening procedures is that of screening mammography. The mammography machine and the facilities to process and interpret films can easily cost over $100,000. Other screening procedures, such as flexible sigmoidoscopy, may also need special facilities, which can limit their inclusion in the CCSP. However, if the CCSP chooses not to include these specialized facilities in its clinical operations, it negates the advantage of providing services outside the primary practitioner's office.

Clinical space of two to four examination rooms can accommodate 15 to 40 patients in an 8-hour day depending on the screening procedure provided and staffing of the clinic. The clinical space used for screening does not have to be dedicated to screening activities full-time. Other clinical services could operate in the space during different times. Sharing space may help offset costs of the CCSP until screening volumes grow to a level that justifies use of the space full-time. It is important that the clinical space be dedicated to screening during the time screening patients are being seen, to ensure the efficient patient flow.

Mobile Unit

> *If the goals of the sponsoring institution of the CCSP include community visibility, community outreach, or ser-*

> *vice to special populations, the CCSP should consider a mobile screening activity. Special populations, such as elderly, rural, or poor groups, may have difficulty getting transportation to a centralized screening office or clinic. This barrier can be eliminated with a mobile cancer screening program.*

For other individuals convenience and time limitations, rather than limited transportation, are the barrier issues. For such individuals, providing mobile screening services to their church or workplace increases the likelihood of their participation in cancer screening.

A mobile screening service allows access to these special groups but requires a large capital expense and considerable maintenance. A mobile service is also less efficient than an office- or clinic-based program. Travel time, setup time, and inefficiencies of scheduling increase the cost of mobile screening programs.

STAFFING
Clinical Staff

> *The CCSP may operate most efficiently and at lowest cost if screening examinations are provided by nonphysician practitioners.*

The types of practitioners most often involved with clinical screening examinations are the physician assistant (PA) and the nurse practitioner (NP). These two disciplines differ in their training programs. Physician assistant programs typically are associated with medical schools, academic health centers, or 4-year colleges, with most programs offering associate's or bachelor's degrees. Nurse practitioner training programs are usually associated with schools of nursing, most of which require a master's degree. There are also several programs in which cross-training between PAs and NPs occurs.[16] Two potentially salient differences between these disciplines are an orientation to health care (medical versus nursing model) and a desire by the NP to practice independent of physicians. However, the roles performed by the PA and the NP in most ambulatory care settings are more similar than different.[17]

Regulation of both PA and NP practice is coordinated at the state level. PA practice is usually regulated under the state's medical practice act, based on physician supervision and delegation of tasks. NP practice is governed by nursing licensure provisions of nursing practice acts in each state.

There are two relevant issues for the CCSP to consider in using the PA and NP for provision of services. The first is whether the clinical screening procedures performed are appropriate to the practitioner. The second issue is the appropriate level of direct supervision needed for the practitioner.

In general, screening examinations provided by a CCSP fall within the types of services appropriately rendered by both the PA and NP. For example, NPs provide screening for colon cancer with flexible sigmoidoscopy (arguably the most complex of the currently recommended screening procedures) at a level of quality equal to physicians.[18]

The level of supervision required by regulation for the PA and the NP may vary from state to state. A description of the differences in regulations of supervision in the state of Florida illustrates this fact. In Florida, PAs are required to have "easy availability and physical presence to the licensed practitioner (supervising physician) for consultation and direction of the actions of the PA." The term *easy availability* is expanded in the law to include ability to communicate by telephone.[17,19] NPs in Florida, on the other hand, enter into a more formal agreement with physician supervisors. The NP establishes a protocol or practice framework in conjunction with the supervising physician. The agreement is specific, defining the duties of the NP and the supervising physician, and must be filed with the state department of nursing. However, no reference to a requirement of proximity or availability of the supervising physician is made in Florida law.[19]

Additional Training

Although both the PA and NP are legally qualified to perform cancer screening tests and have many of the skills necessary to perform these examinations as a result of their training, most often the PA or NP does not have training or experience in all the services offered by the CCSP. It is likely that the PA or NP of a CCSP will need additional training to supplement screening skills. This training may be provided by the medical director of the program, by clinical physicians of the parent organization, or with a formal, structured training program.

The University of Texas M.D. Anderson Cancer Center and Research Institute in Houston has a long-established program that trains nurses to perform comprehensive cancer screening examinations.[20] This 3-week comprehensive module includes both didactic and clinical training in a wide variety of cancer screening examinations, as well as training in cancer risk assessment, education, clinical follow-up, and medical-legal issues. Site-specific training programs (such as the breast cancer module, and the gynecologic cancer module) are also offered.

DATA MANAGEMENT SYSTEMS

A CCSP needs an adequate system to manage scheduling, registration, risk assessment, clinical records, results reporting, clinical follow-up, quality assurance, billing, and financial reporting. Depending on the nature of the parent institution, it may be possible to use existing systems. Alternatively, a data system must be purchased or developed to support the program.

A data system is necessary in a CCSP to manage the large number of screening encounters efficiently and cost-effectively. The system not only should provide typical registration functions, but also should automate as much of the clinical data collection, results reporting, and follow-up as possible. The system should also generate letters, cards, or announcements that can be sent to screenees and their referring physicians, reporting results or reminding them of the time for a return screening examination. When such letters or announcements are personalized, based on the specific risk factors of the individual screenee, there is increased utilization of screening services, particularly by minority women.[21]

QUALITY ASSURANCE

Quality assurance and quality control systems must be developed to support the CCSP. Cancer screening procedures can be separated into two broad categories: (1) tests, such as mammography, Pap test, sigmoidoscopy, and PSA blood tests, and (2) physical examination components, such as clinical breast or digital rectal examination. Screening tests are well defined and often have highly regulated quality assurance protocols. For example, there are national criteria for accreditation of laboratories and mammography screening facilities.[22-24]

> *However, objective technical and professional standards for components of physical examinations are less well defined.*

Nevertheless, these screening components deserve quality assurance protocols.

The minimum quality assurance program ensures that the staff is appropriately licensed and trained and that they receive continuing education. The physical examination components of screening should be clearly defined to ensure that all the practitioners apply the same criteria when performing and documenting the examination. The results reporting of the examination should be standardized to define normal and abnormal results and appropriate follow-up protocols. A training program should be developed to permit the clinical staff to spend time periodically in diagnostic or treatment clinics, and to have the opportunity to confirm the results of a positive clinical examination.

The practitioners should review outcome data on all screenings performed, including follow-up on positive examinations and correlation of surgical biopsy results with screening results. The minimum outcome data to be collected should include (1) number of individuals screened, (2) the number of positive tests, (3) the number and proportion of positive tests with follow-up, (4) the number of cancers detected, (5) the sensitivity of the screening test, (6) the positive predictive value of the screening test, and (7) the stage distribution of detected cancers. Comparisons among practitioners and analysis of both false positive and false negative results should be encouraged.

REIMBURSEMENT

A cancer-related checkup for a 50-year-old woman, as recommended by the ACS, includes screening mammography, breast physical examination, Pap test and pelvic examination, skin examination, stool blood test, and possibly sigmoidoscopy.[15] Of these procedures only screening mammography and Pap tests are currently reimbursed by most indemnity health insurance companies or Medicare. Physical examination components are usually not covered services as screening procedures under traditional health care insurance. On the other hand, health maintenance organizations and other managed care organizations may pay for, and encourage, participation in screening by covered members. Strategies to deliver screening services and receive payments are based on the types of health care financing in the current environment.

Group Contracts

One strategy for delivery of screening services is to avoid the fee-for-service model and emphasize contracted services. The CCSP may contract with managed care providers, health maintenance organizations, or other prepaid, integrated delivery systems. Whereas some of the larger managed care organizations may have cancer screening services incorporated into their care network, others may contract out for screening services, particularly those, such as mammography, that require considerable capital expenditure and regulatory compliance.

Another strategy is to contract directly with employers to provide screening services for employees. Many employers are taking increasingly active roles in managing the expenditure of health care benefits for their employees. Similarly, an increasing number of employers are self-insured for health care expenditures. These employers are often interested in providing comprehensive cancer screening services directly to their employees, particularly if the services can be provided at the worksite.

Grants and Contracts

Another strategy for delivery of cancer screening services is to target specific high-risk, underserved, or uninsured populations, with services reimbursed through grants or contracts with governmental or private sources. Local, regional, or national service and philanthropic sources may fund the cost of cancer screening, but the CCSP must also ensure that proper follow-up and treatment are available. Therefore the costs of follow-up and treatment must be estimated and included in any funding for a screening program that targets these special populations.

Fee for Service

In a traditional fee-for-service environment the CCSP may provide cancer screening services on direct payment basis. Screenees may pay for screening services at the time of their clinical visit. They are provided a receipt with which to claim reimbursement from their insurance company as permitted under their contract. Although this approach is simple in theory, in practice it may not be feasible. Screening mammography, Pap tests, and pelvic examinations are covered by most insurers, including Medicare and Medicaid. Medicare law requires that a bill be submitted by providers, and most other companies have specific rules regarding co-payments in their contractual agreements with providers. To provide screening services to individuals covered by Medicare or other contracted carriers, the CCSP must submit bills for services.

EXAMPLE OF A COMPREHENSIVE CANCER SCREENING PROGRAM

Several types of cancer screening programs have been developed around the country in different settings. These programs take on different configurations depending on the goals of the sponsoring institution. A recent article described a variety of CCSP programs.[25]

One of the programs was developed at St. Joseph's Hospital in Atlanta. This relatively low-volume (approximately 300 comprehensive screenings per year) program uses a commercially available screening data management package (CanScreen) and operates out of two clinic rooms adjacent to an outpatient oncology center. At the other end of the spectrum is the LifeCheq Cancer Prevention Program at the M.D. Anderson Cancer Center in Houston. LifeCheq contracts with companies directly for worksite cancer screening. In the first 2 years of its existence, the LifeCheq program has reached 58 companies and nearly 12,000 employees.[25]

Another cancer screening program is the CCSP I developed at the H. Lee Moffitt Cancer Center and Research Institute (HLMCC&RI) in Tampa, Florida.

Sponsoring Institution

The HLMCC&RI opened in 1986 as a private, not-for-profit organization dedicated to the prevention and cure of cancer. Construction of the $70 million facility was funded largely by proceeds from Florida's state cigarette tax. Located at the University of South Florida (USF), HLMCC&RI is supported by the teaching and research activities of the USF Health Sciences Center, which encompasses the Colleges of Medicine, Nursing, and Public Health. The HLMCC&RI campus encompasses nine buildings, including the six-level 161-bed cancer hospital that houses patient care services and clinical research.

Lifetime Cancer Screening Program

The Lifetime Cancer Screening program was established in 1993, to complement the mission of HLMCC&RI. The mission of Lifetime Cancer Screening is to combine cancer screening services, research, education, and community outreach to support Moffitt Cancer Center's mission. The goals of Lifetime Cancer Screening are to provide state-of-the-art screening services to populations at risk, to provide a platform to conduct clinical, basic science and health services research relating to cancer screening, and to provide a venue for education of students (medical, nursing, public health), medical residents, and other health care practitioners or professionals.

Facilities and Staffing

Lifetime Cancer Screening facilities include a dedicated screening clinic and a mobile screening van. The screening clinic is located in a free-standing business complex adjacent to the USF campus allowing easy access by screenees.

The 6800-square-foot facility includes a dedicated mammography suite, seven examination rooms, a darkroom for film processing, a mammography reading room, a blood draw area, and a group of offices. A conference room accommodates health education classes for the public, and an 800-square-foot garage houses the mobile cancer screening van when it is not on the road.

The mobile unit is equipped to provide comprehensive breast cancer screenings, with a mammography unit, examination room, dressing room, and waiting/education area. The mammography machine on the mobile van can be removed, allowing the van to be adapted to provide other services, such as prostate or skin cancer screenings, when necessary.

Twelve employees comprise the screening program, including an administrative director, three NPs, mammography technologists, a research liaison, a community liaison, and an operations coordinator. The chief of radiology at HLMCC&RI serves as program leader for Lifetime Cancer Screening, and a faculty member from the USF Department of Family Practice provides clinical and research support. An advisory panel composed of physicians, staff, and researchers from HLMCC&RI guides the clinical and research efforts of Lifetime Cancer Screening.

The screening program is supported by community health education department, which conducts cancer prevention and educational outreach in Tampa and the surrounding communities. Six professionals, including four nurses and two health educators, comprise this service. These professionals include a minority outreach educator to serve the African-American community, and a Spanish-speaking outreach coordinator to address the needs of the community's Hispanic populations.

Services Provided in the Clinic

Lifetime Cancer Screening offers site-specific (such as breast or prostate only) or comprehensive (head-to-toe) cancer screenings, appropriate for each individual's gender, age, medical background, family history, and lifestyle. All clinical services are provided by licensed NPs with advanced training in cancer detection. Screening mammography is performed by registered technologists with certified training in mammography. Education is an integral component of all services and is conducted both by NPs and by health educators.

Clinical services provided by Lifetime Cancer Screening include both site-specific and comprehensive screenings. Breast cancer screening includes screening mammography, clinical breast examination, and breast self-examination instruction. Prostate cancer screening includes serum PSA test and digital rectal examination. Gynecologic cancer screening comprises Pap smear and pelvic examination. Skin cancer screening includes a full-body skin examination, risk assessment, and self-examination instruction. Comprehensive cancer screenings include cancer risk assessment and counseling, site-specific screenings appropriate for either men or women, and fecal occult blood test, as well as head and neck cancer screening. Screenees are referred as appropriate for sigmoidoscopy.

The Lifetime mobile cancer screening unit provides services to groups in business and community settings in a seven-county area. Large corporations and small businesses alike have taken advantage of on-site services for their employees. Senior living facilities, women's groups, and churches likewise use mobile services to improve access and encourage screening among their members.

In its first full year of operation Lifetime Cancer Screening provided nearly 7500 combined clinic and mobile screening visits. It is expected that this volume will grow to 12,000 to 15,000 in the next 3 years.

REFERENCES

1. Hayward RSA et al: Preventive care guidelines: 1991, *Ann Intern Med* 114:758, 1991.
2. Eddy DM: What care is "essential"? What services are "basic"? *JAMA* 265:782, 1991.
3. Employee Benefits Research Institute: Sources of health insurance and characteristics of the uninsured: analysis of the March 1991 current population survey, *Issues Brief 123,* Washington, DC, 1992.
4. The NCI Breast Cancer Screening Consortium: Screening mammography: a missed clinical opportunity? *JAMA* 264:54, 1990.
5. Velcher DW, Berg AO, Inui TS: Practical approaches to providing better preventive care: are physicians a problem or a solution? *Am J Prev Med* 4(suppl 4):27, 1988.
6. McPhee SJ, Richard RJ, Solkowitz SN: Performance of cancer screening in a university general internal medicine practice, *J Gen Intern Med* 1:275, 1986.
7. Wender RC: Cancer screening and prevention in primary care: obstacles for physicians, *Cancer* 72:1093, 1993.
8. Use of mammography—the United States, 1990, *MMWR* 39:621, 1990.
9. McPhee SJ, Bird JA: Implementation of cancer prevention guidelines in clinical practice, *J Gen Intern Med* 5:116, 1990.
10. Lewis CE: Disease prevention and health promotion practices of primary care physicians in the United States, *Am J Prev Med* 4(suppl 4):9, 1988.
11. Clark RA: Economic issues in screening mammography, *Am J Roentgenol* 158:527, 1992.
12. Monsees B, Destouet JM: A screening mammography program: staying alive and making it work, *Radiol Clin North Am* 30:211, 1992.
13. Eddy DM: *Common screening tests,* Philadelphia, 1991, American College of Physicians.
14. Fletcher SW et al: Report of the International Workshop on Screening for Breast Cancer, *J Natl Cancer Inst* 85:1644, 1993.
15. American Cancer Society: The American Cancer Society guidelines for the cancer-related checkup, *CA Cancer J Clin* 42:44, 1992.
16. Fowkes VF et al: Assessment of physician assistant (PA), nurse practitioner (NP), and nurse-midwife (CNM) training on meeting the health-care needs of the underserved, Rockville, Md, 1993, US Department of Health and Human Services.
17. Jones PE, Cawley JF: Physician assistants and health system reform: clinical capabilities, practice activities, and potential roles, *JAMA* 271:1266, 1994.
18. Mauls WF: Screening for colorectal cancer by nurse endoscopists, *N Engl J Med* 330:183, 1994.
19. MacDonald JW: Supervision of physician assistants and other health-care professionals, *J Florida Med Assoc* 80:261, 1993.
20. *Comprehensive three week module core curriculum,* Department of Professional Education For Prevention and Early Detection, The University of Texas MD Anderson Cancer Center and Research Institute, Houston, 1994.
21. Skinner CS, Strecher VJ, Hosper H: Physicians' recommendations for mammography: do tailored messages make a difference? *Am J Public Health* 84:43, 1994.
22. *Summary of major provisions of the final rules implementing the clinical laboratory improvement amendments of 1988,* College of American Pathologists and American Society of Clinical Pathologists, Washington, DC, 1992.
23. McLelland R et al: The American College of Radiology accreditation program, *Am J Roentgenol* 157:473, 1991.
24. Pub No 102-539, Mammography Quality Standards Act of 1992.
25. Riley M: Implementing and marketing a cancer prevention and screening program, *Oncol Issues* 7:8, 1993.

LEGISLATIVE EFFORTS TO FUND CANCER SCREENING

14

Connie Mack

NATIONAL CANCER ACT OF 1971

MEDICARE COVERAGE OF BREAST AND CERVICAL CANCER SCREENING

BREAST AND CERVICAL CANCER EARLY DETECTION PROGRAM

MAMMOGRAPHY QUALITY STANDARDS ACT OF 1992

CANCER SCREENING INCENTIVE ACT

FUTURE DIRECTIONS IN FEDERAL CANCER SCREENING

Cancer touches each of our lives in a different, personal way. For myself, the motivation to become involved in the fight against cancer is a personal one. In my family my mother, my wife, our daughter, my brother, and I have all had cancer. It was the death of my brother Michael in 1979 that first motivated me to become involved.

I come from a large family of eight children, and we were all very close. Michael and I attended grade school, high school, and college together. We were fraternity brothers at the University of Florida. Following undergraduate school, Michael attended the University of Florida School of Law.

During his last year of law school, Michael noticed a mole on his head one day as he was combing his hair. He went to a doctor, who diagnosed it as a malignant melanoma. But the cancer did not stop him. He graduated number one in his class with high honors and went on for the next 12 years, making his own special mark in Florida.

My brother Dennis and I spent the last 30 days of Michael's life in his hospital room in Atlanta. That experience had a significant impact on my life in two ways. First, it made me ask myself what life is all about. What's my purpose in life? In what areas should I be involved to make my life more meaningful? For me, it turned out to be my involvement in politics, where I could affect public policy issues and do something to help other people.

Michael's death also motivated me to dedicate my political efforts toward accelerating America's fight against cancer. The first thing I did was to try to better educate myself about this disease by meeting with cancer researchers.

It was during one such meeting in Florida that I received a telephone call from my physician, who asked me to come back to Washington. He had determined that a mole, which had recently been removed, was a malignant melanoma. Had it not been for my familial history with cancer and the experience of meeting with cancer experts, I might not have noticed the spot on my side. I might not have detected it early. And I, too, might have been a victim of this horrible disease. However, because of early detection and prompt treatment, a "thin" melanoma, which is curable, was diagnosed and I am alive and healthy today.

It was just 2 short years later that my wife, Priscilla, came to me and said, "Sit down, Connie, we need to talk." When she told me she had discovered a lump in her breast through self-examination, I went completely numb. The first thought that went through my mind was, "I'm going to lose her." I thought of Michael. I thought of what life would be like without Priscilla by my side.

Because she knew the importance of early detection and the proper way to perform a breast self-examination, Priscilla is alive today. She underwent a mastectomy, chemotherapy, and reconstructive surgery. She is taking tamoxifen as a part of her treatment regimen. She has cleared each obstacle with grace and dignity, and today her prognosis is excellent.

Priscilla's battle with breast cancer had a profound impact on her public life. When I first made the decision to become involved in politics in 1982, Priscilla was very supportive. However, she made two rules. First, she would not give media interviews. Second, she would not give speeches. Today, as a breast cancer survivor, she spends a great deal of her personal time speaking with the media about her experiences with breast cancer and educating women about the importance of breast cancer prevention and early detection.

As a member of the United States Senate, I have worked to ensure that cancer research, education, early detection, and treatment remain priorities within our nation's overall health policy agenda. Starting with the landmark National Cancer Act of 1971, America has invested its time, resources, and talent in the goal of winning the war against cancer.

NATIONAL CANCER ACT OF 1971

With the historic signing of the National Cancer Act[1] in December 1971 by the late President Richard M. Nixon, the United States government embarked on a bold initiative by declaring a virtual war on cancer. It mandated adequate resources, manpower, facilities, and the development of a coordinated national program for the conquest of cancer. This precedent-setting legislation established the foundation for the national cancer program as we know it today.

The National Cancer Act included many important provisions in the areas of research, education, and early detection. It provided for special budget authority for the National Cancer Institute to transmit directly to the President and the Congress a budget, without modifications at other levels of the Executive Branch. Commonly referred to as the *bypass budget,* this document is compiled by cancer researchers and presents funding recommendations based on opportunities and needs in cancer research.

The National Cancer Act also established the National Cancer Panel, a three-member board that communicates progress in cancer research as well as impediments to an effective cancer program directly to the President of the United States. The President also is empowered under the Act to appoint a National Cancer Advisory Board and the director of the National Cancer Institute. No other institute at the National Institutes of Health has a director that is appointed solely at the discretion of the President.

> *The National Cancer Act gave responsibility to the National Cancer Institute to conduct cancer control activities and to establish national research and demonstration centers.*

It also expanded information dissemination activities to provide cancer patients with the most up-to-date information and outreach activities regarding cancer treatment and control options. Finally, the Act mandated a coordinated research effort to include expanding, intensifying, and coordinating federal and nonfederal cancer research efforts, collaborating with industry, and developing a National Cancer Program.

MEDICARE COVERAGE OF BREAST AND CERVICAL CANCER SCREENING

Mammography screening under Medicare, the federal health program for 33 million older Americans, was first included in the ill-fated Medicare Catastrophic Coverage Act of 1988.[3] The benefit never took effect, however, because the law was repealed in 1989.[4]

> *In 1990 biennial Medicare coverage for screening mammography was provided for with a frequency schedule depending on the women's age and risk of developing breast cancer.[5]*

Medicare expenditures for mammography have risen from $170 million in fiscal year 1991 to $360 million in fiscal year 1993 (Table 14-1). Medicare beneficiaries are also eligible to receive Pap tests every 3 years. 1992 expenditures totalled $8.9 million.

There have been several legislative efforts to expand Medicare coverage for cancer screening, including annual mammogram coverage as recommended by the American Cancer Society. In addition, legislation is pending to provide

---

TABLE 14-1

HEALTH AND HUMAN SERVICES CANCER PREVENTION AND EDUCATION FUNDING (DOLLARS IN MILLIONS)

	Fiscal year 1990	Fiscal year 1991	Fiscal year 1992	Fiscal year 1993
Medicare/mammograms	—	170	290	360
CDC breast/cervical screening and education*	5	29	50	72
FDA/MQSA	—	—	—	3
NIH research and education	87	100	155	229
TOTAL	92	299	495	664

From Department of Health and Human Services Office of the Assistant Secretary for Legislation, Health Legislation, January 27, 1994; National Institutes of Health Budget Office, March 10, 1994.
*Includes expenditures related to cervical cancer screening and education. Breakdown of resources allocated between breast and cervical cancer is not available.
CDC, Centers for Disease Control and Prevention; *FDA/MQSA*, U.S. Food and Drug Administration/Mammography Quality Standards Act; *NIH*, National Institutes of Health.

prostate-specific antigen (PSA) testing for prostate cancer. Although there is general support in Congress to pass such legislation, cost factors have limited the ability to expand Medicare coverage in recent years.

BREAST AND CERVICAL CANCER EARLY DETECTION PROGRAM

It was not until 1990 that the Federal government established its first major initiative to provide early cancer detection for non-Medicare patients.

> *The Breast and Cervical Cancer Mortality and Prevention Act of 1990[2] authorized the Centers for Disease Control and Prevention (CDC) to begin a national program to increase cancer screening services to all women, with emphasis placed on outreach to low-income and minority women.*

Under the provisions of this legislation, states that participate in the program must contribute $1 for each $3 of federal funds received in the program, 60% of the funds must be used to pay for screening and follow-up costs, and no more than 10% may be used for administrative purposes. Forty-five states are current participants in the program.

As of September 30, 1994, 177,393 women have received mammography screening under this program; 7% of all participants had abnormal results and were referred for diagnostic follow-up; breast cancer was diagnosed in 752 women. Although the program is flexible and allows states to screen women age 40 to 49, in early 1993 the CDC set forth a goal that 75% of all women screened under this program should be over the age of 50.[6] A total of 277,884 women have received Pap tests for cervical cancer under the program; 5% of all participants had abnormal results and were referred for diagnostic follow-up; cervical cancer has been detected in 8426 women.[6]

The program is now second only to Medicare as the largest federally funded cancer screening program. Currently the CDC is funding comprehensive programs, which include cancer screening, necessary follow-up, education for patients and physicians, community outreach, quality assurance, evaluation, and other important cancer control activities in 18 states. In addition, the CDC program is at work in 27 other states to assist their capacity to carry out full-service programs. Federal appropriations have steadily increased from $4.9 million in fiscal year 1990 to $100 million in fiscal year 1995. In December 1993 the program was reauthorized through fiscal year 1998.

MAMMOGRAPHY QUALITY STANDARDS ACT OF 1992

To address growing consumer concerns regarding the quality of mammograms in the United States, Congress enacted the Mammography Quality Standards Act of 1992 (MQSA).[7] It is intended to establish and enforce national quality standards for mammography in contrast to the prior myriad of differing federal, state, local, and voluntary standards. Before enactment of this landmark legislation, the only federal oversight of mammography was through Medicare's limited quality standards program and the CDC breast and cervical cancer screening program. The U.S. Food and Drug Administration (FDA) had been responsible for regulating the manufacture of mammography equipment, not its use.

Under MQSA the U.S. Department of Health and Human Services (HHS) must develop standards for equipment and personnel in mammography facilities. Enforcement of the standards is achieved through accreditation, certification, and annual inspection. All mammography facilities must receive accreditation from a body approved by HHS before receiving certification. The FDA has been given primary responsibility for the implementation of this law.

To meet the immediate needs for quality assurance, legislation was passed to implement "temporary, but immediately enforceable, interim regulations."[8,9] These temporary regulations were enacted to "expedite the establishment of legally binding initial accreditation and quality standards based on standards currently in use," such as those established by the Health Care Financing Administration.[10] Enforcement of the temporary regulations commenced in October 1994.

The fiscal year 1993 supplemental appropriation provided the FDA with $3 million to begin implementing the new law and further directed the CDC, the National Cancer Institute, and the Health Care Financing Administration to transfer $1 million each to the FDA for this purpose.[11] A total of $13 million has been appropriated for fiscal year 1994 to carry out the provisions of this law.

CANCER SCREENING INCENTIVE ACT

Although strides have been made by the federal government in promoting and implementing cancer screening activities, they have been limited in terms of cancer type and patient population. As a United States Senator, I have often questioned this approach. For example, the government has done little to provide colon and rectal cancer screening, despite the fact that nearly as many Americans will develop colon and rectal cancer as compared with new cases of breast or prostate cancer.[12] More lives will be lost to colon and rectal cancer than any other type of cancer, with the exception of lung cancer.[12] Funding for breast cancer screening is covered under Medicare and some Medicaid programs, but prostate cancer screening is not. In addition, not all Americans are eligible for the federal programs to meet this need.

> *Although 42 states currently have laws requiring insurance companies to pay for mammograms, few have enacted similar laws for other types of cancer.*

After many discussions with cancer researchers, physicians, patients, representatives of consumer organizations, medical economists, and others involved in the fight against cancer, I, along with Senator John Breaux (D-La.), introduced legislation to make cancer screening available to all Americans.

> *The legislation—the Cancer Screening Incentive Act—provides an incentive for all Americans, particularly low-income, uninsured, and underinsured Americans, to take advantage of available early detection procedures. The key element of this legislation is a refundable tax credit for cancer screening of up to $250, depending on income level, for each taxpayer, a spouse, and dependents.*

For taxpayers whose income exceeds the 15% marginal tax rate, the annual credit would be up to $200 per eligible individual.

Certain qualifying procedures such as mammograms, Pap tests, and colon screening examinations have been identified. The Secretary of Health and Human Services, in consultation with cancer research and prevention organizations, would develop the guidelines by which taxpayers may use the cancer screening tax credit. This will include other qualifying procedures, as well as appropriate age and frequency restrictions. Taxpayers would take advantage of the cancer screening credit via a new line on all tax forms, including the 1040-EZ.

Many studies have shown that low-income Americans are at a greater risk for developing cancer and dying from cancer than middle- and upper-income Americans. This is thought to be due to patients who have not had access to health care or screening procedures presenting at diagnosis with a higher stage of disease and subsequent poorer prognosis. These individuals are also least likely to have health insurance that covers early detection tests.

Under my bill, individuals whose household income is no more than 150% of the federal poverty threshold would receive early detection examinations at no cost to the patient. Medical providers would be eligible for tax credits at a reimbursement rate to be determined by the Health Care Financing Administration.

Not only would this simple approach make cancer screening more affordable and less bureaucratic, but also it would send a message that the federal government is encouraging early detection of cancer and is providing an incentive to all Americans to take advantage of current technologies.

FUTURE DIRECTIONS IN FEDERAL CANCER SCREENING

During the 104th Congress a number of bills have been introduced on the subject of health care reform. Many of these proposals do not go into detail regarding specific benefits, such as cancer screening. In most cases the specific benefits offered by the plan are determined by a commission, pending congressional consideration and approval. Other approaches, including those that make reforms in the private health insurance industry, may simply require all public and private insurance companies to provide cancer screening. As Congress attempts to solve the monumental task of reforming our beleaguered health care delivery system, most members believe it is essential that preventive medicine, including cancer screening, be an integral part of the solution.

It is likely that any comprehensive health care reform legislation will be phased in over a number of years. Therefore the demand for federally funded cancer screening will not diminish substantially in the foreseeable future. To the contrary, there will likely be attempts to expand services into other forms of cancer and to provide cancer screening to younger Americans.

As the debate over national health care reform has escalated, I have become increasingly concerned about the effect it will have on our ability to conduct a coordinated national cancer program. If a government-financed delivery system with a large federal bureaucracy is implemented, many in Congress, myself included, believe that funding for research, early detection, education, treatment, and the other cancer-related programs will be significantly diminished.

If, however, the Congress and the President permit the free market to remain as the primary means by which Americans receive health care, I am convinced that our aggressive national cancer program will continue to be the preeminent program in the world.

REFERENCES

1. Public Law 92-218, National Cancer Act of 1971, Dec 23, 1971.
2. Public Law 101-354, Breast and Cervical Cancer Mortality and Prevention Act of 1990, Aug 10, 1990.
3. Public Law 100-360, Medicare Catastrophic Coverage Act of 1988, July 1, 1988.
4. Public Law 101-234, Medicare Catastrophic Coverage Repeal Act of 1989, Dec 13, 1989.
5. Public Law 101-508, Omnibus Budget Reconciliation Act of 1990, Jan 1, 1991.
6. *Update on national breast and cervical cancer early detection program data,* Atlanta, 1995, US Centers for Disease Control and Prevention.
7. Public Law 102-539, Mammography Quality Standards Act of 1992, Oct 27, 1992.
8. Public Law 103-183, Preventive Health Amendments of 1993, Dec 14, 1993.

9. US Congress: *House Report 103-397,* Nov 20, 1993.

10. US Department of Health and Human Services, Food and Drug Administration: Mammography facilities—requirements for accrediting bodies and quality standards and certification requirements, interim rules, *Federal Register* 58:67559, 1993.

11. Public Law 103-50, Making Supplemental Appropriations for the Fiscal Year ending September 30, 1993, July 2, 1993.

12. Wingo PA, Tong T, Bolden S: Cancer statistics 1995, *CA Cancer J Clin* 45:8, 1995.

INDEX